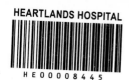

Physical Assessment for Nurse

Second Edition

Physical Assessment for Nurses

Second Edition

Edited by

Carol Lynn Cox
PhD, MSc, MA Ed, PG Dip Ed, BSc (Hons), RN, ENB 254, FHEA
Professor of Nursing, Advanced Clinical Practice
School of Community and Health Sciences
City University, London

Adapted from *Lecture Notes on Clinical Skills* (Third Edition) by:

The late Robert Turner MD, FRCP
Professor of Medicine and Honorary Consultant Physician
Nuffield Department of Clinical Medicine
Radcliffe Infirmary, Oxford

Roger Blackwood MA, FRCP
Consultant Physician, Wexham Park Hospital, Slough
and Honorary Consultant Physician at
Hammersmith Hospital, London

WILEY-BLACKWELL
A John Wiley & Sons, Ltd., Publication

This edition first published 2010
© 2010 Blackwell Publishing Ltd

Blackwell Publishing was acquired by John Wiley & Sons in February 2007.
Blackwell's publishing programme has been merged with Wiley's global Scientific,
Technical, and Medical business to form Wiley-Blackwell.

Registered office
John Wiley & Sons Ltd, The Atrium, Southern Gate, Chichester, West Sussex,
PO19 8SQ, United Kingdom

Editorial offices
9600 Garsington Road, Oxford, OX4 2DQ, United Kingdom
2121 State Avenue, Ames, Iowa 50014-8300, USA

For details of our global editorial offices, for customer services and for information
about how to apply for permission to reuse the copyright material in this book,
please see our website at www.wiley.com/wiley-blackwell.

Library of Congress Cataloging-in-Publication Data
Physical assessment for nurses / edited by Carol Lynn Cox. – 2nd ed.
     p. ; cm.
   Adapted from: Lecture notes on clinical skills (3rd ed.) / Robert Turner,
Roger Blackwood.
   Includes bibliographical references and index.
   ISBN 978-1-4051-8161-7 (pbk. : alk. paper)   1. Nursing assessment.
2. Physical diagnosis.   I. Cox, Carol Lynn.   II. Turner, Robert (Robert Charles),
1938- Lecture notes on clinical skills.
   [DNLM: 1. Nursing Assessment.   WY 100.4 P578 2010]
   RT48.P478 2010
   616.07′5–dc22
                                                                    2009024731

A catalogue record for this book is available from the British Library.

Set in 9.5/11.5 pt Photina MT by Graphicraft Limited, Hong Kong
Printed and bound in Malaysia by KHL Printing Co Sdn Bhd
1   2010

Contents

Prologue: Advanced Practice Nursing

This prologue has been written to describe the development of advanced practice nursing in the UK. It explicates the practice of nurses who have assumed the role of advanced practice nursing. It outlines the events associated with the evolution of advanced practice nursing and reflects on its origins. It follows with the definition, role, educational preparation and Domains of Practice and Competencies (NMC, 2005; RCN, 2008) related to advanced practice nursing. It concludes by considering the profession of advanced practice nursing and its expanding role.

According to the authors of the Advanced Practice Toolkit (www. advancedpractice.scot.nhs.uk/home.aspx), they indicate it has been suggested that 'advanced practice' is simply a broad term that refers to all practice roles at a level above that of initial practice, including under its umbrella both 'specialist' and 'consultant' roles. They believe that this interpretation is unhelpful because it adds little in terms of clarity or consistency. They also postulate that it may further confuse professionals and the public and, as a result, compromise governance in relation to expectations of practitioners and the service as a whole. It is therefore important to have clarity about what 'advanced practice' means. In the section that follows this clarity is provided.

Background

Changes have been occurring rapidly in the National Health Service (NHS) throughout the UK in response to service need and in line with government policy initiatives. In relation to advanced practice roles in nursing, development has been partially due to the *New Deal for Junior Doctors* (NHS Management Executive, 1991) resulting in a reduction in junior hospital doctors' clinical hours and restructuring of the NHS as delineated in *Making a Difference* (DH, 1999) and the *NHS Plan* (DH, 2000) so that healthcare becomes seamless and more orientated toward care in the community.

Recently, with spiralling costs in the NHS and cutbacks and reductions in the workforce, the need for nurses to advance their clinical practice has become acute. Medical and allied health professionals are diminishing in numbers and in some instances are no longer available to provide this care. The reduction of medical and allied health professionals has direct implications for extension of practice by nurses and assumption of advanced clinical practice roles as advanced nurse practitioners and nurse consultants.

Because the provision of healthcare is changing, it is important to consider how nurses working in primary and secondary care can provide more complex/sophisticated care to patients and promote health. This is particularly relevant in relation to the recommendations made by the British Medical Association (BMA, 2002) in which the first point of call for most patients should be an advanced practice nurse rather than a doctor. It is also relevant in relation to the mandates put forward by the Chief Nurse for England in her consultation document of July 2004 (DH, 2004a) and the Nursing and Midwifery Council (NMC) decision following conclusion of its consultation on advanced practice (NMC, 2005) to open a second part of the register to record an Advanced Nurse Practitioner (ANP) qualification.

Origins of advanced practice nursing

It may be argued that advanced practice nursing and educational programmes associated with advanced practice arose not from specific planning efforts or consensus within the profession, but as a response to a demand in healthcare. The impetus for introducing advanced practice nurses in the UK was economic. They evolved out of the economic necessity of service providers, who were experiencing a shortage of doctors in primary and secondary care. Generally, it is postulated in the UK that advanced practice became legitimized with the reduction in junior hospital doctors' hours in acute care (Cox, 2001) and the paper published by the BMA (BMA, 2002). It can be seen that an emphasis on advanced practice nursing occurred in the context of a postmodern culture, with increased professionalization of healthcare, a fundamental emphasis on interprofessional working, an increasingly consumerist approach to health and a move away from the traditional biomedical model of healthcare towards a more holistic approach that has an increased emphasis on improving the healthcare experience for patients (Colyer, 2004). McGee & Castledine (2003) indicate that the early definition of advanced practice published by the United Kingdom Central Council for Nursing, Midwifery and Health Visiting (UKCC, 1994) arose from the recognition that modern healthcare was placing new demands on nurses that required them to extend their practice. The definition provided recognition and subsequent opportunities to develop new roles and assume responsibilities that were 'undreamt of by earlier generations of the profession' (McGee & Castledine, 2003:1).

However, it is postulated here that nurses in the UK were undertaking advanced practice roles for a number of years before this, as can be evidenced by the professional autonomous decisions in which they made a differential diagnosis of a patient's previously undiagnosed problem(s) and developed with the patient an ongoing plan for health that has an emphasis on preventative measures. In the climate of desperate attempts to promote health, the demand arose for nurses to extend their practice. This demand was followed by a response throughout the UK for educational institutions to provide the knowledge, and in some instances generate the knowledge, that addresses the need for appropriately trained advanced practice nurses/advanced nurse practitioners (Horrocks *et al.*, 2002). Nursing's history of demonstrating the ability to function in expanded roles met the demand. The nurse practitioner role developed across Europe, Canada, Australia and New Zealand in the late 1980s (Albarran & Fulbrook, 1999). It has developed extensively in primary care in general practice settings with an accident and emergency department interface. In contrast, the nurse practitioner role in the USA has an extensive history of over 40 years (Daly, 1997). It has repeatedly demonstrated reliable, high-quality, cost-effective care to patients (Daly, 1997; Hillier, 2001). Although in the UK the ANP role has not had as long a history, it is evident from the systematic review undertaken by Horrocks *et al.* (2002) that nurse practitioners provide equivalent care to that of doctors. Horrocks *et al.* (2002) examined randomized controlled trials and observational studies. Their research indicates that advanced practice nurses provide care that leads to increased patient satisfaction as well as having similar health outcomes compared to the care provided by a doctor.

Over the past decade many nurses in the UK have extended their practice and assumed advanced practice roles in order to provide effective care in health and illness. In the present political and professional climate, it is appropriate to provide professional nurses with the opportunity to acquire the education and clinical practice experience that empowers them to take a lead role in advanced practice nursing. However, following on from the NMC consultation (NMC, 2005) and changes occurring globally, the question must be asked: What is advanced practice and what is its role in the provision of healthcare?

Defining advanced practice

In the early 1990s the UKCC defined advanced practice nursing as: *adjusting the boundaries for the development of future practice, pioneering and developing new roles responsive to changing needs and with advancing clinical practice, research and education to enrich professional practice as a whole* (UKCC, 1994:20). McGee & Castledine (2003) indicate that this was the first attempt in the UK to clarify the nature of practice beyond initial registration.

According to Hickey *et al.* (2000), many definitions of advanced practice in nursing have been proposed. The key components in all the definitions that have been published by organizations like the International Council of Nurses (ICN, 2002), the Chief Nurse for England (DH, 2004a), the Nursing and Midwifery Council (NMC, 2005) and the Royal College of Nursing (RCN, 2002, 2008) are the requirement for education at Masters degree level or the ability to demonstrate Masters-level knowledge, patient/family-focused practice and an expanded role. In the UK advanced practice is associated with competencies articulated in the RCN (2008) and the NMC (2005) Domains of Practice.

In February, 2006, the NMC expanded its definition of advanced nursing practice and published 12 core skills that can be expected from an advanced practice nurse (Box 1).

Box 1   Skills of the advanced nurse practitioner (NMC, 2006)

Undertakes a comprehensive patient history
Undertakes physical examinations
Uses expert knowledge and clinical judgement to identify the potential diagnosis
Refers patients for investigations where appropriate
Makes a final diagnosis
Decides on and carries out treatment, including the prescribing of medicines, or refers patients to an appropriate specialist
Uses extensive practice experience to plan and provide skilled and competent care to meet patients' health and social care needs, involving other members of the healthcare team
Ensures the provision of continuity of care including follow-up visits
Assesses and evaluates, with patients, the effectiveness of the treatment and care provided and makes changes as needed
Works independently, although often as part of a healthcare team
Provides leadership
Makes sure that each patient's treatment and care is based on best practice

---

The NMC has published a definition of the ANP that patients and the public can understand. The definition as delineated by the NMC is: *Advanced nurse practitioners are highly experienced, knowledgeable and educated members of the care team who are able to diagnose and treat your healthcare needs or refer you to an appropriate specialist if needed* (NMC, 2006). However, Mayberry & Mayberry (2003) provide a more specific definition of advanced practice nursing which is: *Advanced nursing practice can be defined as a set of skills that involve the undertaking of: taking a clinical history, performing a physical examination, performing appropriate investigations including, for example, proctoscopy and endoscopy, prescribing treatments following agreed protocols based on research or consensus and providing advice and counselling on prognosis and management* (Mayberry & Mayberry, 2003:38).

According to the RCN (2008), an advanced nurse practitioner is: *a registered nurse who has undertaken a specific course of study of at least first degree (Honours) level* and who practises according to the defining role shown in Box 2 (RCN, 2008:3).

Box 2   Definition of the advanced nurse practitioner (RCN, 2008:3)

A registered nurse who has undertaken a specific course of study of at least first degree (Honours) level and who:
- makes professionally autonomous decisions, for which he or she is accountable
- receives patients with undifferentiated and undiagnosed problems and makes an assessment of their healthcare needs, based on highly developed nursing knowledge and skills, including skills not usually exercised by nurses, such as physical examination
- screens patients for disease risk factors and early signs of illness
- makes differential diagnosis using decision-making and problem-solving skills
- develops with the patient an ongoing nursing care plan for health, with an emphasis on preventative measures
- orders necessary investigations, and provides treatment and care both individually, as part of a team, and through referral to other agencies

Therefore it is apparent that: *advanced practice nurses work alongside doctors, practise autonomously and are legally responsible for the care they provide. They make clinical decisions based on investigations and subsequently can treat patients independently* (Cox, 2004: vi–viii).

Role of the advanced practice nurse

According to Jacobs (1998), Rolfe (1998) and McGee & Castledine (2003), advanced practice nursing includes physical examinations, diagnosis and treatment of illnesses, ordering and interpreting tests independently of the doctor, establishing preventive healthcare through health promotion and education, prescribing medications, managing caseloads based on a population perspective that ideally includes individuals, families and/or communities and using business and management strategies for the provision of quality care and efficient use of resources. Their practice includes co-operative and/or collaborative practice arrangements with other healthcare disciplines as well as working in interdisciplinary healthcare teams. Advanced practice nurses are accountable as direct providers of services. Clinical decision making is based on critical thinking, diagnostic reasoning and research.

Advanced practice nurses can have either an acute care (secondary) or a primary care focus which means they can work anywhere. They provide comprehensive health and illness management, consultancy and primary care in a variety of clinical settings (Cox, 2000) and work with doctors and other health professionals in expanded collaborative relationships that influence the care provided by other health professionals. It is seen more often now than ever before that the APN works independently, managing a caseload of patients without supervision, or may work in a team that is consultant led (Brush & Capezuti, 1997; DH, 2006). The model of care provided by the APN has been identified as making an important contribution to quality, cost-effective care (Cox & Hall, 2007).

To summarize, articulation of the remit of an APN according to recent literature and the definitions published by the RCN (2008) and NMC (2005) indicate that the APN possesses advanced assessment, diagnostic, prescriptive and technological skills with a hospital-based acute health/illness perspective and transitional points of health/illness management focus or a community-based primary care focus. They can have either an acute care (secondary) or a primary care focus which means they can work anywhere. They provide comprehensive health and illness management, consultancy and primary care in a variety of clinical settings (Cox, 2000) and work with doctors and other health professionals in expanded collaborative relationships that influence the care provided by other health professionals. It is seen more often now than ever before that the advanced practice nurse works independently managing a caseload of patients without supervision or may work in a team that is consultant led (Brush & Capezuti, 1997; DH, 2006). The model of care provided by the APN has been identified as making an important contribution to quality, cost-effective care (Cox & Hall, 2007). According to Mundinger *et al.* (2000), ANPs provide 60–80% of primary care services as well as or better than general practitioners (GPs) and at a lower cost. Their study found that patients fared just as well when treated by the ANP as they did when treated by a GP.

Educational preparation

According to the Chief Nurse for England (DH, 2004a), advanced practice nurses should be educated at Masters degree level or above. According to the NMC (2005), they should possess Masters-level knowledge and advanced assessment, diagnostic, prescriptive and technological skills as well as research acumen. In their education, which is interprofessional in nature, the central core knowledge, skills, competencies and values of advanced professional and clinical practice experience are acquired in:

- addressing the determinants of health and working with others in the primary, secondary and tertiary care setting to integrate a range of activities that promote, protect and improve the health of the patient/client population served
- functioning in new healthcare settings and interdisciplinary teams that are designed to meet the primary, secondary and tertiary healthcare needs of the public, with an emphasis on high-quality, cost-effective integrated care
- managing and continuously using scientific, technological and patient information that leads to the maintenance of professional competence throughout clinical practice life
- gaining advanced assessment skills used in the provision of care in primary, secondary and tertiary healthcare settings
- diagnosing, screening, treatment and case management of care in primary, secondary and tertiary healthcare settings
- prescribing and supplying drugs, independently and/or according to patient group directions, in primary, secondary and tertiary healthcare settings
- providing emotional support, counselling, referral and discharge in primary, secondary and tertiary healthcare settings.

Learning outcomes within advanced practice programmes are preset with clearly defined objectives for the core competencies that must be achieved as specified by the RCN (2008) and the NMC (2005). The outcomes identify what an individual will know and be able to do at the end of the programme of study. Additional aspects of learning can be individually negotiated through learning contracts. In the main, the programmes are competency based and focus on the knowledge, skills, attributes and outcomes that are informed by practice (McGee & Castledine, 2003). Competencies are informed by theories and hierarchies of skills and knowledge.

With the delineation of the RCN (2008) and NMC (2005) Domains of Practice and Competencies, universities throughout the UK have restructured their programmes to ensure that the essential components of advanced practice are addressed. A variety of advanced practice programmes are now available for nurses who want to become advanced practice nurses. The key component within all the programmes is a clear emphasis on clinical practice that initially builds and then extends as the nurse gains confidence and competence.

RCN (2008) and NMC (2005) Domains of Practice and Competencies

The Domains of Practice and Competencies for the RCN and the NMC can be found on their websites. The NMC (2005) Domains of Practice and Competencies were adapted from the National Organization of Nurse Practitioner

Faculties (NONPF, 1995, 2001) in the USA and the RCN in the UK (RCN, 2002). It is interesting to note that in the UK, in addition to the NONPF (1995, 2001) Domains of Practice and Competencies informing advanced nursing practice, a number of the competencies are evident in the Standards of Proficiency for some of the advanced roles in the allied health professions, such as orthodontists and biomedical scientists (HPC, 2006). The Domains of Practice as specified by the NMC (2005) are:

- the nurse/patient relationship
- respecting culture and diversity
- management of patient illness/health status
- education function
- professional role
- managing and negotiating healthcare delivery systems
- monitoring and ensuring quality of healthcare practice.

The Domains of Practice which have been linked to the NHS Knowledge and Skills Framework (DH, 2004b) dimensions by the RCN (2008) are:

- assessment and management of patient illness/health status
- the nurse/patient relationship
- the education function
- professional role
- managing and negotiating healthcare delivery systems
- monitoring and ensuring quality of advanced healthcare practice
- respecting culture and diversity.

Future directions of advanced clinical practice nursing

Healthcare provision is evolving (BMA, 2002; DH, 2004a, 2006; Horrocks *et al.*, 2002). The Department of Health has mandated the expansion of nursing roles and delineated ways in which knowledgeable, experienced APNs can contribute to the NHS by providing leadership in nursing and service delivery (DH, 2000, 2001, 2006). For example, this may be as an advanced nurse practitioner or nurse consultant. In the UK, APN programmes maintain a commitment to educating nurses who will make substantial contributions to the evolution of healthcare. Although the BMA indicated in its publication on *The Future Health care Workforce* (BMA, 2002) that nurses at advanced practice level would provide expert practice, it is not enough to produce expert nurses. There must be nurses prepared, through appropriate educational programmes, to meet the changing needs of a reformed healthcare system. In addition, it must be remembered that nursing is more than and different from the sum of its parts and must articulate its unique nature and professional perspective within advanced practice. Acquiring and executing tasks that have been traditionally within the purview of medicine does not make nursing more professional as a practice discipline. It is the fact that nurses approach a patient care situation from a very distinct and different perspective to that of medicine. Medicine's approach has always been to diagnose and eradicate a particular disease process. Nursing's perspective is holistic in its approach to caring. In advanced practice nursing, nurses approach the patient care situation from a perspective which addresses the total constellation of care needs of the patient.

Conclusion

In this prologue, advanced practice nursing and its role in the provision of healthcare have been discussed. The events associated with the origins of advanced practice nursing have been reflected upon. The definition, role, educational preparation and Domains of Practice and Competencies (NMC, 2005; RCN, 2008) related to advanced nursing practice have been considered. It was emphasized that advanced practice nursing is more than an aggregation of tasks captured and/or recaptured from other professionals. The acquisition and execution of tasks that have been traditionally within the purview of medicine do not make advanced practice nursing more professional as a practice discipline. Within the practice context, it is seen that advanced practice nurses approach a patient care situation from a distinct and different perspective than that of medicine. They approach the patient care situation from a perspective that addresses the total constellation of care needs of the patient. The skills and knowledge associated with this approach are explicated in the Domains of Practice and Competencies of advanced practice published by the NMC (2005) and the RCN (2008). There must be nurses working at the forefront in primary, secondary and tertiary care who have been prepared as advanced clinical practice nurses to meet the changing needs of the evolving healthcare system. This book is intended to support some of their preparation.

Carol L. Cox, PhD, RN
Professor of Nursing,
Advanced Clinical Practice

References

Advanced Practice Toolkit (2008) www.advancedpractice.scot.nhs.uk/home. aspx.

Albarran, J. & Fulbrook, P. (1999) Advanced nursing practice: an historical perspective. In: Rolfe, G. & Fulbrook, P. (eds) *Advanced Nursing Practice*. Butterworth Heinemann, Oxford: pp 13–32.

British Medical Association (2002) The Future Health care Workforce: Discussion Paper 9. http://web.bma.org.uk/public/pols.

Brush, B. & Capezuti, E. (1997) Professional autonomy: essential for nurse practitioners' survival in the 21st century. *Journal of the American Academy of Nurse Practitioners*, **9**(6): 265–270.

Colyer, H. (2004) The construction and development of health professions: where will it end? *Journal of Advanced Nursing*, **48**(4): 406–412.

Cox, C. (2000) The nurse consultant: an advanced nurse practitioner. *Nursing Times*, **96**(13): 48.

Cox, C. (2001) Advanced nurse practitioners and physician assistants: what is the difference? Comparing the USA and UK. *Hospital Medicine*, **62**(3): 169–171.

Cox, C. (2004) Foreword. In: *Physical Assessment for Nurses*. Blackwell Publishing, Oxford.

Cox, C. & Hall, A. (2007) Advanced practice role in gastrointestinal nursing. *Journal of Gastrointestinal Nursing*, **5**(4): 26–31.

Daly, B. (1997) *The Acute Care Nurse Practitioner*. Springer, New York.

Department of Health (1999) *Making a Difference*. Stationery Office, London.

Department of Health (2000) *The NHS Plan: A Plan for Investment, A Plan for Reform*. Stationery Office, London.

Department of Health (2001) *Implementing the NHS Plan: Modern Matrons, Strengthening the Role of Ward Sisters and Introducing Senior Sisters*. Health Service Circular 2001/10. www.dh.gov.uk/hsc.htm

Department of Health (2004a) *Framework for Developing Nursing Roles: Consultation*. Stationery Office, London.

Department of Health (2004b) *The NHS Knowledge and Skills Framework (NHSKSF) and Its Use in Development Review*. Stationery Office, London.

Department of Health (2006) *Caring for People with Long Term Conditions: An Education Framework for Community Matrons and Case Managers*. www.dh.gov.uk/PublicationsAndStatistics

Hickey, J., Ouimette, R. & Venegoni, S. (2000) *Advanced Practice Nursing: Changing Roles and Clinical Applications*, 2nd edn. Lippincott, New York.

Hillier, A. (2001) The advanced practice nurse in gastroenterology: identifying and comparing care interactions of nurse practitioners and clinical nurse specialists. *Gastroenterology Nursing*, **24**(5): 239–245.

Horrocks, S., Anderson, E. & Salisbury, C. (2002) Systematic review of whether nurse practitioners working in primary care can provide equivalent care to doctors. *British Medical Journal*, **324**(6): 819–823.

Health Professions Council (2006) *Health Professions Council Standards of Proficiency*. www.hpc-uk.org/publications/standards/index.asp

International Council of Nurses (2002) ICN announces position on advanced nursing roles, Geneva, 31 October 2002. International Council of Nurses, Geneva. www.icn.ch/pr19_02.htm

Jacobs, S. (1998) Advanced nursing practice in New Zealand: 1998. *Nursing Praxis in New Zealand*, **13**(3): 4–11.

Mayberry, K. & Mayberry, J. (2003) The status of nurse practitioners in gastroenterology. *Clinical Medicine*, **3**(1): 37–40.

McGee, P. & Castledine, G. (2003) *Advanced Nursing Practice*, 2nd edn. Blackwell Publishing, Oxford.

Mundinger, M., Kane, R., Lenz, R. *et al.* (2000) Primary care outcomes in patients treated by nurse practitioners or physicians: a randomized trial. *Journal of the American Medical Association*, **283**(1): 59–68.

NHS Management Executive (1991) *Junior Doctors: The New Deal*. NHS Management Executive, London.

Nursing and Midwifery Council (2005) *Annex 1: Domains of Practice and Competencies. NMC Consultation on a Proposed Framework for Post-Registration Nursing*. Nursing and Midwifery Council, London.

Nursing and Midwifery Council (2006) A revision of the definition of advanced nurse practice so that it can be accessible to patients and the public. www.nmc-uk.org

National Organization of Nurse Practitioner Faculties (1995) *Advanced Nursing Practice: Curriculum Guidelines and Programme Standards for Nurse Practitioner Education*, 2nd edn. National Organization of Nurse Practitioner Faculties, Washington, DC.

National Organization of Nurse Practitioner Faculties (2001) *Revised Advanced Nursing Practice: Curriculum Guidelines and Programme Standards for Nurse Practitioner Education*. National Organization of Nurse Practitioner Faculties Education Committee, Washington, DC.

Rolfe, G. (1998) Advanced practice and the reflective nurse: developing knowledge out of practice. In: Rolfe, G. & Fulbrook, P. (eds) *Advanced Nursing Practice*. Butterworth Heinemann, Oxford: pp219–228.

Royal College of Nursing (2002) *Nurse Practitioners – An RCN Guide to the Nurse Practitioner Role, Competencies and Programme Accreditation*. Royal College of Nursing, London.

Royal College of Nursing (2008) *Advanced Nurse Practitioners – An RCN Guide to the Advanced Nurse Practitioner Role, Competencies and Programme Accreditation*. Royal College of Nursing, London.

United Kingdom Central Council for Nursing, Midwifery and Health Visiting (1994) *The Future of Professional Practice – The Council's Standards for Education and Practice Following Registration*. United Kingdom Central Council for Nursing, Midwifery and Health Visiting, London.

Preface

Over the past decade, the role of the nurse has changed. It has evolved from basic practice in which the nurse was an assistant to the doctor into an independent practitioner with specialist/advanced practice qualifications. These nurses are expected to know how to provide expert holistic health-oriented care for culturally diverse populations. Specialist/advanced practice nurses view the patient as an individual with physical as well as emotional, psychological, intellectual, social, cultural and spiritual needs. A comprehensive assessment of the patient is the foundation upon which healthcare decisions are made. The best way to develop assessment skills is to learn them systematically. The systematic approach involves taking a full health history, performing a physical examination and reviewing diagnostic texts/laboratory data. Use of the nursing process is essential in clinical decision making that leads to the formulation of a differential diagnosis and final diagnosis.

This text for specialist/advanced practice nurses is based on Turner & Blackwood's *Lecture Notes on Clinical Skills* that was written for medical students. It is intended to be used as a pocket book that can be reviewed near the patient in the clinical setting. In general, the pages are arranged with simple instructions on the left, with important aspects requiring action marked with a bullet (●). Subsidiary lists are marked with a dash (–). On the right are brief details of clinical situations and diseases that are relevant to abnormal findings.

Turner & Blackwood's *Lecture Notes on Clinical Skills* has been used in the Oxford Clinical Medical School for over 25 years and is viewed as an essential guide for nurses beginning the journey to becoming specialist/advanced practitioners. Although some doctors may use slightly different techniques in taking a history and physical examination, it is recommended that nurses embarking on a career as specialist/advanced practice nurses use the techniques suggested in this text because they provide a sound approach for developing and employing clinical decision making.

Carol L. Cox, PhD, RN
Professor of Nursing,
Advanced Clinical Practice

Acknowledgements

Special thanks are extended to Robert Turner and Roger Blackwood for granting permission for their text, *Lecture Notes on Clinical Skills*, to be revised as a text for nurses. In addition, I am grateful to my students for encouraging me to revise this text so that they could have an accessible pocket book for reference purposes in the clinical setting. This book has benefited from their suggestions as well as from those of nurse consultants and medical colleagues with whom I practise. Any faults or omissions in the text are entirely my own.

Figures 2.33, 2.34, 2.41, 3.5, 3.9, 3.10, 3.11, 3.12, 3.13, 3.21, 4.1, 4.2, 4.3, 4.4, 4.5, 4.6, 4.11, 4.13 and 4.14 are reproduced with permission of City University from *Advanced Practice: Physical Assessment* (1997), Carol Lynn Cox. City University London, St Bartholomew School of Nursing and Midwifery, ISBN 1900804255, Reprinted 2002.

The visual acuity reading charts (Appendices 1 and 2) are reproduced courtesy of Keeler Ltd.

The colour illustrations are reproduced courtesy of the Department of Medical Illustration, Heatherwood and Wexham Park Hospitals Trust (2.4, 2.14–2.20, 2.27, 2.28, 2.30, 2.35, 2.36, 2.43–2.46, 2.49, 9.6, 9.42), King Edward VII Hospital, Windsor (2.6, 2.7, 2.10, 2.12, 2.23, 2.37, 5.3), Department of Medical Illustration, John Radcliffe Hospital, Oxford (2.13, 2.25, 2.39, 3.20), Department of Medical Illustration, Radcliffe Infirmary, Oxford (2.38, 2.48).

Contributors

Graham M. Boswell, PhD, MA Ed, BA (Hons), BSc (Hons) RGN, RNT
Senior Lecturer, Department of Adult Nursing, City University, London
Chapter 9: Examination of the Nervous System

Patrick Callaghan, PhD, MSc, BSc (Hons), RN
Professor of Mental Health Nursing and Chartered Health Psychologist
University of Nottingham and Nottinghamshire Health Care NHS Trust,
Nottingham, England
Chapter 8: Mental Health Assessment

Carol L. Cox, PhD, MSc, MA Ed, PG Dip Ed, BSc (Hons), RN, FHEA
Professor of Nursing, Advanced Clinical Practice, Department of Applied
Biological Sciences, City University, London
Chapter 1: History Taking
Chapter 2: General Examination
Chapter 3: Examination of the Cardiovascular System
Chapter 4: Examination of the Respiratory System
Chapter 13: Assessment of Disability Including Care of the Older Adult
Chapter 14: Basic Examination, Notes and Diagnostic Principles
Chapter 15: Presenting Cases and Communication
Chapter 17: The 12-Lead Electrocardiogram
Chapter 18: Interpretation of Investigations

Jennifer Edie, MA Ed, TDCR, DMU
Deputy Dean, School of Community and Health Sciences, City University,
London
Chapter 16: Imaging Techniques and Clinical Investigations

Helen Gibbons, MSc, PG Dip Ophth, BA (Hons), RGN
Research Practitioner, Department of Applied Biological Sciences,
City University, London and Moorfields Eye Hospital NHS Foundation Trust,
London
Chapter 10: Ophthalmic Examination

Carol L. Cox, PhD, MSc, MA Ed, PG Dip Ed, BSc (Hons), RN, CCRN
Professor of Nursing, Advanced Clinical Practice, Department of Applied Biological Sciences, City University, London
and

Polly Lee, MSc, BA (Hons) RSCN, RGN, RM, Dip N, ILTM
Lecturer in Children's Nursing, Department of Midwifery and Child Health, City University, London
Chapter 12: Assessment of the Child

Victoria Lack, MSc, PG Dip (Academic Practice), BN, DN Cert, RGN, FNP
Lecturer in Practice Nursing, Department of Public Health and Primary Care, City University, London
Chapter 7: Examination of the Female Reproductive System

Antonia Lynch, MSc (ANP), RN
Consultant Nurse, Emergency Department, Barts and the London NHS Trust, Whitechapel, London
Chapter 20: Common Emergency Treatments

Anthony McGrath, MSc, PGCE, BA (Hons) RMN, RGN, RNT
Principal Lecturer, Adult Nursing, University of Bedfordshire, Aylesbury, England
Chapter 5: Examination of the Abdomen
Chapter 6: Examination of the Male Genitalia

Nicola L. Whiteing, MSc, BSc (Hons), RN, ANP
Lecturer in Nursing, Department of Adult Nursing, City University, London
Chapter 11: Examination of the Musculoskeletal System

Christopher Richard Young, FIBMS, DLM
Department Manager, Clinical Laboratories, Newham Healthcare NHS Trust, London
Chapter 19: Laboratory Results – Reference Values

INTRODUCTION
The First Approach

General principles

It is important that the nurse understands that for the purpose of assessment and diagnosis, she is framing her approach to the patient from the perspective of the medical model. However, she must recognize that as a nurse, she employs the medical model within her practice, but is not practising medicine.

General objectives

When the student (or nurse) approaches a patient there are **four initial objectives**.

- **Obtain a professional rapport with the patient and gain her confidence.**
- **Obtain all relevant information that allows assessment of the illness, and provisional diagnoses.**
- **Obtain general information regarding the patient, her background, social situation and problems. In particular, it is necessary to find out how the illness has affected her, her family, friends, colleagues and her life.**

  A holistic assessment of the patient is of the utmost importance.
- **Understand the patient's own ideas about her problems, her major concerns and what she expects from the hospital admission, outpatient or general practice consultation.**

  Remember, medicine is just as much about worry as disease. Whatever the illness, whether chest infection or cancer, anxiety about what may happen is often uppermost in the patient's mind. **Listen attentively**.

The following notes provide a guide as to how one obtains the necessary information.

Specific objectives

In taking a history or conducting a physical examination there are **two complementary aims**:

- **Obtain all possible information about a patient and her illness (a database) from both subjective and objective perspectives.**
- **Solve the problem as to the diagnoses.**

Analytical approach

For each symptom or sign, one needs to think of a differential diagnosis and of other relevant information (from the history, physical examination or investigative tests) that will be needed to support or refute possible diagnoses. A good history, physical examination and investigation include these two facets and can be viewed as either positive (support) or negative (refute) findings. To achieve a formal diagnosis, following differential diagnosis, critical thinking/clinical decision making is used to examine positive and negative findings. Nurses frequently find that using the first two components of the SOAP (Subjective, Objective, Assessment and Plan) format (Clark, 1999) can help them formulate their diagnosis. The nurse should never approach the patient with just a set series of rote questions.

Frequently within the nurse-led preassessment clinic, ambulatory service (outpatient) clinics or in the general practice setting, standard assessment forms, either paper or electronic, will be used as a guide to history taking. These tools provide the necessary basis for a later, more inquisitive approach that should develop as knowledge about the patient's problem is acquired. Key to the process of achieving a diagnosis and formulating a plan of care is listening carefully to the patient, taking time, not assuming a diagnosis when the patient initially expresses her chief complaint, and understanding one's own values, attitudes and beliefs as they relate to diverse patient populations.

The subjective and objective components of the SOAP format provide the basis for diagnosis. Within the subjective component, the patient's perspective of her problem/illness is stated in her own words. This is often listed as the patient's chief complaint. In addition, the patient's 'subjective' view of her health history (e.g. childhood diseases and immunizations), as well as family history, present medications, how and when the patient takes the medications and chronological ordering of sequelae leading to the presenting problem, are documented. The objective component comprises the nurse's physical examination and investigative tests. Assessment involves the formulation of a diagnosis from the history, physical examination and investigative tests. Plan involves the development of the plan of care for the patient as well as where, when, how and by whom the plan will be implemented.

Self-reliance – getting started

The nurse must take her own history, make her own examination and write her own clinical records. After 1 month she should be sufficiently proficient that her notes could become the final record. The nurse should add a summary including her assessment of the problem list, provisional diagnoses and preliminary investigations. Initially these will be incomplete and occasionally incorrect. Nevertheless, the exercise will help to inculcate an enquiring approach and to highlight areas in which further questioning, investigation or reading is needed.

What is important when you start?

At the basis of all practice is clinical competence. No amount of knowledge will make up for poor technique.

Over the first few weeks it is essential to learn the basics of history taking and physical examination. This involves:
- **how to relate to patients**
- **how to take a good history efficiently, knowing which question to ask next and avoiding leading questions**
- **how to examine patients in a logical manner, in a set routine that will mean you will not miss an unexpected sign.**

You would be surprised how often nurses/students can fail an exam not because of lack of knowledge but because they have not mastered elementary clinical skills. These notes are written to try and help you to identify what is important and to help relate findings to common clinical situations.

There is nothing inherently difficult about history taking and physical examination. You will quickly become clinically competent if you:
- apply yourself
- initially learn the skills that are appropriate for each situation.

Common sense

Common sense is the cornerstone of good practice.
- **Always be aware of the patient's needs.**
- **Always evaluate what important information is needed:**
  - **to obtain the diagnosis**
  - **to provide appropriate treatment**
  - **to ensure continuity of care at home.**

Many mistakes are made by being side-tracked by aspects that are not important. Remain focused on the patient.

Learning

Your clinical skills and knowledge can soon develop with good organization.
- **Take advantage of seeing many patients** in acute care (hospital and ambulatory clinics) and in primary care (the community). It is particularly helpful to be present when patients are being admitted as emergencies or are being seen in a clinic or general practice setting for the first time.

- **Obtain a wide experience of clinical diseases**, how they affect patients and how they are managed.

   The more patients you can clerk yourself, the sooner you will become proficient and the more you will learn about patients and their diseases.

Building up knowledge

At first, history taking and physical assessment seem like a huge subject and each fact you learn seems to be an isolated piece of information. How will you ever be able to learn what is required? You will find after a few months that the information related to each system interrelates with other systems. The pieces of the jigsaw puzzle begin to fit together and then your confidence will increase. Although you will need to learn many facts, it is equally important to acquire the attitude of questioning, reasoning and knowing when and where to go to seek additional information.

- **Choose a medium-sized textbook in which you can read up about each disease you see or each problem you encounter.**

   Attaching knowledge to individual patients is a great help in acquiring and remembering facts. To practise history taking and physical assessment without a textbook is like a sailor without a chart, whereas to study books rather than patients is like a sailor who does not go to sea.

Understand the scientific background of disease, including the advances that are being made and how these could be applied to improve care.

- **Regularly read the editorials or any articles that interest you** in general medical and nursing journals.

   Even if at first you are not able to put the information into context, these articles will keep you in touch with new developments that add interest. However, it is not sensible to delve too deeply into any one subject when you are just beginning.

Relationships

Good relationships with patients and clinical colleagues are essential. You should maintain a natural, sincere, receptive and supportive relationship with your patients and clinical colleagues. Your ultimate goal in working with patients and clinical colleagues is to achieve good care.

Your role as an advanced practice nurse

The role of the advanced practice nurse extends the boundaries of professional nursing practice. The skills and practices associated with the advanced practice nursing role involve advanced clinical assessment techniques, interpretation of diagnostic tests including diagnostic imaging, implementing and monitoring therapeutic regimes, prescribing pharmacological interventions, initiating and receiving appropriate referrals, and discharge of patients. The Nursing and Midwifery Council (NMC) elected to record advanced practice nursing as an advanced nurse practitioner qualification on the register in 2005. These qualifications will be recorded on the second tier of the register associated with advanced practice. Specific competencies have been developed by the NMC (2005) and Royal College of Nursing (2002, 2008) that you must be able demonstrate in order to practise as an advanced practice nurse.

The Royal College of Nursing delineated domains of practice associated with the nurse practitioner role in April 2002 and extended this to advanced nurse practitioner in 2008. The domains of practice published by the RCN in 2008 are:

- assessment and management of patient illness/health status
- the nurse/patient relationship
- the education function
- professional role
- managing and negotiating healthcare delivery systems
- monitoring and ensuring quality of advanced healthcare practice
- respecting culture and diversity.

Undertaking a comprehensive history, physical examination and interpreting diagnostic tests as well as prescribing care are represented within the domains published by the Royal College of Nursing. It is essential that you develop sound skills within the framework delineated above in order to be competent at specialist/advanced practice level.

References

Clark, C. (1999) Taking a history. In: Walsh, M., Crumbie, A. & Reveley, S. (eds) *Nurse Practitioners, Clinical Skills and Professional Issues*. Butterworth Heinemann, Oxford.

Nursing and Midwifery Council (NMC) (2005) *Annex 1: Domains of Practice and Competencies*. NMC consultation on a proposed framework for postregistration nursing. Nursing and Midwifery Council, London.

Royal College of Nursing (RCN) (2002) *Nurse Practitioners – An RCN Guide to the Nurse Practitioner Role, Competencies and Programme Accreditation*. Royal College of Nursing, London.

Royal College of Nursing (RCN) (2008) *Advanced Nurse Practitioners – An RCN Guide to the Advanced Nurse Practitioner Role, Competencies and Programme Accreditation*. Royal College of Nursing, London.

CHAPTER 1

History Taking

General procedures

Introduction

The patient's history is the major subjective source of data about his health status. Physiological, psychological and psychosocial information (including family relationships and cultural influences) can be obtained which will inform you about the patient's perception of his current health status and lifestyle. It will give you insight into actual and potential problems as well as providing a guide for the physical examination.

Approaching the patient

- **Put the patient at ease by being confident and quietly friendly.**
- **Greet the patient: 'Good morning, Mr Smith'. (Address the patient formally and use his full name until he has given you permission to address him less formally.)**
- **Shake the patient's hand or place your hand on his if he is ill. (This action begins your physical assessment. It will give you a baseline indication of the patient's physical condition. For example, cold, clammy, diaphoretic or pyrexial.)**
- **State your name and title/role.**
- **Make sure the patient is comfortable.**
- **Explain that you wish to ask the patient questions to find out what happened to him.**

Start the history taking by stating something like 'I will start the history by asking you some questions about your health'. (Always begin with general questions and then move to more specific questions.) Inform the patient how long you are likely to take and what to expect. For example, after discussing what has happened to the patient, explain that you would like to examine him (Fig. 1.1).

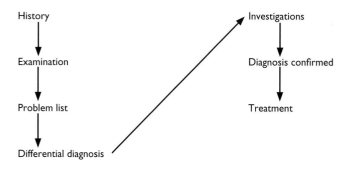

Fig. 1.1 Usual sequence of events.

Importance of the history

- It identifies:
  - what has happened
  - the personality of the patient
  - how the illness has affected him and his family
  - any specific anxieties
  - the physical and social environment.
- It establishes the nurse/patient relationship.
- It often gives the diagnosis.

Find the principal symptoms or symptom. Ask one of the following questions:
  - **'How may I help you?'**
  - **'What has the problem been?'**
  - **'Tell me why have you come to the surgery today?'** or **'Tell me why you came to see me today?'**

Effective history taking involves allowing the patient to talk in an unstructured way whilst you maintain control of the interview. Use language that the patient can understand and avoid the use of medical jargon. Avoid asking questions that can be answered by a simple 'yes' or 'no'. Ask questions that require a graded response – for example, 'Describe how your headache feels'. Avoid using multiple-choice questions that may confuse the patient. Ask one question at a time. Avoid asking questions like: 'What's wrong?' or 'What brought you here?'. Use clarification to confirm your understanding of the patient's problem. Avoid forming premature conclusions about the patient's problem and above all remain non-judgemental in your demeanour. Avoid making judgemental statements.

- **Let the patient tell his story in his own words as much as possible. At first listen and then take discreet notes as he talks.**

When learning to take a history, there can be a tendency to ask too many questions in the first 2 minutes. After asking the first question, you should normally allow the patient to talk uninterrupted for up to 2 minutes.

Do not worry if the story is not entirely clear or if you do not think the information being given is of diagnostic significance. If you interrupt too early, you run the risk of overlooking an important symptom or anxiety.

You will be learning about what the patient thinks is important. You have the opportunity to judge how you are going to proceed. Different patients give histories in very different ways. Some patients will need to be encouraged to enlarge on their answers to your questions; with others, you may need to ask specific questions and to interrupt in order to prevent too rambling a history. Think consciously about the approach you will adopt. If you need to interrupt the patient, do so clearly and decisively.

- **Try, if feasible, to conduct a conversation rather than an interrogation, following the patient's train of thoughts.**

You will usually need to ask follow-up questions on the main symptoms to obtain a full understanding of what they were and of the chain of events.

- **Obtain a full description of the patient's principal complaints.**
- **Enquire about the sequence of symptoms and events.**

Beware pseudo-medical terms, e.g. 'gastric flu'; instead, enquire what happened. Clarify by asking what the patient means.

- **Do not ask leading questions.**

A central aim in taking the history is to understand patients' symptoms from their own point of view. It is important not to tarnish the patient's history by your own expectations. For example, do not ask a patient whom you suspect might be thyrotoxic: 'Do you find hot weather uncomfortable?'. This invites the answer 'yes' and then a positive answer becomes of little diagnostic value. Instead, ask the open question: 'Do you particularly dislike either hot or cold weather?'.

- **Be sensitive to a patient's mood and non-verbal responses.**

For example, hesitancy in revealing emotional content. Use reflection so that the patient will expand on his discussion.

- **Be understanding, receptive and matter of fact without being sympathetic. Display and express empathy rather than sympathy.**
- **Avoid showing surprise or reproach.**
- **Clarify symptoms and obtain a problem list.**
- **When the patient has finished describing the symptom or symptoms:**
  - **briefly summarize the symptoms**
  - **ask whether there are any other main problems.**

    For example, say, 'You have mentioned two problems: pain on the left side of your tummy, and loose motions over the last six weeks. Before we talk about those in more detail, are there any other problems I should know about?'.

Usual sequence of history

- **principal complaints, e.g. chest pain, poor home circumstances**
  - history of present complaint

- details of current illness
- enquiry of other symptoms (see Functional enquiry)
- **present medications/allergies**
- **past history**
- **family history**
- **personal and social history**

If one's initial enquiries make it apparent that one section is of more importance than usual (e.g. previous relevant illnesses or operation), then relevant enquiries can be brought forward to an earlier stage in the history (e.g. past history after finding principal complaints).

History of present illness

- **Start your written history with a single sentence** summing up what your patient is complaining of. It should be like the banner headline of a newspaper. For example: c/o chest pain for 6 months. (You may choose to state the patient's chief complaint in the patient's own words when documenting.)
- **Determine the chronology of the illness by asking:**
  - 'How and when did your illness begin?' or
  - 'When did you first notice anything wrong?' or
  - 'When did you last feel completely well?'
- **Begin by stating when the patient was last perfectly well. Describe symptoms in chronological order of onset.**
  - Both the **date of onset** and the **length of time** prior to being seen by you should be recorded. Symptoms should never be dated by the day of the week as this later becomes meaningless.
- **Obtain a detailed description of each symptom by asking:**
  - 'Tell me what the pain was like', for example. Make sure you ask about all symptoms, whether they seem relevant or not.
- With all symptoms, obtain the following details:
  - **duration**
  - **onset – sudden or gradual**
  - **what has happened since:**
    - **constant or periodic**
    - **frequency**
    - **getting worse or better**
  - **precipitating or relieving factors**
  - **associated symptoms**
- **If pain is a symptom**, also determine the following:
  - **site**
  - **radiation**
  - **character**, e.g. ache, pressure, shooting, stabbing, dull
  - **severity**, e.g. 'Did it interfere with what you were doing? Does it keep you awake? Have you ever had this type of pain before? Does the pain make you sweat or feel sick?

Avoid technical language when describing a patient's history. Do not say 'the patient complained of melaena' but rather 'the patient complained of passing loose, black, tarry motions'.

Supplementary history

When patients are unable to give an adequate or reliable history, the necessary information must be obtained from friends or relations. A history from a person who has witnessed a sudden event is often helpful.

When the patient does not speak English, arrange for an interpreter to translate for the patient. Bear in mind that Barkauskas *et al.* (2002) indicate that if possible, family members and patients' young children should not be used as interpreters. Family members will frequently tell you what they think the patient's problem is rather than what the patient thinks his problem is. Because some questions that you may ask the patient are sensitive in nature, children should not be asked to interpret for their parents.

Functional enquiry

This is a checklist of symptoms not already discovered.

Do not ask questions already covered in establishing the principal symptoms. This list may detect other symptoms.

- **Modify your questioning according to the nature of the suspected disease, available time and circumstances.**

     If during the functional enquiry a positive answer is obtained, full details must be elicited. **Asterisks (*) denote questions that must nearly always be asked.**

General questions

Ask about the following points:

- ***appetite**: 'What is your appetite like? Do you feel like eating?'
- ***weight**: 'Have you lost or gained weight recently?'
- ***general well-being**: 'Do you feel well in yourself?'
- ***feelings of sadness or depression** (to rule out feelings of suicide.) 'Do you feel sad or depressed?'
- **fatigue**: 'Are you more or less tired than you used to be?'
- **fever or chills**: 'Have you felt hot or cold? Have you shivered?'
- **night sweats**: 'Have you noticed any sweating at night or any other time?'
- **aches or pains**
- **rash**: 'Have you had any rash recently? Does it itch?'
- **lumps and bumps**

Cardiovascular and respiratory system

Ask about the following points:
- ***chest pain**: 'Have you recently had any pain or discomfort in the chest?'
  The most common causes of chest pain are:
  - *ischaemic heart disease*: severe constricting, central chest pain radiating to the neck, jaw and left arm; *angina*: pain frequently precipitated by exercise or emotion and relieved by rest; *myocardial infarction*: the pain may come on at rest, be more severe and last hours
  - *pleuritic pain*: sharp, localized pain, usually lateral; worse on inspiration or cough
  - *anxiety or panic attacks*: a very common cause of chest pain. Enquire about circumstances that bring on an attack
- ***shortness of breath**: 'Are you breathless at any time?'
  Breathlessness (dyspnoea) and chest pain must be accurately described. The degree of exercise that brings on the symptoms must be noted (e.g. climbing one flight of stairs, after 0.5 km (1/4 mile) walk).
- **shortness of breath on lying flat** (*orthopnoea*): 'Do you get breathless in bed? What do you do then? Does it get worse or better on sitting up? How many pillows do you use? Can you sleep without them?'
- **waking up breathless**: 'Do you wake at night with any symptoms? Do you gasp for breath? What do you do then?'
  Orthopnoea (breathless when lying flat) and *paroxysmal nocturnal dyspnoea* (waking up breathless, relieved on sitting up) are features of *left heart failure*.
- ***ankle swelling**
  Common in *congestive cardiac failure* (*right heart failure*).
- **palpitations**: 'Are you aware of your heart beating?'
  Palpitations may be:
  - single thumps (*ectopics*)
  - slow or fast
  - regular or irregular
  Ask the patient to tap them out.
  Paroxysmal tachycardia (sudden attacks of palpitations) usually starts and finishes abruptly.
- ***cough**: 'Do you have a cough? Is it a dry cough or do you cough up sputum? When do you cough?'
- **sputum**: 'What colour is your sputum? How much do you cough up?'
  Green sputum usually indicates an *acute chest infection*. Clear sputum daily during winter months suggests *chronic bronchitis*. Frothy sputum suggests *left heart failure*.

- ***blood in sputum** (*haemoptysis*): 'Have you coughed up blood?'
  Haemoptysis must be taken very seriously. Causes include:
    - carcinoma of bronchus
    - pulmonary embolism
    - mitral stenosis
    - tuberculosis
    - bronchiectasis
- **blackouts** (*syncope*): 'Have you had any blackouts or faints? Did you feel light-headed or did the room go round? Did you lose consciousness? Did you have any warning? Can you remember what happened?'
- ***smoking**: 'Do you smoke? How many cigarettes do you smoke each day?'

Gastrointestinal system

Ask about the following points:
- **nausea**: 'Are there times when you feel sick?'
- **vomiting**: 'Do you vomit? What is it like?'
  'Coffee grounds' vomit suggests altered blood.
  Old food suggests *pyloric stenosis*.
  If blood, what colour is it – dark or bright red?
- **difficulty in swallowing** (*dysphagia*): 'Do you have difficulty swallowing? Where does it stick?'
  For solids: often organic obstruction.
  For fluids: often neurological or psychological.
- **indigestion**: 'Do you have any discomfort in your stomach after eating?'
- **abdominal pain**: 'Where is the pain? How is it connected to meals or opening your bowels? What relieves the pain?'
- ***bowel habit**: 'How often do you open your bowels?' or 'How many times do you open your bowels per day? Do you have to open your bowels at night?' (often a sign of true pathology)
  If *diarrhoea* is suggested, the number of motions per day and their nature (blood? pus? mucus?) must be established.
  'What are your motions like?' The stools may be pale, bulky and float (fat in stool – *steatorrhoea*) or tarry from digested blood (*melaena* – usually from upper gastrointestinal tract).
  Bright blood on the surface of a motion may be from *haemorrhoids*, whereas blood within a stool may signify *cancer* or *inflammatory bowel disease*.
- **jaundice**: 'Is your urine dark? Are your stools pale? What tablets have you been taking recently? Have you had any recent injections or transfusions? Have you been abroad recently? How much alcohol do you drink?'

Jaundice may be:
  - **obstructive** (dark urine, pale stools) from:
    - carcinoma of the head of the pancreas
    - gallstones
  - **hepatocellular** (dark urine, pale stools may develop) from:
    - *ethanol* (cirrhosis)
    - drugs or transfusions (viral hepatitis)
    - drug reactions or infections (travel abroad, viral hepatitis or amoebae)
  - **haemolytic** (unconjugated bilirubin is bound to albumin and is not secreted in the urine)

Genitourinary system

Ask about the following points:
  - **dysuria**: pain on urination – usually burning (often a sign of infection/cystitis)
  - **loin pain**: 'Any pain in your back?'
    Pain in the loins suggests pyelonephritis.
  - ***urine**: 'Are your waterworks all right? Do you pass a lot of water at night? Do you have any difficulty passing water? Is there blood in your water?' (suggests haematuria)
    Polyuria and *nocturia* occur in *diabetes.*
    Prostatism results in slow onset of urination, a poor stream and terminal dribbling.
  - **sex**: 'Any problems with intercourse or making love?'
  - ***menstruation**: 'Any problems with your periods? Do you bleed heavily? Do you bleed between periods?'
    Vaginal bleeding between periods or after the menopause raises the possibility of *cervical* or *uterine cancer.*
    Menstrual cycle: last menstrual period (LMP) and length of bleeding. (Normal cycle is 21–35 days. Normal period is between 5 and 8 days with between 70 and 200 ml of blood loss.) If indicated, ask about intermenstrual, postmenopausal or postcoital bleeding.
  - **vaginal discharge** (if present, ask about colour, consistency and odour; does it cause itching?)
  - **pain on intercourse** (*dyspareunia*)

Nervous system

Ask about the following points:
  - ***headache**: 'Do you ever have any headaches? Where are they? (location) When do you get headaches? What are they like?' (quality/intensity)

Headaches often originate from tension and can be either frontal or occipital. Occipital headache on waking in the early morning may be due to *raised intracranial pressure* (e.g. from a *tumour* or *malignant hypertension*). Ask if the headache is associated with flashing lights (*amaurosis fugax*).

- **vision**: 'Do you have any blurred or double vision?'
- **hearing**: ask about tinnitus, deafness and exposure to noise
- **dizziness**: 'Do you have any dizziness or episodes when the world goes round (*vertigo*)?'

   Dizziness with light-headed symptoms, when sudden in onset, may be *cardiac* (enquire about palpitations). When slow, onset may be *vasovagal 'fainting'* or an *internal haemorrhage*.
   Vertigo may be from *ear disease* (*labyrinthitis/infection, Ménière's disease*; enquire about deafness, earache or discharge) or *brainstem dysfunction*.

- **unsteady gait**: 'Any difficulty walking or running?'
- **weakness** (consider ME or *myasthenia gravis*)
- **numbness** or increased sensation: 'Any patches of numbness?'
- **pins and needles**
- **sphincter disturbance**: 'Any difficulties holding your water/bowels?' (sign of spinal cord compression; ask about back injury)
- **fits or faints**: 'Have you had any funny episodes?'

   The following details should be sought from the patient:
   - **duration**
   - **frequency and length of attacks**
   - **time of attacks, e.g. if standing, at night**
   - **mode of onset and termination**
   - **premonition or aura, light-headed or vertigo**
   - **biting of tongue, loss of sphincter control, injury, etc.**

   Grand mal epilepsy classically produces sudden unconsciousness without any warning and on waking, the patient feels drowsy with a headache and sore tongue, and has been incontinent.

Mental health

Ask about the following points:
- **depression**: 'How is your mood? Happy or sad? If depressed, how bad? Have you lost interest in things? Can you still enjoy things? How do you feel about the future? Has anything happened in your life to make you sad or depressed? Do you feel guilty about anything?'. If the patient seems depressed: 'Have you ever thought of suicide? How long have you felt like this? Is there a specific problem? Have you felt like this before?'

- **active periods**: 'Do you have periods in which you are particularly active?'

> Susceptibility to depression may be a personality trait. In *bipolar affective disease*, swings to *mania* (excess activity, rapid speech and excitable mood) can recur. Enquire about interest, concentration, irritability, sleep difficulties.

- **anxiety**: 'Have you worried a lot recently? Do you get anxious? In what situations? Are there any situations you avoid because you feel anxious? Do you worry about your health? Any worries in your job or with your family? Any financial worries? Do you have panic attacks? What happens?'
- **sleep**: 'Any difficulties sleeping? Do you have difficulty getting to sleep? Do you wake early?'

> Difficulties of sleep are commonly associated with depression or anxiety.

Refer to Chapter 8 for more comprehensive information on mental health assessment.

The eye

Ask about the following points:

- **eye pain, photophobia or redness**: 'Have the eyes been red, uncomfortable or painful?'
- painful red eye, particularly with photophobia, may be serious and due to:
  > *iritis* – anterior/posterior uveitis must be treated as a medical emergency (it may be related to *ankylosing spondylitis, Reiter's disease, sarcoid, Behçet's disease*)
  > *scleritis (systemic vasculitis)*
  > *corneal ulcer*
  > *acute glaucoma*
- painless red eye may be:
  > *episcleritis*
  > temporary and of no consequence
  > *systemic vasculitis*
- sticky red eye may be *conjunctivitis* (usually infective)
- itchy eye may be *allergic*, e.g. *hay fever*
- gritty eye may be dry (sicca or *Sjögren's syndrome*)
- **clarity of vision**: 'Has your vision been blurred?'
  - blurring of vision for either near or distance alone may be an error of focus, helped by spectacles
  - loss of central vision (or of top or bottom half) in one eye may be due to a *retinal or optic nerve disorder*
  - transient complete blindness in one eye lasting for minutes – *amaurosis fugax* (fleeting blindness)

suggests retinal arterial blockage from embolus
may be from *carotid atheroma* (listen for bruit)
may have a cardiac source
- subtle difficulties with vision, difficulty reading – problems at the chiasm or visual path behind it:
complete *bitemporal hemianopia – tumour* pressure on chiasm
homonymous
hemianopia: posterior cerebral or optic radiation lesion
    - usually *infarct* or *tumour*; rarely complains of 'half vision' but may have difficulty reading
- **diplopia**: 'Have you ever seen double?'
Diplopia may be due to:
    - *lesion* of the motor cranial nerves III, IV or VI
    - *third nerve palsy*
causes double vision in all directions
often with dilation of the pupil and ptosis
    - *fourth nerve palsy*
causes doubling looking down and in (as when reading) with images separated horizontally and vertically and tilted (not parallel)
    - *sixth nerve palsy*
causes horizontal, level and parallel doubling
worse on looking to the affected side
    - *muscular disorder*
e.g. thyroid-related (see below)
myasthenia gravis (weakness after muscle use, antibodies to nerve endplates)

Locomotor system

Ask about the following points:
- **pain, stiffness, or swelling of joints**: 'When and how did it start? Have you injured the joint?'
There are innumerable causes of *arthritis* (painful, swollen, tender joints) and *arthralgia* (painful joints). Patients may incorrectly attribute a problem to some injury.
Osteo-arthritis is a joint 'wearing out' and is often asymmetrical, involving weight-bearing joints such as the hip or knee. Exercise makes the joint pain worse.
Rheumatoid arthritis is a generalized autoimmune disease with symmetrical involvement. In the hands, fusiform swelling of the interphalangeal joints is accompanied by swollen metacarpophalangeal joints. Large joints are often affected. Stiffness is worse after rest, e.g. on waking, and improves with use.

Gout usually involves a single joint, such as the first metatarsophalangeal joint, but can lead to gross hand involvement with asymmetrical uric acid lumps (*tophi*) by some joints, and in the tips of the ears.

Septic arthritis is a single, hot, painful joint.
- **functional disability**: 'How far can you walk? Can you walk up stairs? Is any particular movement difficult? Can you dress yourself? (Observe how the patient is dressed.) How long does it take? Are you able to work? Can you write?' (In the physical examination observe how the patient walks and his manual dexterity.)

Thyroid disease

Ask about the following points:
- **weight change**
- **reaction to the weather**: 'Do you dislike hot or cold weather?'
- **irritability**: 'Are you more or less irritable compared with a few years ago?'
- **diarrhoea/constipation**
- **palpitations**
- **dry skin or greasy hair**: 'Is your skin dry or greasy? Is your hair dry or greasy?'
- **depression**: 'How has your mood been?'
- **croaky voice**

> *Hypothyroid* patients put on weight without increase in appetite, dislike cold weather, have dry skin and thin, dry hair, a puffy face, a croaky voice, are usually calm and may be depressed.
>
> *Hyperthyroid* patients may lose weight despite eating more, dislike hot weather, perspire excessively, have palpitations, a tremor, and may be agitated and tearful. Young people have predominantly nervous and heat intolerance symptoms, whereas old people tend to present with cardiac symptoms. (Exophthalmos may be present.)

Past history

- **All previous illnesses or operations**, whether apparently important or not, must be included.

  > For instance, a casually mentioned attack of influenza or chill may have been a manifestation of an occult infection.
- The importance of a past illness may be determined by finding out **how long the patient was in bed or off work**.
- **Complications of any previous illnesses** should be carefully enquired into and here, leading questions are sometimes necessary.

General questions

Ask about the following:
- 'Have you had any serious illnesses?'
- 'Have you had any emotional or nervous problems?'
- 'Have you had any operations or admissions to hospital?'
- 'Have you ever:
  - had yellow skin (jaundice), fits (epilepsy), TB, high blood pressure (hypertension), low blood pressure (hypotension), rheumatic fever, kidney problems or diabetes?
  - travelled abroad?
  - had allergies?'
- 'Have any medicines ever upset you?'

   Allergic responses to drugs may include an itchy rash, vomiting, diarrhoea or severe illness, including jaundice. Many patients claim to be allergic but are not. An accurate description of the supposed allergic episodes is important.
- Other questions can be included when relevant such as: **'Have you ever had a heart attack?'**
- **Additional questions can be asked** depending on the patient's previous responses such as:
  - if the patient has high blood pressure, ask about kidney problems, if relatives have hypertension or whether he eats liquorice
  - if a possible heart attack, ask about hypertension, diabetes, diet, smoking, family history of heart disease
  - if the patient's history suggests cardiac failure, you must ask if he has had *rheumatic fever*

Patients may have had examinations for life insurance or the armed forces.

Family history

The family history gives clues to possible predisposition to illness (e.g. heart attacks) and whether a patient may have reason to be particularly anxious about a certain disease (e.g. mother died of cancer).

Death certificates and patient knowledge are often inaccurate. Patients may be reluctant to talk about relatives' illnesses if they were mental diseases, epilepsy or cancer. It will be useful to construct a genogram of the patient's family history for quick referral.

General questions

Ask about the following:
- '**Are your parents alive?** Are they fit and well? What did your parents die from?'

- 'Have you any brothers or sisters? Are they fit and well?'
- 'Do you have any children? Are they fit and well?'
- 'Is there any family history of:
  - heart trouble?
  - diabetes?
  - high blood pressure?'

These questions can be varied to take account of the patient's chief complaint.

Personal and social history

You need to find out what kind of person the patient is, what his home circumstances are and how his illness has affected him and his family. Your aim is to understand the patient's illness in the context of his personality and his home environment.

If in hospital or following day surgery, can the patient convalesce satisfactorily at home and at what stage? What are the consequences of his illness? Will advice, information and help be needed? An interview with a relative or friend may be very helpful.

General questions

Ask about the following:

- **family**: 'Is everything all right at home? Do you have any family problems?'

   It may be appropriate to ask: 'Is your relationship with your partner/husband/wife all right? Is sex all right?'. Problems may arise from physical or emotional reasons, and the patient may appreciate an opportunity to discuss worries. Note that a patient's sexual preference and sexual orientation may be different.

- **accommodation**: 'Where do you live? Is it all right?'
- **job**: 'What is your job? Could you tell me exactly what you do? Is it satisfactory? Will your illness affect your work?'
- **hobbies**: 'What do you do in your spare time? Do you have any social life? What is your social life like?'
- **alcohol**: 'How much alcohol do you drink?'

   Alcoholics usually underestimate their daily consumption. (Normally intake should not exceed 21 units per week for a male and 14 units per week for a female.) It may be helpful to go through a 'drinking day'. If there is a suspicion of a drinking problem, you can ask: 'Do you ever drink in the morning? Do you worry about controlling your drinking? Does it affect your job, home or social life?'.

- **smoking**: 'Do you smoke?' Have you ever smoked? Why did you give up? How many cigarettes, cigars or pipefuls of tobacco do you smoke a day?'

  This is particularly relevant for heart or chest disease, but must always be asked.
- **drugs**: 'Do you take any recreational drugs? If so, what do you take?'
- **prescribed medications**: 'What pills are you taking at the moment? Have you taken any other pills in the last few months?'

  This is an extremely important question. A complete list of all drugs and doses must be obtained.

If relevant, ask about any pets, visits abroad, previous or present work exposure to coal dust, asbestos, etc.

The patient's ideas, concerns and expectations

Make sure that you understand the patient's main ideas, concerns and expectations. Ask, for example:

- **What do you think is wrong with you?**
- **What are you expecting to happen to you whilst you are in the surgery or in hospital?**
- **Is there something particular you would like us to do?**
- **Have you any questions?**

The patient's main concerns may not be your main concerns. The patient may have quite different expectations of his visit to the surgery, the hospital admission or outpatient appointment from what you assume. If you fail to address the patient's concerns, he is likely to be dissatisfied, leading to a difficult nurse/patient relationship and possible non-compliance.

Strategy

Having taken the history, you should:

- **have some idea of possible diagnoses (in 90–95% of cases the patient will tell you what his problem is whilst you are taking the history)**
- **have made an assessment of the patient as a person**
- **know which systems you wish to concentrate on when examining the patient.**

Further relevant questions may arise from abnormalities found on examination or investigation.

Reference

Barkauskas, V., Baumann, L. & Darling-Fisher, C. (2002) *Health and Physical Assessment*, 3rd edn. Mosby, London.

CHAPTER 2

General Examination

Introduction

An initial assessment of the patient will have been made whilst taking the history. The **general appearance of the patient** will be your first observation. Subsequently, the order of your examination will vary based on the subjective information provided in the patient's history.

The system to which the presenting symptoms refer is generally examined first. Otherwise, devise your own routine, examining each part of the body in turn, covering all systems as required. An example is:

- **general appearance**
- **alertness, mood, general behaviour**
- **hands and nails**
- **skin**
- **radial pulse**
- **axillary nodes**
- **cervical lymph nodes**
- **facies, eyes, tongue**
- **jugular venous pulse/distension**
- **heart**
- **breasts**
- **respiratory**
- **abdomen, including femoral pulses**
- **rectal or pelvic examination**
- **musculoskeletal**
- **nervous system including fundi (if not examined with the eyes as noted above).**

Whichever part of the body you are examining, always use the same routine*:

1. **inspection**
2. **palpation**
3. **percussion**
4. **auscultation.**

(*The routine will vary in examination of the abdomen, with auscultation following inspection.)

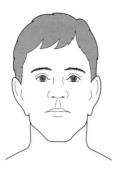

Fig. 2.1 Carefully observe the patient.

General inspection (Fig. 2.1)

The beginning of the examination is a careful observation of the patient as a whole. Note the following.
- **Does the patient look ill?**
  - what age does he look?
  - febrile, dehydrated?
  - alert, confused, drowsy?
  - co-operative, happy, sad, resentful?
  - fat, muscular, wasted?
  - in pain or distressed?

Hands

- **Temperature:**
  - unduly cold hands – ? *low cardiac output*
  - unduly warm hands – ? *high-output state*, e.g. *thyrotoxicosis*
  - cold and sweaty – ? anxiety or other causes of *sympathetic over-reactivity*, e.g. *hypoglycaemia*
- Peripheral cyanosis
- **Raynaud's syndrome** (Fig. 2.2)

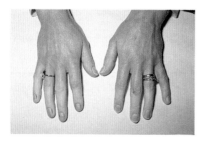

Fig. 2.2 Raynaud's syndrome – white/blue fingers induced by cold.

- ● **Nicotine stains**
- ● **Nails:**
  - – bitten
  - – leuconychia – white nails
    Can occur in *cirrhosis*
  - – koilonychia – misshapen, concave nails (Figs 2.3, 2.4)
    Can occur in *iron deficiency anaemia*
  - – clubbing – loss of angle at base of nail (Figs 2.5–2.7)

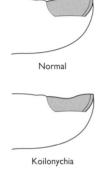

Normal

Koilonychia

Fig. 2.3 A normal nail and a nail with koilonychia.

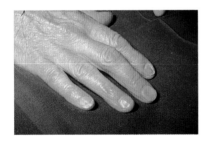

Fig. 2.4 Koilonychia from iron deficiency – spoon-shaped nails.

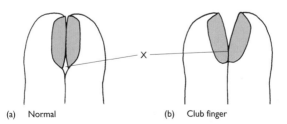

(a)   Normal   (b)   Club finger

Fig. 2.5 A normal finger (a) and a club finger (b).

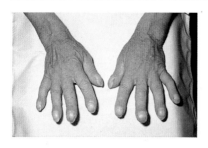

Fig. 2.6 Finger clubbing – gross with carcinoma of bronchus.

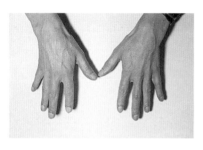

Fig. 2.7 Congenital cyanotic heart disease – dusky, cyanotic hands with mild clubbing.

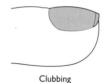

Clubbing

Fig. 2.8 Nail clubbing.

Nail clubbing (Fig. 2.8) occurs in specific diseases:
- heart: infectious *endocarditis, cyanotic congenital heart disease*
- lungs: *carcinoma of the bronchus (chronic infection: abscess; bronchiectasis, e.g. cystic fibrosis; empyema); fibrosing alveolitis* (not chronic bronchitis)
- liver: *cirrhosis*
- *Crohn's disease*
- *congenital*
- splinter haemorrhages (Figs 2.9, 2.10)

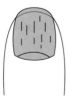

Splinter
haemorrhages

Fig. 2.9 Splinter haemorrhages.

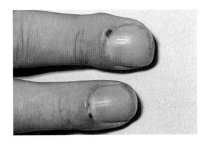

Fig. 2.10 Nailfold infarcts from polyarteritis – small black areas, often associated with splinter haemorrhages in nails.

Occur in *infectious endocarditis* but are more common in people doing manual work.
- pitting – *psoriasis*
- onycholysis – separation of nail from nail bed; *psoriasis, thyrotoxicosis*
- paronychia – pustule in lateral nailfold
● **Palms:**
  - erythema – can be normal, also occurs with *chronic liver disease, pregnancy* (Fig. 2.11)
  - Dupuytren's contracture (Fig. 2.12) – tethering of skin in palm to flexor tendon of fourth finger; can occur in *cirrhosis*

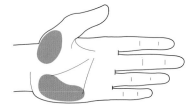

Fig. 2.11 Palmar erythema.

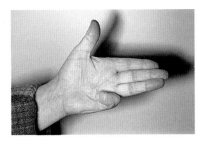

Fig. 2.12 Dupuytren's contraction – thickened palmar skin attached to the tendons.

● **Joints:**
  - symmetrical swellings occur in *rheumatoid arthritis* (Fig. 2.13)
  - asymmetrical swellings occur in *gout* (Fig. 2.14) and *osteo-arthritis*

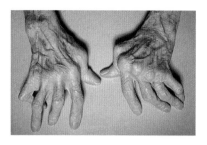

Fig. 2.13 Rheumatoid arthritis – symmetrically enlarged metacarpophalangeal and interphalangeal joints, with secondary wasting of interossei muscles and subluxation of fingers from snapped dorsal tendons.

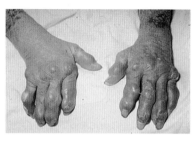

Fig. 2.14 Gout – asymmetrical swelling of joints with subcutaneous 'tophi' of uric acid deposits.

Skin

Inspection of skin

- Distribution of any lesions
- Examine close up with palpation of skin
- Remember mucous membranes, hair and nails
- **Colour:**
  - pigmented apart from racial pigmentation or suntan (Fig. 2.15) – examine buccal mucosa
  - if appears jaundiced, examine sclerae
  - if pale, examine conjunctivae for anaemia

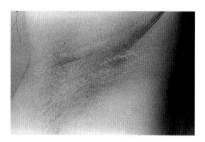

Fig. 2.15 Acanthosis nigricans in the armpit – thickened epidermis from gross insulin resistance which also occurs on the neck.

- **Skin texture:**
  - ? normal for age (becomes thinner from age 50)
  - thin, e.g. *Cushing's syndrome, hypothyroid, hypopituitary, malnutrition, liver or renal failure*

- thick, e.g. *acromegaly, androgen excess*
- dry, e.g. *hypothyroid*
- tethered or puckered e.g. *scleroderma* of fingers, attached to underlying breast tumour
- **Rash:**
  - what is it like? (describe precisely)

Inspection of lesions

- distribution of lesions:
  symmetrical or asymmetrical
  peripheral or mainly on trunk
  maximal on light-exposed sites
  pattern of contact with known agents, e.g. shoes, gloves, cosmetics
- number and size of lesions
- look at an early lesion
- discrete or confluent
- pattern of lesions, e.g. linear, annular, serpiginous (like a snake), reticular (like a net), star shaped (melanoma)
- is edge well demarcated?
- colour (melanomas have atypical pigmentation in the epidermis such as shades of grey, white, red, blue, brown and black)
- surface, e.g. scaly, shiny

Palpation of lesions

- flat, impalpable – *macular* (Fig. 2.16)
- raised
  papular: in skin, localized
  plaque: larger, e.g. >0.5 cm
  nodules: deeper in dermis, persisting more than 3 days
  wheal: oedema fluid, transient, less than 3 days
  vesicles: contain fluid (Fig. 2.17)
  bullae: large vesicles, e.g. >0.5 cm
  pustular

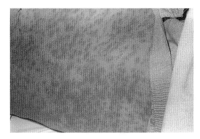

Fig. 2.16 Ampicillin rash – patchy red macules that blanch on pressure.

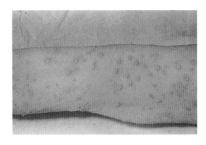

Fig. 2.17 Chicken pox – peripheral circumscribed, erythematous papules with central blister.

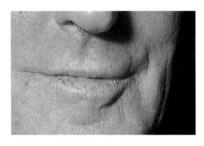

Fig. 2.18 Osler–Weber–Rendu syndrome – telangiectasia on the lip in a patient with haematemesis.

- deep in dermis – *nodules*
- temperature
- tender?
- blanches on pressure – most erythematous lesions, e.g. *drug rash, telangiectasia* (Fig. 2.18), dilated capillaries
- does not blanch on pressure

> *Purpura* or *petechiae* are small discrete microhaemorrhages approximately 1 mm across, red, non-tender macules.
> If palpable, suggests *vasculitis* (Fig. 2.19).
> *Senile purpura* local haemorrhages are from minor traumas in thin skin of hands or forearms. Flat purple/brown lesions.

- hard
- sclerosis, e.g. *scleroderma* of fingers (Fig. 2.20)
- infiltration, e.g. *lymphoma* or *cancer*
- scars

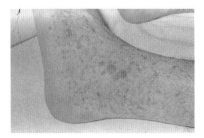

Fig. 2.19 Henoch–Schönlein syndrome – macular/papular rash including petechiae that do not blanch on pressure.

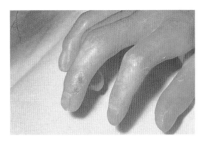

Fig. 2.20   Scleroderma – thick shiny skin and limiting joint movements with ulcers from subcutaneous calcification.

Enquire about the time course of any lesion

- 'How long has it been there?'
- 'Is it fixed in size and position? Does it come and go?'
- 'Is it itchy, sore, tender or anaesthetic?'

Knowledge of the differential diagnosis will indicate other questions:

- dermatitis of hand – contact with chemicals or plants, wear and tear
- ulcer of toe – *arterial disease, diabetes mellitus, neuropathy*
- pigmentation and ulcer of lower medial leg – *varicose veins*

Table 2.1   Common skin diseases

Disease	Description
Acne	Pilar-sebaceous follicular inflammation – papules and pustules on face and upper trunk, blackheads (*comedones*), cysts.
Basal cell carcinoma (rodent ulcer) (Fig. 2.21)	Shiny papule with rolled border and capillaries on surface. Can have a depressed centre or ulcerate.

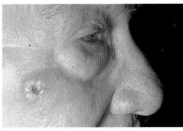

Fig. 2.21   Rodent ulcer – raised, shiny papule with telangiectasia on the surface with a central ulcer.

Bullae	Blisters due to burns, infection of the skin, allergy or, rarely, autoimmune diseases affecting adhesion within epidermis (*pemphigus*) or at the epidermal–dermal junction (*pemphigoid*).

Table 2.1 *(continued)*

Disease	Description
Café-au-lait patches	Permanent discrete brown macules of varying size and shape. If large and numerous (6 or >6 café-au-lait spots) requires evaluation – suggests neurofibromatosis (Fig. 2.22).

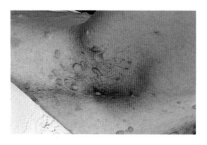

Fig. 2.22 Neurofibromatosis type 1 (von Recklinghausen's disease) – multiple cutaneous fibroma.

Drug eruptions (Fig. 2.23)

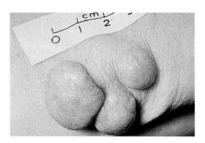

Usually macular, symmetrical distribution. Can be urticaria, eczematous and various forms, including erythema multiforme or erythema nodosum (see below).

Fig. 2.23 Tuberous xanthoma of elbows in homozygous familial hypercholesterolaemia – also occurs in tendons and signifies very high cholesterol levels.

Eczema (Fig. 2.24)

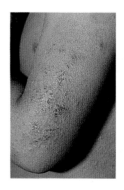

Atopic dermatitis: dry skin, red, plaques, commonly on the face, antecubital and popliteal fossae, with fine scales, vesicles and scratch marks secondary to *pruritus* (itching). Often associated with *asthma* and *hayfever*.
Family history of atopy.
Contact dermatitis: may be irritant or allergic.
Red, scaly plaques with vesicles in acute stages.

Fig. 2.24 Eczema on upper arm – diffuse erythema and scratch marks, with small blisters and fine scales that cannot be seen on this photo.

Table 2.1 (*continued*)

Disease	Description
Erythema multiforme	Symmetrical, widespread inflammatory 0.5–1 cm macules/papules, often with central blister. Can be confluent. Usually on hands and feet. Due to: *drug reactions* *viral infections* *no apparent cause* *Stevens–Johnson syndrome* – with mucosal desquamation involving genitalia, mouth and conjunctivae, with fever.
Erythema nodosum (Fig. 2.25)	Tender, localized, red, diffusely raised, 2–4 cm nodules in anterior shins. Due to: *streptococcal infection*, e.g. with *rheumatic* *fever* *primary tuberculosis* and other infections *sarcoid* *inflammatory bowel disease* *drug reactions* *no apparent cause.*

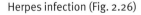
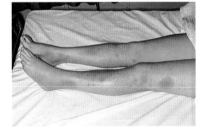

Fig. 2.25 Erythema nodosum – approximately 5–10 cm across, swellings in dermis of shins with red, warm surfaces.

Fungus	Red, annular, scaly area of skin. When involving the nails, they become thickened with loss of compact structure.
Herpes infection (Fig. 2.26)	Clusters of vesicopustules which crust, recurs at the same site, e.g. lips, buttocks.

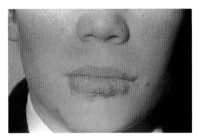

Fig. 2.26 Herpes simplex on lips ('cold sores') – these can erupt with other illnesses.

Table 2.1 *(continued)*

Disease	Description
Impetigo	Spreading pustules and yellow crusts from staphylococcal infection.
Malignant melanoma	Usually irregular pigmented (grey, white, red, blue, brown and black), papule or plaque, superficial or thick with irregular edge, enlarging with tendency to bleed.
Psoriasis (see Fig. 2.49)	Symmetrical eruption: chronic, discrete, red plaques with silvery scales. Gentle scraping easily induces bleeding. Often affects scalp, elbows and knees. Nails may be pitted. Familial and precipitated by streptococcal sore throats or skin trauma.
Scabies	Mite infection: itching with 2–4 mm tunnels in epidermis, e.g. in webs of fingers, wrists, genitalia.
Squamous cell carcinoma	Warty localized thickening, may ulcerate.
Urticaria	Transient wheal with surrounding erythema. Lasts around 24 hours. Usually due to allergy to food or drugs, e.g. aspirin, or physical, e.g. dermographism, cold.
Vitiligo	Permanent demarcated, depigmented white patches due to autoimmune disease.

Mouth

- **Look at the tongue:**
  - cyanosed, moist or dry

    Cyanosis is a reduction in the oxygenation of the blood, with more than 5 g/dl deoxygenated haemoglobin.

    Central cyanosis (Fig. 2.27) (blue tongue) denotes a right-to-left shunt (unsaturated blood appearing in systemic circulation):
    - congenital heart disease, e.g. *Fallot's tetralogy*
    - lung disease, e.g. *obstructive airways disease.*

    Peripheral cyanosis (Fig. 2.28) (blue fingers, pink tongue) denotes inadequate peripheral circulation.

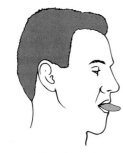

Central cyanosis

Fig. 2.27 Central cyanosis.

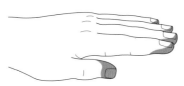

Peripheral cyanosis

Fig. 2.28 Peripheral cyanosis.

A dry tongue can mean salt and water deficiency (often called 'dehydration') but also occurs with mouth breathing.
- **Look at the teeth:**
    - caries (exposed dentine), poor dental hygiene, false
- **Look at the gums:**
    - bleeding, swollen
- **Look at the throat:**
    - tonsils
    - pharynx: swelling, redness, ulceration
- **Smell patient's breath:**
    - ketosis
    - alcohol
    - foetor
    constipation, appendicitis
    musty in liver failure
        Ketosis is sweet-smelling breath occurring with *starvation* or *severe diabetes*.
        Hepatic foetor is a musty smell in *liver failure*.

Eyes

- **Look at the eyes:**
    - *sclera*, icterus
        The most obvious demonstration of *jaundice* is the yellow sclera (Fig. 2.29).

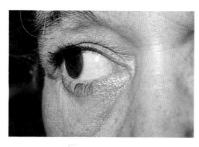

Fig. 2.29   Jaundice – yellow sclerae.

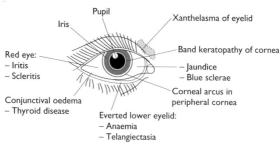

Fig. 2.30   The eye.

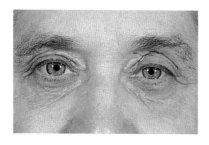

Fig. 2.31   Xanthelasma, cholesterol deposits – suggests raised lipids in younger persons, but lipids are often normal in the elderly.

- lower lid conjunctiva, anaemia

  Anaemia: If the lower lid is everted, the colour of the mucous membranes can be seen. If these are pale, the haemoglobin is usually <9 g/dl.

- eyelids: white/yellow deposit, *xanthelasma* (Figs 2.30, 2.31)
- puffy eyelids

  general oedema, e.g. *nephrotic syndrome*

  thyroid eye disease (Fig. 2.32), hyper or hypo

  myxoedema (Fig. 2.33)

- red eye

  iritis (*uveitis* – anterior/posterior. This is a medical emergency.)

  conjunctivitis

  scleritis or *episcleritis*

  acute glaucoma (This is a medical emergency.)

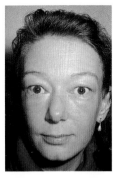

Fig. 2.32 Thyrotoxicosis – wide palpebral fissures in a tense person.

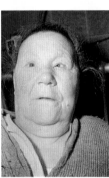

Fig. 2.33 Myxoedema – puffy face, thin dry hair and dry skin in a sluggish person.

- white line around cornea, *arcus senilis*
  common and of little significance in the elderly
  suggests *hyperlipidaemia* in younger patients (Fig. 2.34)
- white-band keratopathy-hypercalcaemia
  sarcoid
  parathyroid tumour or *hyperplasia*
  lung oat cell tumour
  bone secondaries
  vitamin D excess intake
  Hypercalcaemia may give a horizontal band across exposed medial and lateral parts of cornea.

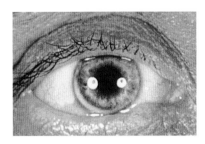

Fig. 2.34 Corneal arcus – same age relationship as xanthelasma.

– white growth of bulbar conjunctival tissue

  Pterygium (Usually occurs from the nasal side toward the centre of the cornea. It may interfere with vision if it covers the pupil.)

Examine the fundi

This is often done as part of the neurological system when examining the cranial nerves (see Chapter 9) or as a separate examination (see Chapter 10). It is replicated here as features are also covered in the general examination.

- **Use an ophthalmoscope**
  - The patient should be sitting. Remove spectacles from yourself and the patient.
  - Begin by setting the lens dioptre dial at 0 if you do not use spectacles. If you are myopic, you should start with the 'minus' lenses. Set the lens dioptre at −4 to begin, which is indicated as a red number. If you are hyperopic you should use the 'plus' lenses which are indicated by black numbers. Keep your index finger on the dial to permit easy focusing. Hold the ophthalmoscope about 30 cm from the patient, shine the light into the patient's pupil, identify the red reflex (from the retina) and approach the patient at an angle of 15°. Approach on the same horizontal plane as the equator of the patient's eye. This will bring you straight to the patient's optic disc. After observing the disc, examine the peripheral retina fully by following the blood vessels to and back from the four main quadrants.
  - Hold the ophthalmoscope in your right hand in front of your right eye to examine the patient's right eye, and your left eye to examine the patient's left eye. Try to hold your breath when using the ophthalmoscope. Do not breathe into the patient's face.
  - If the patient's pupils are small, dilate with 1% tropicamide, 1 drop per eye. Works in 15–20 minutes and lasts 2–4 hours. Warn the patient that his vision will be blurred for approximately 4 hours. Do **not** dilate if neurological observation of pupils is needed.
  - The patient should be told he cannot drive, if his pupils have been dilated, for at least 4–6 hours.
- **Look at the optic disc**
  - normally pink rim with white 'cup' below surface of disc
  - *optic atrophy*
    - disc pale: rim no longer pink
      multiple sclerosis
      after optic neuritis
      optic nerve compression, e.g. *tumour*
  - papilloedema
    - disc pink, indistinct margin
    - cup disappears

- dilated retinal veins
  increased cerebral pressure, e.g. *tumour*
  accelerated hypertension
  optic neuritis, acute stage
- glaucoma – enlarged cup, diminished rim
- new vessels – new fronds of vessels coming forward from disc
  ischaemic diabetic retinopathy

● **Look at arteries**
  - arteries narrowed in hypertension, with increased light reflex along top of vessel
    Hypertension grading:
    1 narrow arteries
    2 'nipping' (narrowing of veins by arteries)
    3 flame-shaped haemorrhages and cotton-wool spots
    4 papilloedema
  - occlusion artery – pale retina
  - occlusion vein – haemorrhages

● **Look at the retina**
  - hard exudates (shiny, yellow circumscribed patches of lipid)
    diabetes
  - cotton-wool spots (soft, fluffy white patches) (Figs 2.35, 2.36)
    microinfarcts causing local swelling of nerve fibres
    diabetes
    hypertension
    vasculitis
    human immunodeficiency virus (HIV)
  - small, red dots
    microaneurysms – retinal capillary expansion adjacent to capillary closure
    diabetes
  - haemorrhages
    - round 'blots': haemorrhages deep in retina larger than micro-aneurysms
      diabetes
    - flame-shaped: superficial haemorrhages along nerve fibres
      hypertension
      gross anaemia
      hyperviscosity
      bleeding tendency
    - Roth's spots (white-centred haemorrhages)
      microembolic disorder
      subacute bacterial endocarditis
  - pigmentation
    - widespread
      retinitis pigmentosa

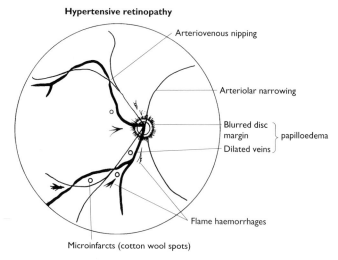

Hypertensive retinopathy

- Arteriovenous nipping
- Arteriolar narrowing
- Blurred disc margin ⎫ papilloedema
- Dilated veins ⎭
- Flame haemorrhages
- Microinfarcts (cotton wool spots)

Diabetic retinopathy

- Intraretinal new vessels
- Microaneurysms
- Disc neovascularization (new vessels)
- Optic disc with normal central "cup"
- Vein with segmental dilation
- Blot haemorrhages
- Central fovea
- Circinate hard exudates (in a circle)

Fig. 2.35 Hypertensive retinopathy and diabetic retinopathy.

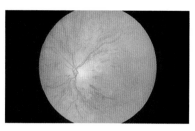

Fig. 2.36 Hypertensive retinopathy – narrow arteries, flame haemorrhages and an early papilloedema with an indistinct disc margin.

- localized
  choroiditis (clumping of pigment into patches)
  drug toxicity, e.g. chloroquine
- tigroid or tabby fundus: normal variant in choroid beneath retina
- peripheral new vessels
  ischaemic diabetic retinopathy
  retinal vein occlusion
- medullated nerve fibres – normal variant, areas of white nerves radiating from optic disc

Examine for palpable lymph nodes (Fig. 2.37)

- In the neck:
  - above clavicle (posterior triangle)
  - medial to sternomastoid area (anterior triangle)

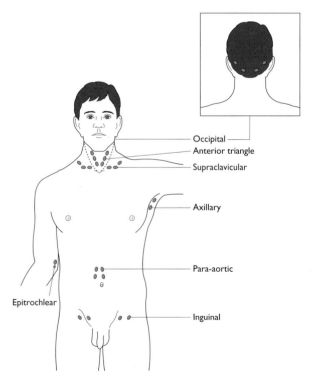

Fig. 2.37 Lymph nodes.

- submandibular (can palpate submandibular gland)
- occipital

    These glands are best felt by sitting the patient up and examining from behind. A left supraclavicular node can occur from the spread of a gastrointestinal malignancy (Virchow's node).

- In the axillae:
    - abduct the arm, insert your hand along the lateral side of axilla, and adduct the arm, thus placing your fingertips in the apex of the axilla. Palpate gently
- In the epitrochlear region:
    - medial to and above elbow
- In the groins:
    - over inguinal ligament
- In the abdomen:
    - usually very difficult to feel; some claim to have felt para-aortic nodes

        Axillae often have soft, fleshy lymph nodes.

        Groins often have small, shotty nodes.

        Generalized large, rubbery nodes suggest *lymphoma*.

        Localized hard nodes suggest *cancer*.

        Tender nodes suggest *infection*.
- If many nodes are palpable – examine spleen and look for anaemia. *Lymphoma or leukaemia?*

Lumps

- If there is an unusual lump, **inspect first and palpate later**:
    - **site**
    - **size** (measure in centimetres)
    - **shape**
    - **surface, edge**
    - **surroundings**
    - **fixed or mobile**
    - **consistency**, e.g. cystic or solid, soft or hard, fluctuance
    - **tender**
    - **pulsatile**
    - **auscultation**, e.g. thyroid 'hum' from increased vascularity
    - **transillumination**

        A *cancer* is usually hard, non-tender, irregular, fixed to neighbouring tissues, and possibly ulcerating skin.

        A *cyst* may have:

        - **fluctuance**: pressure across cyst will cause it to bulge in another plane

- **transillumination**: a light can be seen through it (usually only if room is darkened).
- Look at neighbouring lymph nodes. May find:
  - spread from cancer
  - inflamed lymph nodes from infection

Heart

Routine examination

For the full examination refer to Chapter 3, Examination of the Cardiovascular System.

- **Inspect precordium**
  - observe PMI (usually 5th ICS in an adult may be the 6th ICS left of McLinan older adult)
  - look for heaves
- **Palpate precordium**
  - heaves or thrusts
  - thrills (palpable murmurs/vibrations)
- **Percuss precordium**
  - heart will enlarge in congestive heart failure and cardiomegaly
  - apex may shift laterally to the left and be located in the 6th ICS
- **Auscultate:** S_1, S_2 (? S_3, S_4, clicks, snaps or murmurs)
  - rate
  - rhythm (regular, regularly irregular, irregular)
- **Assess** JVD/JVP (Fig. 2.38)

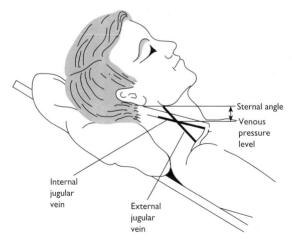

Fig. 2.38 Position for assessment of JVD/JVP. Reproduced with permission.

Breasts

If you are a male nurse, arrange a female chaperone, particularly when the patient is a young adult, shy or nervous.

Routine examination

- Examine the female breasts **when you examine the precordium.**
- **Inspect for asymmetry**, obvious lumps, inverted nipples, skin changes.
- **Palpate each quadrant of both breasts** with the flat of the hand (fingers together, nearly extended with gentle pressure exerted from metacarpophalangeal joints, avoiding pressure on the nipple).
- If there are any possible lumps, proceed to a more complete examination.

Full breast examination

When patient has a symptom or a lump has been found:
- **Inspect**
  - **With the patient sitting up, ask her to raise her hands above her head, put hands on hips, rotate shoulders forward and then with hands on hips to lean forward** (so that you can examine under the breast). Look anteriorly and laterally.
  - **inspect for asymmetry** or obvious lumps
    - differing size or shape of breasts
    - nipples – symmetry
    - rashes, redness (abscess)
      Breast cancer is suggested by:
      - asymmetry
      - skin tethering or puckering
      - *peau d'orange* (oedema of skin)
      - nipple deviated or inverted.
- **Palpate** (Fig. 2.39)
  - patient lying flat on one pillow with one arm under her head and other at her side (right arm under head to examine right breast and left arm under head to examine left breast)
  - **examine each breast with flat of hand, each quadrant in turn** (ensure that you examine well below each breast and into the tail of Spence)
  - examine bimanually if the breast is large
  - examine any lump as described above in the general examination of skin and lymph nodes
  - is lump attached to skin or muscles?
  - examine lymph nodes (axilla, infraclavicular and supraclavicular)
  - feel liver

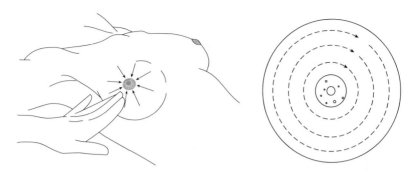

Fig. 2.39　Breast examination. Reproduced with permission.

Respiratory system

Routine examination

For the full examination refer to Chapter 4, Examination of the Respiratory System.

- **Inspect:**
  - symmetry (? flail, tracheal deviation)
  - scars/lesions
  - respiratory rate
  - ? nasal flaring
- **Palpate:**
  - thoracic integrity
  - lumps/bumps
  - crepitations
  - fremitus
- **Percuss:**
  - anteriorly
  - posertiorly
  - laterally
  - ? dullness on percussion (consolidation or tumour)
- **Auscultate:**
  - tracheobronchial sounds
  - bronchovesicular sounds
  - vesicular sounds
  - ? adventitious sounds

Thyroid

- **Inspect**: then ask the patient to swallow, having given him a glass of water. Is there a lump? Does it move upwards on swallowing?

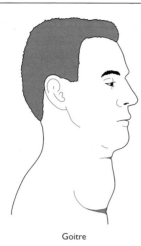

Goitre   **Fig. 2.40** Goitre.

- **Palpate bimanually**: stand behind the patient and palpate with fingers of both hands. Is the thyroid of normal size, shape and texture? (Avoid the throttling position when examining behind the patient as this may frighten him.)
- If a lump is felt:
    - is thyroid multinodular?
    - does lump feel cystic?

    > The thyroid is normally soft. If there is a goitre (swelling of thyroid) (Fig. 2.40), assess if the swelling is:
    > - localized, e.g. *thyroid cyst*, *adenoma* or *carcinoma*
    > - generalized, e.g. *autoimmune thyroiditis*, *thyrotoxicosis*
    > - multinodular.
    >
    > A swelling does not mean the gland is under- or overactive. In many cases the patient may be euthyroid. The thyroid becomes slightly enlarged in pregnancy.
- **Ask patient to swallow** – does thyroid rise normally?
- Is thyroid fixed?
- **Can you get below the lump**? If not, percuss over upper sternum for retrosternal extension
- **Are there cervical lymph nodes**?
- **If there is a possibility of the patient being thyrotoxic (see Fig. 2.32), look for**:
    - warm hands
    - perspiration
    - tremor
    - tachycardia, sinus rhythm or atrial fibrillation
    - wide, palpable fissure or lid lag
    - thyroid 'hum' – bruit (on auscultation)

Endocrine exophthalmos (may be associated with thyrotoxicosis):
- conjunctival oedema: *chemosis* (seen by gentle pressure on lower lid, pushing up a fold of conjunctiva when oedema is present)
- proptosis: eye pushed forwards (look from above down on eyes)
- deficient upward gaze and convergence
- diplopia
- papilloedema.

- **If there is a possibility of the patient being hypothyroid (see Fig. 2.33), look for:**
  - dry hair and skin
  - xanthelasma
  - puffy face
  - croaky voice
  - delayed relaxation of supinator or ankle jerks

Other endocrine diseases

Acromegaly (Fig. 2.41)

- enlarged soft tissue of hands, feet, face
- coarse features, thick, greasy skin, large tongue (and other organs, e.g. thyroid)
- bitemporal hemianopia (from tumour pressing on optic chiasma)

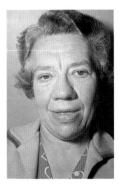

Fig. 2.41 Acromegaly – coarse features with thick lips, enlarged nose and thickened skin.

Hypopituitarism

- no skin pigmentation
- thin skin
- decreased secondary sexual hair or delayed puberty
- short stature (and on X-ray, delayed fusion of epiphyses)
- bitemporal hemianopia if pituitary tumour

Addison's disease

- increased skin pigmentation, including non-exposed areas, e.g. buccal pigmentation
- postural hypotension
- if female, decreased body hair

Cushing's syndrome (Fig. 2.42)

- truncal obesity, round, red face with hirsutism
- thin skin and bruising, pink striae, hypertension
- proximal muscle weakness

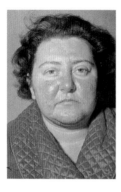

Fig. 2.42 Cushing's syndrome – plethoric, round face.

Diabetes

Diabetic complications include:
- skin lesions
  Necrobiosis lipoidica – ischaemia in skin, usually on shins, leading to fatty replacement of dermis, covered by thin skin.
- ischaemic legs (Fig. 2.43)

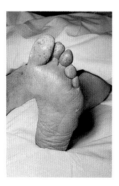

Fig. 2.43 Ischaemic toes from acute arterial insufficiency – white toes becoming blue, with erythematous reaction at demarcation.

- diminished foot pulses
- skin shiny blue, white or black
- no hairs, thick nails
- ulcers (Fig. 2.44)

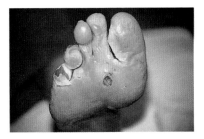

Fig. 2.44   Diabetic foot – shiny, dry skin with ulcer from abnormal pressure point from motor neuropathy and painless, unsuspected blister on toe.

- peripheral neuropathy
- absent leg reflexes
- diminished sensation
- thick skin over unusual pressure points from dropped arch
- autonomic neuropathy
- dry skin
- mononeuropathy
- lateral popliteal nerve – footdrop
- III or VI – diplopia
- asymmetrical muscle wasting of the upper leg
- retinopathy (Fig. 2.45)

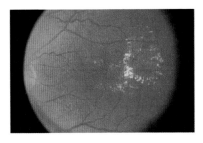

Fig. 2.45   Diabetic retinopathy – hard exudates in a ring (circinate).

Abdominal

The abdomen is divided into four imaginary quadrants with components distributed as shown in Table 2.2.

Table 2.2 Distribution of components in the four imaginary quadrants of the abdominal system (see Fig. 2.46)

Right upper quadrant	**Left upper quadrant**
RUQ	LUQ
Liver	Stomach
Gallbladder	Spleen
Head of pancreas	Body of pancreas
Right kidney	Left kidney
Large intestine	Large intestine
Small intestine	Small intestine
Right lower quadrant	**Left lower quadrant**
RLQ	LLQ
Appendix	
Right ovary	Left ovary
Large intestine	Large intestine
Small intestine	Small intestine
Uterus	
Bladder	

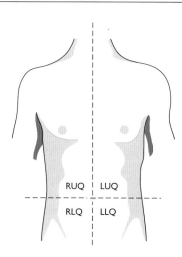

Fig. 2.46 The four imaginary quadrants of the abdominal system. Reproduced with permission.

Routine examination

For the full examination refer to Chapter 5, Examination of the Abdomen.

- **Inspect:**
  - symmetry (? concave or convex)
  - scars/lesions (? evidence of liver disease)
- **Auscultate:**
  - four quadrants (Fig. 2.46)

- **Palpate:**
  - nine quadrants (light and deep palpation)
  - lumps/bumps (? presence of tumour)
- **Percuss:**
  - nine quadrants
  - tympani
  - ? central dullness and lateral tympani (ovarian tumour)
  - ? central tympani and lateral dullness (ascites – assess for shifting dullness)
  - consider rectal/vaginal examination

Musculoskeletal

Normally you would examine the joints briefly when examining neighbouring systems. If a patient specifically complains of joint symptoms or an abnormal posture or joint is noted, a more detailed examination is needed. (Refer to Chapter 11).

General habitus

- Note the following:
  - is the patient unduly tall or short? (measure height and span)
  - are all limbs, spine and skull of normal size and shape?
    - normal person:
      height = span
      crown to pubis = pubis to heel
    - long limbs:
      Marfan's syndrome
      eunuchoid during growth
    - *collapsed vertebrae*:
      span > height
      pubis to heel > crown to pubis
  - is the posture normal?
  - curvature of the spine:
    kyphosis
    lordosis
    scoliosis
    gibbus
  - is the gait normal?
    Observing the patient walking is a vital part of examination of the locomotor and neurological systems.
    Painful gait, transferring weight quickly off a painful limb, bobbing up and down – an abnormal rhythm of gait.

Painless abnormal gait may be from:
short leg (bobs up and down with equal-length steps)
stiff joint (lifts pelvis to prevent foot dragging on ground)
weak ankle (high stepping gait to avoid toes catching on ground)
weak knee (locks knee straight before putting foot on the ground)
weak hip (sways sideways using trunk muscles to lift pelvis and to swing leg through)
unco-ordinated gait (arms are swung as counterbalances)
hysterical or malingering causes.
Look for abnormal wear on shoes.

Inspection

Inspect the joints before you touch them.
- Look at:
  - skin
    redness – inflammation
    scars – old injury
    bruising – recent injury
  - soft tissues
    muscle wasting – old injury
    swelling – injury/inflammation
  - bones
    deformity – compare with other side (Fig. 2.47)
      varus: bent out from midline (bowleg)
      valgus: bent in towards midline
- Assess whether an isolated joint is affected or if there is polyarthritis.
- If there is polyarthritis, note if it is symmetrical or asymmetrical.
- Compare any abnormal findings with the other side.

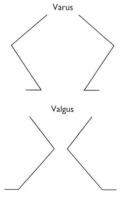

Varus

Valgus

Fig. 2.47   Varus and valgus bone deformity.

Arthritis – swollen, hot, tender, painful joint.
Arthropathy – swollen but not hot and tender.
Arthralgia – painful, e.g. on movement, without being swollen.
Swelling may also be due to an effusion, thickening of the periarticular tissues, enlargement of the ends of bones (e.g. *pulmonary osteopathy*) or complete disorganization of the joint without pain (*Charcot's joint*).

Palpation

- Before you touch any joint ask the patient to tell you if it is painful.
- Feel for:
  - warmth
  - tenderness
    - watch patient's face for signs of discomfort
    - locate signs of tenderness – soft tissue or bone
  - swelling or displacement
  - fluctuation (effusion)
        An inflamed joint is usually generally tender. Localized tenderness may be mechanical in origin, e.g. ligament tear. Joint effusion may occur with arthritis or local injury.

Movement

Test the range of movement of the joint both actively and passively. This must be done **gently**.
- **Active** – how far can the patient move the joint through its range?
  Do not seize limb and move it until patient complains.
- **Passive** – if range is limited, can you further increase the range of movement?
        Abduction: movement from central axis.
        Adduction: movement to central axis.
- Is the passive range of movement similar to the active range?
        Limitation of the range of movement of a joint may be due to pain, muscle spasms, contracture, inflammation or thickening of the capsules or periarticular structures, effusions into the joint space, bony or cartilaginous outgrowths or painful conditions not connected with the joint.
- **Resisted movement** – ask patient to bend joint while you resist movement. How much force can be developed?
- **Hold your hand round the joint** whilst it is moving. A grating or creaking sensation (*crepitus*) may be felt.
        Crepitus is usually associated with *osteo-arthritis*.

Summary of signs of common illnesses

Osteoarthritis
- 'wear and tear' of a specific joint – usually large joints
- common in elderly or after trauma to joint
- often involves joints of the lower limbs and is asymmetrical
- often in the lumbar or cervical spine
- aches after use, with deep, boring pain at night
- Heberden's nodes – osteophytes on terminal interphalangeal joints

Rheumatoid arthritis (see Fig. 2.13)
Characteristically:
- a polyarthritis
- symmetrical, inflamed if active
- involves proximal interphalangeal and metacarpophalangeal joints of hands with ulnar deviation of fingers
- involves any large joint
- muscle wasting from disuse atrophy
- rheumatoid nodules on extensor surface of elbows
- may include other signs, e.g. with splenomegaly it is *Felty's syndrome*

Gout (see Fig. 2.14)
Characteristically:
- asymmetrical
- inflamed first metatarsophalangeal joint (big toe) – *podagra* (Fig. 2.48)
- involves any joint in hand, often with tophus – hard round lump of urate by joint
- tophi on ears

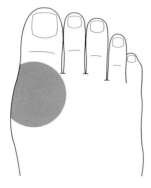

Fig. 2.48   Podagra.

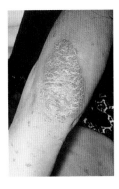

Fig. 2.49 Psoriasis – circumscribed plaque with scales.

Psoriasis (Fig. 2.49)

– particularly involves terminal interphalangeal joints, hips and knees
– often with pitted nails of psoriasis as well as skin lesions

Ankylosing spondylitis

– painful, stiff spine
– later fixed in flexed position
– hips and other joints can be involved

CHAPTER 3

Examination of the Cardiovascular System

General examination

Introduction

The purpose of examining the cardiovascular system is to assess the function of the heart as a pump and the arteries and veins throughout the body in transporting oxygen and nutrients to the tissues and transporting waste products and carbon dioxide from the tissues. Your assessment of the cardiovascular system is important because cardiovascular disease is the most prevalent healthcare problem in the United Kingdom. Over 250 000 deaths per year are attributed to cardiovascular disease (Hatchett & Thompson, 2007).

- **Examine**
  - clubbing of fingernails
      Clubbing in relation to the heart suggests *cyanotic heart disease* (see Fig. 2.7).
  - cold hands with blue nails – poor perfusion, peripheral cyanosis
  - under the tongue, and at the gum line for central cyanosis (in light-skinned patients the colour will be bluish purple, in dark skinned patients the colour will be grey)
  - conjunctivae for anaemia
  - signs of dyspnoea or distress
      Assess the degree of breathlessness by checking if *dyspnoea* occurs on undressing, talking, at rest or when lying flat (*orthopnoea*).
  - xanthomata:
    - *xanthelasma* (common) – intracutaneous yellow cholesterol deposits occur around the eyes – normal or with *hyperlipidaemia* (Fig. 3.1; see Fig. 2.31)
    - *xanthoma* (uncommon):
      hypercholesterolaemia – tendon deposits (hands and Achilles tendon) (Fig. 3.2) or tuberous xanthomata at elbows (see Fig. 2.23)
      hypertriglyceridaemia – eruptive xanthoma, small yellow deposits on buttocks and extensor surfaces, each with a red halo

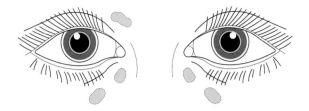

Fig. 3.1 Xanthelasma.

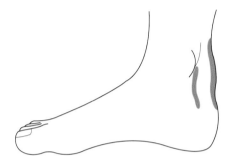

Fig. 3.2 Xanthoma.

Palpate the radial pulse

Feel the radial pulse just medial to the radius, with two forefingers (Fig. 3.3).

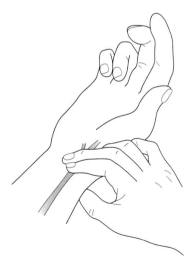

Fig. 3.3 Taking a radial pulse.

- **Pulse rate:**
  Take for one minute (some clinicians count the pulse for 15 seconds and multiply by four; however, this does not reflect an accurate pulse rate, particularly if the patient has arrhythmias):
  - *tachycardia* >100 beats/min
  - *bradycardia* <50 beats/min
- **Rhythm:**
  - regular
  normal variation on breathing: *sinus arrhythmia*
  - regularly irregular
  pulsus bigeminus, coupled extrasystoles (digoxin toxicity)
  Wenckebach (type I second-degree heart block; the P–R interval lengthens until a P-wave is finally not conducted and the sequence starts again)
  - irregularly irregular
  atrial fibrillation
  premature ventricular contractions (PVC), ventricular extrasystoles/ ventricular ectopic beats (VE)
  Check apical rate by auscultation whilst palpating the pulse for true heart rate, as ventricular premature beats are not transmitted to radial pulse.
- **Waveform of the pulse** (Fig. 3.4):
  - normal (1)
  - slow rising and plateau – moderate or severe *aortic stenosis* (2)
  - collapsing pulse – pulse pressure greater than diastolic pressure, e.g. *aortic incompetence*, elderly *arteriosclerotic* patient or *gross anaemia* (3)
  - bisferiens – moderate *aortic stenosis* with severe *incompetence* (4)
  - pulsus paradoxus – pulse weaker or disappears on inspiration, e.g. *constrictive pericarditis, tamponade, status asthmaticus* (5)
- **Volume:**
  - small volume – *low cardiac output*
  - large volume
  carbon dioxide retention
  thyrotoxicosis
- **Stiffness of the vessel wall:**
  - in the elderly, a stiff, strongly pulsating, palpable 5–6 cm radial artery indicates *arteriosclerosis*, a hardening of the walls of the artery that:
    - is common with ageing
    - is not atheroma
    - is associated with systolic hypertension
- **Pulsus alternans:**
  A difference of 20 mmHg systolic blood pressure between consecutive beats signifies poor left ventricular function. This needs to be measured with a sphygmomanometer.

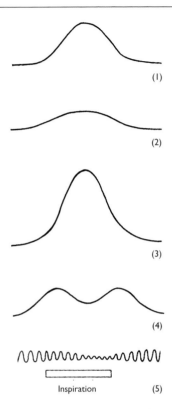

(1)

(2)

(3)

(4)

Inspiration   (5)   **Fig. 3.4**   Waveform of the pulse.

Take the blood pressure

- Wrap the cuff neatly and tightly around either upper arm.
- Gently inflate the cuff until the radial artery is no longer palpable.
- Using the stethoscope, listen over the brachial artery for the pulse to appear as you drop the pressure slowly (3–4 mm/s) (Fig. 3.5).
- Systolic blood pressure: **appearance of sounds**
  - **Korotkoff phase 1**
- Diastolic blood pressure: **disappearance of sounds**
  - **Korotkoff phase 5**
  Use large cuff for fat arms (circumference >30 cm) so that inflatable cuff >1/2 arm circumference.
  Beware auscultatory gap with sounds disappearing in midsystole. If sounds go to zero, use Korotkoff phase 4.
  In adults, ~ >140/85 mmHg or more is the current guideline in non-diabetic patients and ~ >130/80 mmHg in diabetic patients.

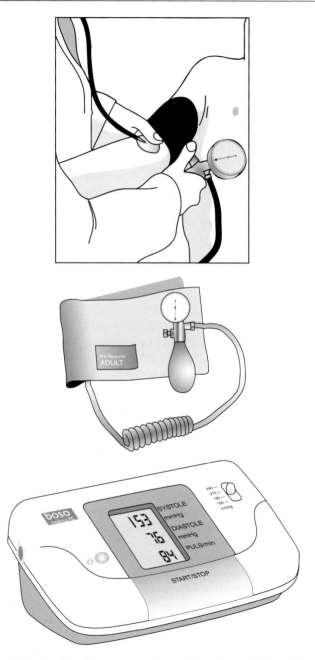

Fig. 3.5 Taking the blood pressure and types of equipment that can be used. Reproduced with permission.

The patient may be nervous when first examined and the blood pressure may be falsely high. Take it again at the end of the examination.

Wide pulse pressure (e.g. 160/30 mmHg) suggests *aortic incompetence.*

Narrow pulse pressure (e.g. 95/80 mmHg) suggests *aortic stenosis.* Difference of >20 mmHg systolic between arms suggests *arterial occlusion,* e.g. *dissecting aneurysm* or *atheroma.*

Difference of 10 mmHg is found in 25% of healthy subjects.

The variable pulse from atrial fibrillation means a precise blood pressure cannot easily be obtained.

Jugular venous pulse (frequently called pressure)

- **Observe the height of the jugular venous pulsation (JVP).**
  Position the patient lying at approximately 45° to the horizontal with his head on pillows. Shine a torch at an angle across the neck.
- **Look at the veins in the neck**. Use tangential lighting.
  - internal jugular vein not directly visible: pulse diffuse, medial or deep to sternomastoid
  - external jugular vein: pulse lateral to sternomastoid. Only informative if pulsating
- **Assess vertical height** in centimetres above the manubriosternal angle, using the pulsating external jugular vein or upper limit of internal jugular pulsation (Fig. 3.6).

The **external jugular vein** is often more readily visible but may be obstructed by its tortuous course, and is less reliable than the internal jugular pulse (Fig. 3.7).

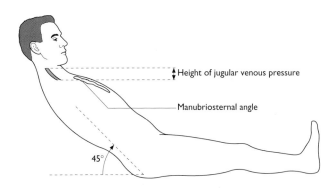

Height of jugular venous pressure

Manubriosternal angle

45°

Fig. 3.6   Assessing height of JVP.

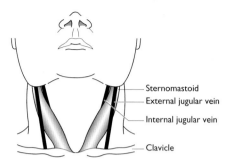

Fig. 3.7 The veins of the neck.

The **internal jugular vein** is sometimes very difficult to see. Its pulsation may be confused with the carotid artery but it:
- has a complex pulsation
- moves on respiration and decreases on inspiration except in tamponade
- cannot be palpated
- can be obliterated by pressure on base of neck
- demonstrates right heart pressure

    The **hepatojugular reflux** is checked by firm pressure with the flat of the right hand over the liver, while watching the JVP.

    Compression on the dilated hepatic veins increases the JVP by 2 cm.

    If the JVP is found to be raised above the manubriosternal angle and pulsating, it implies *right heart failure*. Look for the other signs, i.e. pitting oedema and large tender liver. Sometimes the JVP is so raised it can be missed, except that the ears waggle.

    Dilated neck veins with no pulsation suggest *non-cardiac obstruction* (e.g. carcinoma bronchus causing superior caval obstruction or a kinked external jugular vein).

    If venous pressure rises on inspiration (it normally falls), suspect *constrictive pericarditis* or *pericardial effusion* causing *tamponade*.
- **Observe the character of JVP.** Try to ascertain the waveform of the JVP (Fig. 3.8). It should be a double pulsation consisting of:
  - a-wave atrial contraction – ends synchronous with carotid artery pulse c
  - v-wave atrial filling – when the tricuspid valve is closed by ventricular contraction – with and just after carotid pulse

        Large a-waves are caused by obstruction to flow from the right atrium due to stiffness of the right ventricle from hypertrophy:
        pulmonary hypertension
        pulmonary stenosis
        tricuspid stenosis.
        Absent a-wave in *atrial fibrillation.*

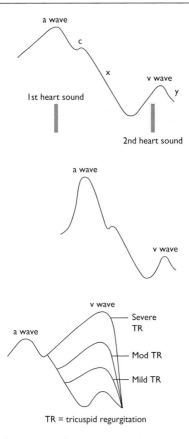

Fig. 3.8 Assessing the JVP waveform.

Large v-waves are caused by regurgitation of blood through an *incompetent tricuspid valve* during ventricular contraction.

A sharp y descent occurs in *constrictive pericarditis.*

Cannon waves (giant a-waves) occur in *complete heart block* when the right atrium occasionally contracts against a closed tricuspid valve.

Musset's sign

- **Observe the patient's ability to hold his head still.**
  Slight rhythmic bobbing of the head in time with the heartbeat may accompany high back pressure caused by aortic insufficiency or aortic aneurysm.

The precordium

- **Inspect the precordium for abnormal pulsation.**
  A large left ventricle may easily be seen on the left side of the chest, some-times in the axilla.
- **Palpate the apex beat (point of maximal impulse – PMI)** (Fig. 3.9).
  - Feel for the point furthest out and down where the pulsation can still be distinctly felt. In the adult this is normally felt in the 5th intercostal space (ICS) midclavicular line (MCL). In the older adult this may shift to the 6th ICS just left of the MCL.
  - If you are unable to palpate the PMI, lean the patient forward and turn him onto his left side. (This will slightly shift the heart forward in the chest so that it is easier to feel.)

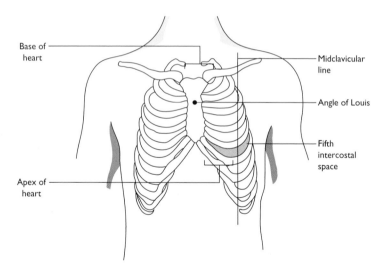

Fig. 3.9 Location of PMI at the apex. Reproduced with permission.

- **Measure the position** (Fig. 3.10).
  - Determine the space, counting down from the 2nd ICS which lies below the 2nd rib (opposite the manubriosternal angle) where the PMI is felt.
  - Measure laterally in centimetres from the midline.
  - Describe the apex beat in relation to the MCL, anterior axillary line and midaxillary line.
- **Assess character:**
  Try to judge if an enlarged heart is:
  - **feeble** (dilated) or
  - **stronger** than usual (left or right ventricle hypertrophy or both).

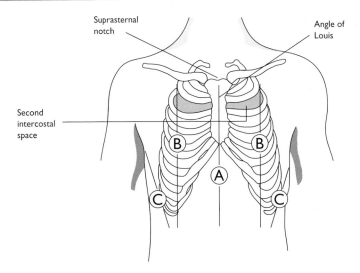

Suprasternal notch

Angle of Louis

Second intercostal space

Fig. 3.10 (a) Midsternal. (b) Midclavicular. (c) Anterior axillary. Reproduced with permission.

Thrusting displaced apex beat occurs with volume overload: an active, large stroke volume ventricle, e.g. *mitral* or *aortic incompetence, left-to-right shunt* or *cardiomyopathy.*

Sustained apex beat occurs with pressure overload in *aortic stenosis* and *gross hypertension.* Stroke volume is normal or reduced.

Tapping apex beat (palpable first heart sound) occurs in *mitral stenosis.*

Diffuse pulsation asynchronous with apex beat occurs with a *left ventricular aneurysm* – a dyskinetic apex beat.

Impalpable – obesity, overinflated chest, pericardial effusion.

- **Palpate firmly the left border of the sternum.**
  - Use the flat of your hand.
    A heave suggests *right ventricular hypertrophy* (Fig. 3.11).
- **Palpate all over the precordium** with the flat of hand for thrills (palpable murmurs).

N.B. If by now you have found an abnormality in the cardiovascular system, think of possible causes before you listen.

For example, if left ventricle is forceful:
  - ? hypertension – was blood pressure (BP) raised?
  - ? aortic stenosis or incompetence – was pulse character normal? will there be a murmur?
  - ? mitral incompetence – will there be a murmur?
  - ? thyrotoxicosis or anaemia

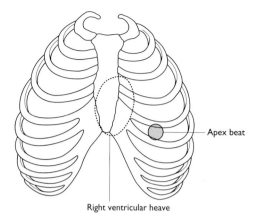

Fig. 3.11   Palpation position for right ventricular heave.

Auscultation

- **Listen over the five main areas of the heart** and in each area with both the bell and diaphragm of the stethoscope. The bell will transmit soft sounds (S_3 and S_4) that are lost when the diaphragm is used. The diaphragm transmits loud harsh sounds. Concentrate in order on:
  - **heart sounds**
  - **added sounds**
  - **murmurs**

Keep to this order when listening or describing what you have heard, or you will miss or forget important findings.

The five main areas are (Fig. 3.12):
  - **apex, mitral area** in the 5th ICS MCL (and left axilla if there is a murmur) = S_1 (mitral = M_1)
  - **tricuspid area** in the 4th ICS left sternal boarder = S_1 (tricuspid = T_1)
  - **aortic area** in the 2nd ICS right of the sternum (and neck if there is a murmur) = S_2 (aortic = A_2)
  - **pulmonary area** in the 2nd ICS left of the sternum = S_2 (pulmonic = P_2)
  - **Erb's point** in the 3rd ICS left of the sternum = best location to hear murmurs across chambers

    These areas represent where heart sounds and murmurs associated with these valves are best heard. They do not represent the surface markings of the valves.

    If you hear little, turn the patient onto his left side and listen over the apex (having palpated for it).

    Note that because the diaphragm filters out low-frequency sounds, the bell should be used for mitral stenosis, which is a low-frequency sound.

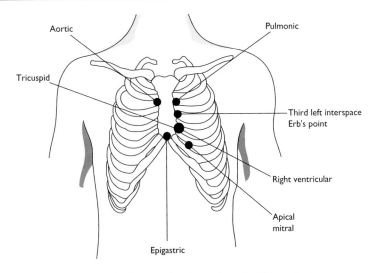

Fig. 3.12   Ausculation site landmarks. Reproduced with permission.

Normal heart sounds

I (S₁) Sudden cessation of mitral and tricuspid flow due to valve closure. (Use both the bell and diaphragm in auscultation.)
   – loud in *mitral insufficiency (stenosis)*
   – soft in *mitral incompetence, aortic insufficiency (stenosis), left bundle branch block*
   – variable in *complete heart block* and *atrial fibrillation*

II (S₂) Sudden cessation of aortic and pulmonary flow due to valve closure – usually split (see below). (Use both the bell and diaphragm in auscultation.)
   – loud in *hypertension*
   – soft in *aortic* or *pulmonary insufficiency (stenosis)* (heard best with the bell)
   – wide normal split – *right bundle branch block*
   – wide fixed split – *atrial septal defect*

Added sounds (Fig. 3.13)

III (S₃) First phase – rapid ventricular filling sound in early diastole (S₃). (Heard best with the bell lightly held. Pressure on the bell will extinguish the sound.)

Common in children and young adults. In these instances it is known as a physiological S₃. It is heard in hyperkinetic states producing an increased cardiac output (CO). Examples include

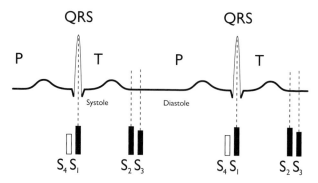

Fig. 3.13 Relationship of heart sounds to the electrocardiogram. Reproduced with permission.

hyperthyroidism, exercise, pregnancy and anxiety-related tachycardia. It can also be heard in mitral and tricuspid insufficiency ischaemia, advanced CHF and left-to-right shunts. When it is heard in middle-aged adults it is considered abnormal. You should suspect *left ventricular heart failure, fibrosed ventricle* or *constrictive pericarditis*. When it originates in the left ventricle (LV), it is best heard at the apex with the patient on his left side exhaling. When it originates in the right ventricle (RV), it is best heard at Erbs point.

IV (S_4) Second phase – atrial contraction (atrial kick) inducing ventricular filling towards the end of diastole (S_4). (Heard best with the bell lightly held. Pressure on the bell will extinguish the sound.)

A physiological S_4 may be heard in middle-aged adults who have thin-walled chests, especially after exercise. It occurs when there is an overload of either the left or right ventricle when diastolic pressure is increased. In the adult, suspect hyperthyroidism, pulmonary hypertension, aortic or pulmonary insufficiency, myocardial infarction or heart failure. In the older adult, suspect hypertensive cardiovascular disease, coronary artery disease, pulmonary hypertension, aortic or pulmonary insufficiency, myocardial ischaemia, infarction, congestive heart failure. It may be the first evidence of cardiovascular disease. If it is heard over LLSB it is probably RV in origin. If it is heard over the apex it is probably LV in origin.

Canter rhythm (often termed **gallop**) with tachycardia gives the following cadences:

S_3: frequently indicated as sounding like **Ken** — **tucky** (k = first heart sound). Note that S_3 comes after S_2.

S_4: frequently indicated as sounding like **Tenne** – **ss**ee (n = first heart sound). Note that S_4 comes before S_1.

Clicks and snaps

Normally the opening of a heart valve is silent. Ejection clicks arise from abnormal aortic or pulmonary valves when they open. These occur in early systole and may be mistaken for splitting. An opening snap is associated with an abnormal mitral or tricuspid valve and is heard best in diastole.

Opening snap
- Mitral valve normally opens silently after S_2.
- In *mitral insufficiency (stenosis)*, sudden movement of rigid valve makes a snap, after S_2 (Fig. 3.14).

Ejection click
- Aortic valve normally opens silently after S_1.
- In *aortic insufficiency (stenosis* or *sclerosis)*, the valve can open with a click after S_1.

Splitting of second heart sound ($S_2 = a_2p_2$)

Ask the patient to take deep breaths in and out. Blood is drawn into the thorax during inspiration and then on to the right ventricle. There is temporarily more blood in the right ventricle than the left ventricle, and the right ventricle takes fractionally longer to empty.

Splitting is best heard during inspiration. If the patient is breathless, **do not** ask him to **hold** his breath in or out when assessing splitting.

Physiological splitting may occur in children and young people. In older people, a delay in closure of p_2 (p_2 comes after a_2) may be associated with right heart failure or pulmonary hypertension.

Paradoxical splitting occurs in *aortic insufficiency (stenosis)* and *left bundle branch block*.

In both these conditions (Fig. 3.15) the left ventricle takes longer to empty, thus delaying a_2 until after p_2. During inspiration p_2 occurs later and the sounds draw closer together.

Knock and rub

A loud low-frequency diastolic noise best known as a knock can be heard in constrictive pericarditis. A pericardial friction rub is a high-pitched frequency noise, heard loudest in systole but frequently present in diastole as well. A rub may vary from hour to hour, and when a significant pericardial effusion occurs the rub will disappear (Brown *et al.*, 2002).

Murmurs

Use the diaphragm of the stethoscope for most high-pitched sounds or murmurs (e.g. aortic incompetence) and the bell for low-pitched murmurs (e.g. mitral insufficiency – stenosis). Note the following.

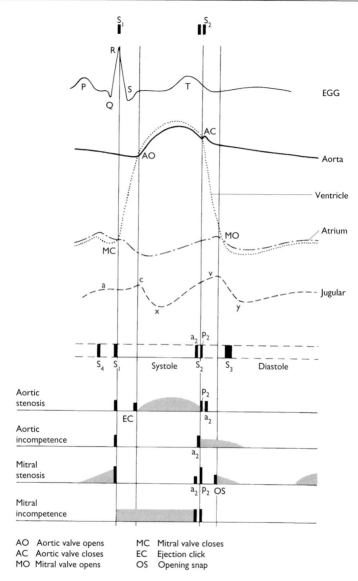

AO	Aortic valve opens	MC	Mitral valve closes
AC	Aortic valve closes	EC	Ejection click
MO	Mitral valve opens	OS	Opening snap

Fig. 3.14 Relation of murmurs to pressure changes and valve movements.

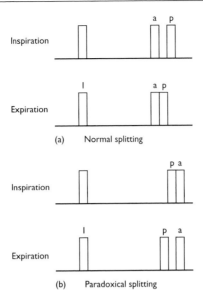

Fig. 3.15 (a) Normal and (b) paradoxical splitting.

- **Timing systolic** or **diastolic** (compare with finger on carotid pulse) (see Fig. 3.14).
- **Site and radiation,** e.g.:
  - mitral incompetence > axilla
  - aortic insufficiency (stenosis) > carotids and apex
  - aortic incompetence > sternum
- **Character:**
  - loud or soft
  - pitch, e.g. squeaking or rumbling, 'scratchy' = pericardial or pleural
  - length
  - pansystolic, throughout systole
  - early diastolic, e.g. aortic or pulmonary incompetence
  - midsystolic, e.g. aortic insufficiency (stenosis) or flow murmur
  - mid-diastolic, e.g. mitral insufficiency (stenosis)
- **Relation to posture:**
  - sit forward – aortic incompetence louder
  - lie left side – mitral insufficiency (stenosis) louder
- **Relation to respiration:**
  - inspiration increases the murmur of a right heart lesion
  - expiration increases the murmur of a left heart lesion
  - variable – pericardial rub
- **Relation to exercise:**
  - increases the murmur of mitral insufficiency (stenosis)

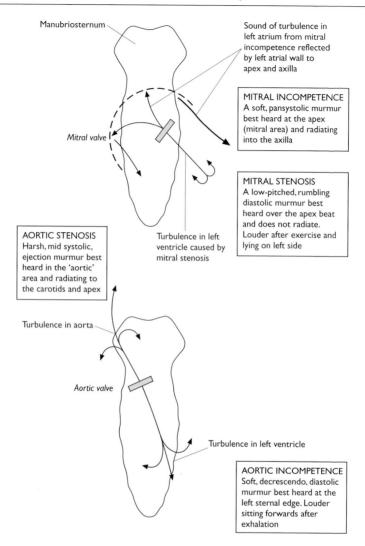

Fig. 3.16   Radiation of sound from turbulent blood flow.

Optimal position for hearing murmurs (Fig. 3.16)
- **Mitral insufficiency (stenosis)** – the patient lies on left side, arm above head; listen with bell at apex as this is a diastolic murmur. Murmur is louder after exercise, e.g. repeated touching of toes from lying position that increases cardiac output.

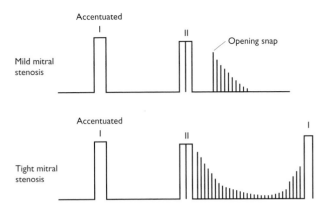

Fig. 3.17 Diastolic murmurs in mitral stenosis.

- **Aortic incompetence (regurgitation)** – the patient sits forward after deep inspiration; listen with diaphragm at lower left sternal edge.

N.B. Murmurs alone do not make the diagnosis. Take other signs into consideration, e.g. arterial or venous pulses, blood pressure, apex or heart sounds. Also consider the status of the patient when deciding treatment. Does the patient look or state that he feels compromised? Is he breathless, for example?

Loudness is often not proportional to severity of disease, and in some situations length of murmur is more important, e.g. mitral insufficiency (stenosis) (Fig. 3.17).

- For completion:
  - **auscultate base of lungs** for inspiratory and expiratory crackles from left ventricular failure
  - **palpate liver** – smooth, tender, enlarged in right heart failure
  - **palpate peripheral pulses** (? stronger in lower extremities than upper)
  - **peripheral oedema** – ankle/sacral (? right ventricular failure)

Summary of timing of murmurs

Ejection systolic murmur

aortic insufficiency (stenosis or *sclerosis)* (same murmur, due to stiffness of valve cusps and aortic walls, with normal pulse pressure); *aortic insufficiency (sclerosis)* is present in 50% of 50 year olds
pulmonary insufficiency (stenosis)
atrial septal defect
Fallot's syndrome – right outflow tract obstruction

Pansystolic murmur

> *mitral incompetence (regurgitation)*
> *tricuspid incompetence (regurgitation)*
> *ventricular septal defect*

Late systolic murmur

> *mitral valve prolapse – due to incompetence* (frequently this sound is termed a systolic 'click')
> *hypertrophic cardiomyopathy*
> *coarction aorta* (extending in diastole to a 'machinery murmur')

Early diastolic murmur

> *aortic incompetence (regurgitation)*
> *pulmonary incompetence (regurgitation)*
> Graham Steell murmur in *pulmonary hypertension*

Mid–late diastolic murmur

> *mitral insufficiency (stenosis)*
> *tricuspid insufficiency (stenosis)*
> Austin Flint murmur in *aortic incompetence*
> *left atrial myxoma* (variable – can also give other murmurs)

Signs of left and right ventricular failure

Left heart failure

- dyspnoea
- basal crackles on inspiration and expiration
- fourth heart sound, or third in older patients
● Sit the patient forward and listen at the bases of the lungs with the diaphragm of the stethoscope for fine inspiratory and expiratory crackles.

> Fine crackles heard on inspiration only are caused by alveoli opening on inspiration. If a patient has been recumbent for a while, alveoli tend to collapse in the normal lung. On taking a deep breath, fine inspiratory crackles will be heard. This is termed atelectasis. These do not mean the patient has fluid in his alveoli or pulmonary oedema. Ask the patient to take a deep breath and then cough. The crackles should clear. If crackles are present on inspiration and expiration, this is indicative of fluid in the alveoli. With medium to coarse crackles, consider pulmonary oedema and request a chest X-ray for confirmation.

Right heart failure

- raised JVP
- enlarged tender liver (see Chapter 5)
- pitting oedema
- With the patient sitting forward, look for swelling over the sacral area. If there is, push your thumb into the swelling and see if you leave an indentation (pitting oedema). If you do, determine the severity of the oedema in terms of seconds it takes for the pitting to disappear.
- Check both ankles for pitting oedema.
    Oedema (fluid) collects at the most dependent part of the body. A patient who is mostly sitting will have ankle oedema while a patient who is lying will have predominantly sacral oedema.

Functional result

- Having ascertained the basic pathology (e.g. *myocardial infarction, aortic insufficiency -stenosis, pericarditis*), make an assessment of the functional result.
    - **history:** how far the patient can walk, etc.
    - **examination:** evidence of:
        - cardiac enlargement (hypertrophy or dilation)
        - heart failure
        - arrhythmias
        - pulmonary hypertension
        - cyanosis
        - endocarditis
    - **investigations:** for example:
        - chest X-ray
        - electrocardiogram (ECG)
        - treadmill exercise test with ECG for ischaemia
        - echocardiograph – sonar 'radar' of heart, for muscle and ventricle size, muscle contractility and ejection fraction, valve function
        - 24-hour ECG tape for arrhythmias
        - cardiac catheterization for pressure measurements, blood oxygenation and angiogram
        - radio-active scan – to image live, ischaemic or dead cardiac muscle

Summary of common illnesses

Mitral stenosis

- small pulse – fibrillating?
- JVP only raised if heart failure

- RV ++ LVo tapping apex
- loud S_1; loud p_2 if pulmonary hypertension
- opening snap (os)
- mid-diastolic murmur at apex only (low-pitched rumbling)
- severity indicated by early opening snap and long murmur
- best heard with the patient in left lateral position, in expiration with the bell of the stethoscope, particularly after exercise has increased cardiac output
- presystolic accentuation of murmur (absent if atrial fibrillation and stiff cusps)
- sounds 'ta ta rooofoo T'
  from S_2 os murmur S_1

Mitral incompetence

- fibrillating?
- JVP only raised if heart failure
- RV+LV++ systolic thrill
- soft S_1; loud p_2 if pulmonary hypertension
- pansystolic murmur apex > axilla

Mitral valve prolapse

- midsystolic 'click', late systolic murmur
  - posterior cusp – murmur apex > axilla
  - anterior cusp – murmur apex > aortic area

There are three stages; see Fig. 3.18.

Aortic stenosis

- plateau pulse – narrow pulse pressure
- JVP only raised if heart failure
- LV++ systolic thrill
- soft a_2 with paradoxical split (± ejection click)
- harsh midsystolic murmur, apex and base, radiating to carotids
  - note discrepancy of forceful apex and feeble arterial pulse
  - the longer the murmur, the tighter the stenosis; loudness does not necessarily imply severity

Aortic incompetence

- water-hammer pulse – wide pulse pressure; pulse visible in carotids
- JVP only raised if heart failure
- LV++ with dilation

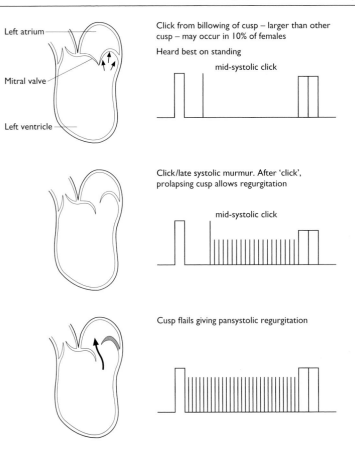

Fig. 3.18 Stages of mitral valve prolapse.

- – (ejection click)
- – early diastolic murmur base > lower sternum (also ejection systolic murmur from increased flow)
    - – (sometimes Austin Flint murmur – see below)
    - – heard best with patient leaning forward, in expiration
    - – the longer the murmur, the more severe the regurgitation

Tricuspid incompetence

- – JVP large v-wave
- – RV++, no thrill
- – soft pansystolic murmur at maximal tricuspid area
- – increases on inspiration

Austin Flint murmur

- mid-diastolic murmur (like mitral stenosis) in aortic incompetence due to regurgitant stream of blood on anterior cusp mitral valve

Graham Steell murmur

- pulmonary early diastolic murmur (functional pulmonary incompetence) in mitral stenosis or other causes of pulmonary hypertension

Atrial septal defect

- JVP only raised if failure or tricuspid incompetence
- RV++ LVo
- widely fixed split second sound
- pulmonary systolic murmur (tricuspid diastolic flow murmur)

Ventricular septal defect

- RV+ LV+
- pansystolic murmur on left sternal edge (loud if small defect!)

Patent ductus arteriosus

- systolic > diastolic 'machinery' or continuous murmur below left clavicle

Metal prosthetic valves

- loud clicks with short flow murmur
- aortic systolic
- mitral diastolic
- need anticoagulation

Tissue prosthetic valves

- porcine xenograft or human homograft
- tend to fibrose after 7–10 years, leading to stenosis and incompetence
- may not require anticoagulation

Pericardial rub

- scratchy (sounds like two pieces of leather rubbing together), superficial noise heard in systole and diastole
- brought out by stethoscope pressure, and sometimes variable with respiration

Infectious endocarditis (diagnosis made from blood cultures)

- febrile, unwell, anaemia
- splinter haemorrhages on nails (see Fig. 2.10)
- Osler's nodes
- cardiac murmur
- splenomegaly
- haematuria

Rheumatic fever

- flitting arthralgia
- erythema nodosum or erythema marginatum
- tachycardia
- murmurs
- *Sydenham's chorea* (irregular, uncontrollable jerks of limbs, tongue)

Clues to diagnosis from facial appearance

- *Down's syndrome* from 21 trisomy
    - ventricular septal defect
    - patent ductus arteriosus
- *thyrotoxicosis* – atrial fibrillation
- *myxoedema* from hypothyroid – cardiomyopathy
- dusky, congested face – *superior vena cava obstruction*
- red cheeks in infraorbital region in mitral facies from mitral stenosis

Clues to diagnosis from general appearance

- *Turner's syndrome* from sex chromosomes XO
    - female, short stature, web of neck
    - coarctation of aorta
- Marfan's syndrome
    - tall patient with long, thin fingers
    - aortic regurgitation

Peripheral arteries

- **Feel all peripheral pulses** (Fig. 3.19). Lower limb pulses are usually felt after examining the abdomen.

    Diminished or absent pulses suggest *arterial stenosis* or *occlusion*. The lower limb pulses are particularly important if there is a history of *intermittent claudication*.

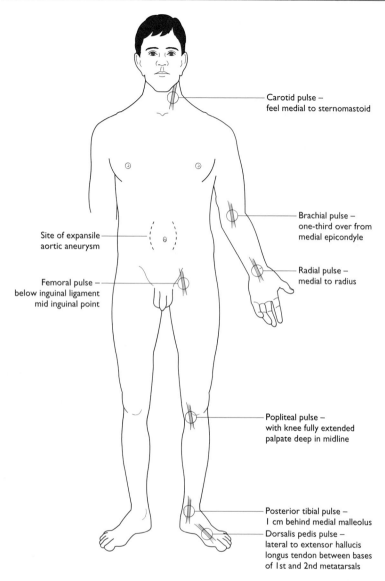

Fig. 3.19   Sites of peripheral pulses.

Auscultation of the carotid and femoral vessels is useful if there is a suspicion that these arteries are stenosed. A bruit is heard if the stenosis causes turbulent flow.

Coarctation of the aorta delays the femoral pulse after the radial pulse.

Peripheral vascular disease

- white or blue discoloration
- ulcers with little granulation tissue and slow healing (Fig. 3.20)

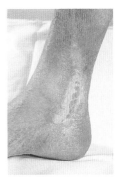

Fig. 3.20 Healing varicose ulcer – classic site in lower leg medially with pigmentation from venous stasis.

- shiny skin, loss of hairs, thickened dystrophic nails
- absent pulses
- Buerger's test of severity of arterial insufficiency
- loss of autoregulation of blood flow
- patient lying supine, lift leg up to 45° – positive test: pallor of foot; venous guttering
- hang legs over side of bed: note time to capillary and venous filling; reactive hyperaemia; subsequent cyanosis

Diabetes, when present, also signs from **neuropathy**:
- dry skin with thickened epidermis
- callus from increased foot pressure over abnormal sites, e.g. under tarsal heads in midfoot, secondary to motor neuropathy and change in distribution of weight (see Fig. 2.42)
- absent ankle reflexes
- decreased sensation

Aortic aneurysm

- Musset's sign (observe the patient's ability to hold his head still)
- central abdominal pulsation visible or palpable
- need to distinguish from normal, palpable aorta in midline in thin people
  - aortic aneurysm is expansible to each side as well as forwards
  - a systolic bruit may be audible (Fig. 3.21)
  - associated with femoral and popliteal artery aneurysms

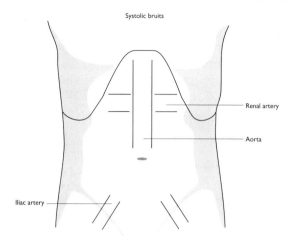

Systolic bruits

Renal artery

Aorta

Iliac artery

Fig. 3.21 Site of systolic bruit in aortic aneurysm. Reproduced with permission.

Varicose veins

- Varicose veins and herniae are examined **when the patient is standing**, possibly at the end of the whole examination at the same time as the gait.

  > Majority are associated with incompetent valves in the long saphenous vein or short saphenous vein.
  >
  > Long saphenous – from femoral vein in groin to medial side of lower leg.
  >
  > Short saphenous – from popliteal fossa to back of calf and lateral malleolus.

- **Observe:**
  - swelling ⎫
  - pigmentation ⎬ indicates chronic venous insufficiency
  - eczema ⎭
  - inflammation – suggests thrombophlebitis
- **Palpate:**
  - soft or hard (thrombosed)
  - tender – thrombophlebitis
  - cough impulse – implies incompetent valves. Incompetent valves can be confirmed by the **Trendelenburg test**:
    - Elevate leg to empty veins.
    - Occlude long saphenous vein with a tourniquet around upper thigh.
    - Stand patient up.

- If veins fill rapidly, this indicates incompetent thigh perforators below the tourniquet.
- If, after release of tourniquet, veins fill rapidly, this indicates incompetent saphenofemoral junction.

If veins fill immediately on standing, then incompetent valves are in thigh or calf, so do the **Perthes test**:

- As for Trendelenburg, but on standing let some blood enter veins by temporary release of groin pressure.
- Ask patient to stand up and down on toes.
- Veins become less tense if:
  - muscle pump is satisfactory
  - perforating calf veins are patent with competent valves

System-oriented examination

Examine the cardiovascular system

- hands – ? moist, cold, clammy, palmar erythema
- nails – leuconychia, splinter haemorrhages, capillary refill
- radial pulse – rate, rhythm, waveform, volume, state of artery
- blood pressure
- eyes – anaemia
- area around eyes – xanthelasma
- mouth – central cyanosis
- JVP – height, waveform
- apex beat – PMI site, character
- auscultate
- at apex – PMI (with thumb/finger on carotid artery for timing)
- heart sounds
- added sounds
- murmurs
- in neck over carotid artery – each area of precordium with diaphragm
- aortic incompetence – lean forward in full expiration with diaphragm
- mitral stenosis – lay patient on left side and listen at apex with bell
- listen to the bases of lungs for crackles
- examine for hepatomegaly
- peripheral oedema and peripheral pulses

Table 3.1 Intracardiac values and pressures

Intracardiac values

Cardiac Output (CO)	4–8 l/min
Cardiac Index (CI)	2.4–4.2 l/min/m²
Stroke Volume (SV)	60–120 ml
Stroke Volume Index (SVI)	35–70 ml/beat/m²
Left Cardiac Work (LCW)/Left Cardiac Work Index (LCWI)	3.4–4.2 kg m/m²
Left Ventricular Stroke Work (LVSW)/Left Ventricular Stroke Work Index (LVSWI)	LVSW = 50–60 gm-m/m²
Right Cardiac Work (RCW)/Right Cardiac Work Index (RCWI)	RCW = 0.54–0.66 km-m/m²
Right Ventricular Stroke Work (RVSW)/Right Ventricular Stroke Work Index (RVSWI)	RVSWI = 7.9–9.7 gm-m/m²
Systemic Vascular Resistance (SVR)	900–1600 dyn/sec/cm⁵
Pulmonary Vascular Resistance (VR)	20–120 dyn/sec/cm⁵
Mixed Venous Saturation (SvO₂)	75%
Delivery of Oxygen (DO₂)	900–1100 ml/min
Consumption of Oxygen (VO₂)	200–290 ml/min
Oxygen Extraction Ratio (OER)	0.22–0.30

Intracardiac pressures

Central Venous Pressure (CVP)	0 – +8 mmHg (right atrial level)
Right Ventricle (RV)	0 – +8 mmHg diastolic
	+15 – +30 mmHg systolic
Pulmonary Capillary Wedge Pressure (PCWP)	
	+5 – +15 mmHg
Left Atrium (LA)	+4 – +12 mmHg
Left Ventricle (LV)	+4 – +12 mmHg diastolic
	+90 – +140 mmHg systolic
Aorta	+90 – +140 mmHg systolic
	+60 – +90 mmHg diastolic
	+70 – +105 mmHg mean

References

Brown, E., Collis, W., Leung, T. & Salmon, A. (2002) *Heart Sounds Made Easy.* Churchill Livingstone, Edinburgh.

Hatchett, R. & Thompson, D. (2007) The sociological and human impact of coronary heart disease. In: *Cardiac Nursing: A Comprehensive Guide,* 2nd edn. Churchill Livingstone, Edinburgh.

CHAPTER 4

Examination of the Respiratory System

General examination

Introduction

The respiratory assessment constitutes an essential aspect in evaluating the patient's health. Functions of the respiratory system involve the exchange of oxygen and carbon dioxide in the lungs and tissues and regulation of the acid/base balance. Changes in the respiratory system affect other systems.

Examine the patient for:
- **signs of respiratory distress** (tachypnoea, dyspnoea, nasal flaring, use of accessory muscles, cyanosis)
- **nicotine** on fingers
- **clubbing**: respiratory causes include:
  - intrathoracic tumours:
    carcinoma of bronchus
    mesothelioma
  - bronchiectasis
  - lung abscess
  - empyema
  - fibrosing alveolitis
  - COPD (e.g. emphysema)
  - mixed venous to arterial shunts
  - chronic hepatic fibrosis
- **evidence of respiratory failure:**
  - **hypoxia**: central cyanosis
  - **hypercapnia**: drowsiness, confusion, papilloedema, warm hands, bounding pulse, dilated veins, coarse tremor/flap
- **respiratory rate**: count per minute
- **pattern of respiration:**
  Cheyne–Stokes:
  - alternating hyperventilation and apnoea
  - severe increased intracranial pressure
  - left ventricular failure
  - high altitude

Biot's – ataxic breathing: unpredictable irregularity (respirations may be shallow or deep and are interrupted by periods of apnoea – seen in neurological disease/disorders)

hyperventilation or Kussmaul respiration: increases in both rate and depth (hyperpnoea is an increase in depth only – seen in exercise, anxiety and metabolic acidosis; Kussmaul is hyperventilation associated with metabolic acidosis)

tachypnoea: rapid, shallow breathing >24 breaths per minute (seen in restrictive lung disease, pleuritic chest pain and elevated diaphragm)

air trapping: present in pulmonary diseases (as air is trapped in the lungs, respiratory rate rises and breathing becomes shallow)

- **positional dyspnoea:**
  - orthopnoea (congestive heart failure, severe asthma, emphysema, mitral valve disease, chronic bronchitis, neurological disease)
  - trepopnoea (congestive heart failure: patient is more comfortable breathing whilst lying on one side)
  - platypnoea (neurological disease, cirrhosis causing intrapulmonary shunts, hypovolaemia, status postpneumonectomy)
- **obstructive airways disease:**
  - pursed-lip breathing: expiration against partially closed lips
  - chronic obstructive airways disease to delayed closure of bronchioles
  - use of accessory muscles: sternomastoids, strap muscles and platysmus
- **wheezing:**
  - bronchospasm
  - asthma
  - allergy
  - congestive heart failure
- **stridor:** partial obstruction of trachea
  - **hoarse voice:** abnormal vocal cords or *recurrent laryngeal palsy*
- **cough:**
  - haemoptysis (coughing up blood)
  - sputum production (chronic/productive related to chronic bronchitis, bronchiectasis, abscess, bacterial pneumonia, tuberculosis)
  - dry/hacking (viral infection, interstitial lung disease, allergies, tumour
  - barking (epiglottal disease such as croup)
  - morning ('smoker's cough')
  - nocturnal (postnasal drip, congestive heart failure)
  - when eating or drinking (neuromuscular disease of the upper oesophagus)
- **sleep apnoea:** characterized by daytime fatigue, sleepiness, disruptive snoring, episodic upper airway obstruction, nocturnal hypoxaemia (Swartz, 2006).

First examine the front of the chest fully and then similarly examine the back of the chest.

- **Landmarks to locate the lungs** (Figs 4.1–4.3):

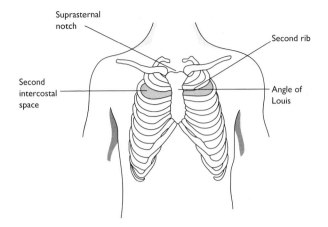

Fig. 4.1 Anterior and posterior landmarks to locate the lungs. Reproduced with permission.

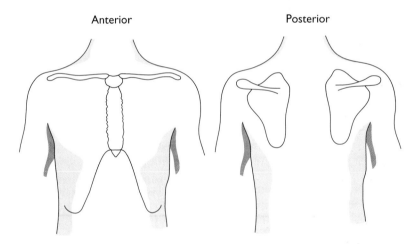

Fig. 4.2 Anterior and posterior landmarks to locate the lungs. Reproduced with permission.

- manubrium of the sternum
- sternal angle (angle of Louis)
- sternum
- xiphoid process
- sternal notch
- costal angle
- clavicles
- scapulae
- spinous processes.

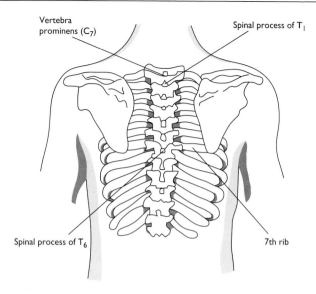

Vertebra prominens (C₇)

Spinal process of T₁

Spinal process of T₆

7th rib

Fig. 4.3 Anterior and posterior landmarks to locate the lungs. Reproduced with permission.

- **Demarcation lines of the thorax** (Figs 4.4–4.6):
  - used to identify and describe the location/condition of underlying organs/sounds.

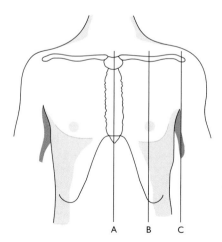

A   B   C

Fig. 4.4 Demarcation lines of the thorax. (a) Midsternal line.
(b) Midclavicular line. (c) Anterior axillary line (left) or left anterior line.
Reproduced with permission.

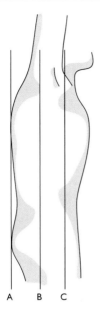

Fig. 4.5 Demarcation lines of the thorax. (a) Posterior axillary line. (b) Midaxillary line. (c) Anterior axillary line. Reproduced with permission.

A B C

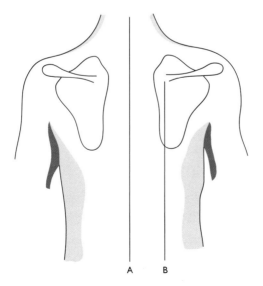

A B

Fig. 4.6 Demarcation lines of the thorax. Reproduced with permission.

Inspection of the chest

- **Rest the patient comfortably in the bed at 45°:**
  - compare hemithoraces; progress from the neck down
  - distended neck, puffy blue face and arms
  - superior mediastinal obstruction
  - tracheal shift
- **Inspect the shape of the chest:**
  - colour, contour and condition of the skin (ecchymosis, lesions, scars, e.g. from previous surgery)
  - asymmetry: diminution of one side or possible flail
    lung collapse
    fibrosis
  - deformity: check spine (Fig. 4.7)
  - pectus excavatum: sunken sternum
  - pectus carinatum: 'pigeon breast'
  - barrel chest
  - **obstructive airways disease**
    - barrel chest: lower costal recession on deep inspiration; cricoid cartilage close to sternal notch; chest appears to be fixed in inspiration

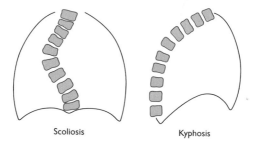

Scoliosis   Kyphosis

Fig. 4.7   Check for deformity of the spine.

Palpation

- **Check integrity of the thorax (palpate ribs, clavicles, sternum and scapulae for abnormalities):**
  - crepitations (e.g. fracture or unstable sternum)
  - pain
- **Check mediastinum position:**
  - **trachea** – check position: palpate with a single finger in the midline and determine if it slips preferentially to one side or the other (Fig. 4.8)
- **Lymph nodes**, supraclavicular fossae/axillae – *tuberculosis, lymphoma, cancer of the bronchus*, infraclavicular and parasternal

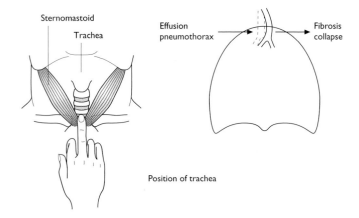

Fig. 4.8 Checking the mediastinum position of the trachea.

- **Apex beat** – may be displaced because of enlarged heart and not a shift in the mediastinum
- **Unequal movement of chest:**
    - Look from the end of the examination table/couch or bed.
    - Classic method of palpation to discern respiratory excursion (Fig. 4.9):
        - extend your fingers and anchor fingertips far laterally around chest wall whilst your extended thumbs meet in the midline
        - on inspiration, assess whether there is asymmetrical movement of thumbs from the midline (movement should be equal to 1–2 cm)

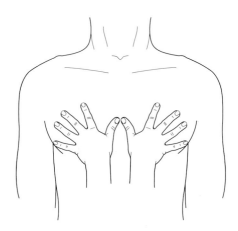

Fig. 4.9 Respiratory excursion.

- – Alternative method of palpation to discern respiratory excursion:
- – lay a hand comfortably on either side of the chest and, using these as a gauge, assess if there is diminution of movement on one side during inspiration

N.B. Diminution of movement on one side indicates pathology on that side. In older adults respiratory excursion may be minimal to absent as the anterior–posterior dimension of the thorax expands and lateral movement diminishes.

- ● **Palpate intercostal spaces for abnormalities:**
  - – lumps, surgical emphysema
- ● **Tactile fremitus:**
  - – vocal fremitus (assessed when pathology is suspected)

Percussion

- ● Percuss with the middle finger (hammer finger) of one hand against the middle phalanx of the middle finger of the other, laid flat on the chest. The hammer finger should strike at right angles and the wrist of the hammer finger hand should flick with each strike (Fig. 4.10). See Table 4.1 for discrimination of sounds.

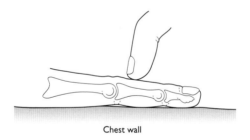

Chest wall

Fig. 4.10   Position for percussion.

Table 4.1   Discrimination of sounds

Sound	Relative intensity	Relative pitch	Relative duration
Flatness	Soft	High	Short
Dullness	Medium	Medium	Medium
Resonance	Loud	Low	Long
Hyper-resonance	Very loud	Lower	Longer
Tympani	Loud	Hollow	Hollow

- **Percuss both sides of the chest for resonance**, at top, middle and lower segments. Compare sides and if different, also compare the front and back of chest (Fig. 4.11).

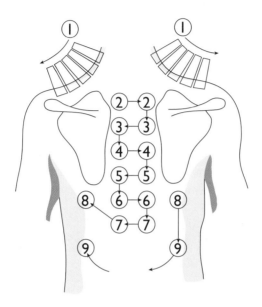

Fig. 4.11 Percussion sequence of the chest. Reproduced with permission.

- If a dull area exists, map out its limits by percussing from a resonant to the dull area.
- Percuss the level of the diaphragm from above downwards.

    Increased resonance may occur in:
    - pneumothorax
    - emphysema

    Decreased resonance may occur in:
    - *effusion:* very dull, sometimes called stony dullness
    - *solid lung*
    - consolidation
    - alveolar collapse
    - abscess
    - neoplasm

    Remember the surface markings of the lungs when percussing. Thus, the lower lobe predominates posteriorly and the upper lobe predominates anteriorly (Fig. 4.12).

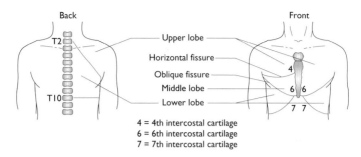

4 = 4th intercostal cartilage
6 = 6th intercostal cartilage
7 = 7th intercostal cartilage

Fig. 4.12   Percuss the diaphragm from above downwards. These markings are at full inspiration. Under normal examination conditions the hepatic dullness extends to the fifth intercostal cartilage.

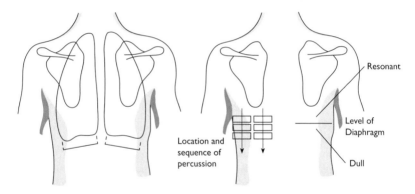

Fig. 4.13   Determination of diagphramatic excursion. Reproduced with permission.

● Determine diaphragmatic excursion (Fig. 4.13) by percussing the level of the diaphragm from above downwards. Start with the patient breathing normally. Percuss downward from the bottom of the scapula in the intercostal spaces from tympani to dullness. When dullness is heard, mark this space. Ask the patient to take a deep breath and hold it. Percuss from the marked space (tympani) to dullness. Diaphragmatic excursion should be greater on the left than on the right. (Position of the liver diminishes excursion on the right. Position of the heart increases excursion on the left.)
  – *decrease in excursion indicative of diaphragmatic paralysis (seen following cardiothoracic surgery and abdominal surgery or trauma/injury)*

Auscultation

- **Before listening, ask the patient to cough up any sputum** which may create adventitious sounds.
- Use either the diaphragm or bell of the stethoscope, dependent on the condition/physique of the patient, and listen starting at the top (apex), then moving to the middle and bottom (base) of both sides of the chest, and then in the axilla. Auscultate downwards in approximately 5 cm distances (Fig. 4.14).

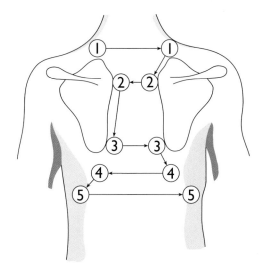

Fig. 4.14 Sequence for auscultation. Reproduced with permission.

Ask the patient to breathe through his mouth moderately deeply. It helps to demonstrate this yourself.

The bell of the stethoscope is used to hear low-pitched sounds. Hold the bell lightly on the patient's skin. If pressure is put on the bell, a diaphragm will be created and the ability to hear low-pitched sounds will be lost. In cachectic, thin patients, patients with prominent ribs or if the chest is hairy, use of the bell is more effective. Protruding ribs make placement of the stethoscope diaphragm difficult as pressure must be applied to the diaphragm in order to use it effectively (Swartz, 2006).

It is not acceptable to listen to the chest through clothing. The bell/diaphragm must always be in direct contact with the patient's skin.

Table 4.2   Characteristics of sounds

Breath sound	Duration of inspiration and expiration	Pitch of expiration	Intensity of expiration	Sample location
Vesicular	Inspiration longer than expiration	Low	Soft	Most of lungs
Bronchovesicular	Inspiration and expiration are equal	Medium	Medium	Near bronchi, e.g. below the clavicles and between the scapulae, especially on the right
Bronchial	Expiration longer than inspiration	Medium-high (dependent on location)	Usually high (dependent on location)	Over the lower part of the trachea
Tracheal/tubular	Expiration longer than inspiration	High	High/harsh	Over the upper part of the trachea

- **Listen for normal breath sounds** (Table 4.2), comparing both sides:
  - **vesicular:** breath sounds heard over most of the lung tissue
  - **bronchovesicular:** heard near the bronchi (e.g. below the clavicles and between the scapulae, especially on the right)
  - **bronchial:** patent bronchi plus conducting tissue
  - **tracheal/tubular:** sounds similar to sounds with stethoscope over trachea
- **Listen for added sounds (adventitious sounds)**, and note if inspiratory or expiratory (Fig. 4.15):

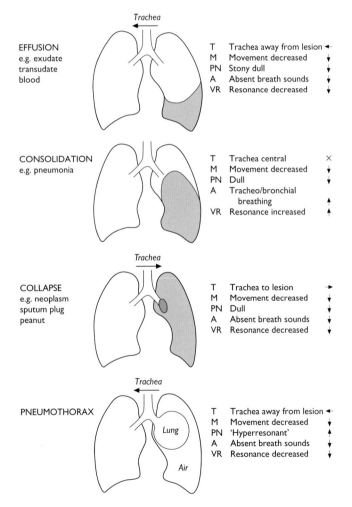

Fig. 4.15 Auscultation of adventitious sounds.

- **tracheal/tubular or bronchial:** sounds heard in an area other than
  the upper or lower trachea
  consolidation (usually pneumonia)
  neoplasm
  fibrosis
  abscess
- **diminution:** indicates either no air movement (e.g. obstructed
  bronchus) or air or fluid preventing sound conduction
  effusion
  pneumothorax
  emphysema
  collapse – obstruction
- **crackle** (outdated terms include rales, crepitations and creps): caused
  by either the alveoli popping open on inspiration (indicative of atelecta-
  sis) or fluid in the lungs (in which the crackling sound is heard on inspiration and expiration)
  - fine – heart failure, alveolitis or if late on inspiration, indicative of
    pulmonary fibrosis
  - medium – infection or fluid in the alveoli
  - coarse – air bubbling through fluid in the alveoli and larger bron-
    chioles, e.g. bronchiectasis or pulmonary oedema
- wheeze (outdated terms include sibilant rale, musical rale, sonorous
  rale or low-pitched wheeze): caused by rapid air flow through a con-
  stricted airway
  - asthma – note the presence of air trapping
  - bronchitis
  - pulmonary oedema
  - congestive heart failure
- **ronchus:** transient airway plugging caused by mucous secretions
  - bronchitis
- **pleural rub:** caused by *pleurisy* (inflammation of the pleura due to
  pneumonia or pulmonary infarction); sounds like two pieces of leather
  rubbing together

Vocal fremitus/resonance

Should be assessed when pathology is suspected.

Speech creates vibrations that can be evaluated through feeling and
hearing. The presence or absence of fremitus can provide useful information
about the density of underlying lung tissue and the chest cavity. Conditions
that increase density increase the transmission/frequency of tactile fremitus.
Conditions that decrease the transmission of sound waves decrease tactile
fremitus.

- **Ask the patient to repeat '99'** whilst you palpate the patient's chest with either the ulnar surface or palms of both of your hands simultaneously in the same general areas as auscultation. The frequency of vibrations is greater over areas of consolidation. Compare both sides.
- **You can also auscultate** for vocal resonance. Ask the patient to say 'e'. At the surface of an *effusion* the word 'e' takes on a bleating character like a goat, which is called **aegophony**. If vocal resonance is gross, **whispered pectoriloquy** can be elicited by asking the patient to whisper '1, 2, 3' repeatedly. The whispered sound when auscultated will be loud and pronounced rather than soft and muffled.

N.B. Vocal fremitus, breath sounds and vocal resonance all depend on the same criteria and vary together.

To determine further clues, check:

- chest movement asymmetry
- mediastinum displacement
- percussion (Barkauskas *et al.*, 2002; Bickley & Szilagyi, 2007; Epstein *et al.*, 2008; Hatton & Blackwood, 2003; Jarvis, 2008; Seidel *et al.*, 2006; Swartz, 2006; Talley & O'Connor, 2006).

Sputum

Examination of the sputum is unpleasant but important. Normally 75–100 ml of sputum is secreted daily by the bronchi. Describe according to colour, consistency, quantity, presence or absence of blood or pus and number of times brought up during the day and night.

- Look for:
  - **colour** (in yellow or green it may be infected)
  - **consistency** (if all mucus it may be saliva)
  - **quantity** (increased grossly in bronchiectasis)
  - **blood** (cancer, tuberculosis, embolus)

Ideally the sputum should be examined under the microscope for:

- bacteria
- pus cells
- eosinophils
- plugs
- asbestos

Functional result

Make an assessment of the functional result.

- **History – exertion/exercise:** for example, how far the patient can walk and how many stairs can be climbed

- **Examination:**
  - **Po₂ ↓**: central cyanosis
    - confusion
  - **Pco₂ ↑**: peripheral signs
    - warm periphery
    - dilated veins
    - bounding pulse
    - flapping tremor
    - central signs
    - drowsy
    - papilloedema
    - small pupils
- Check by arterial blood gases.
- **Tests** (usually undertaken for COPD):
  - **force of expiration**: blowing out a lighted match about 15 cm from the mouth and with the mouth wide open is easy as long as the patient's peak flow is above approximately 80 l/min (normal 300–500 l/min)
  - **expiration time**: an assessment of airways obstruction can be made by timing the period of full expiration through wide-open mouth following a deep breath; this should be less than 2 seconds when normal
  - **chest expansion**: expansion from full inspiration to full expiration should be more than 5 cm; reduced if hyperinflation of the chest is due to chronic obstructive airways disease
  - **peak flow**: a measure of airways obstruction is the peak rate of flow of air out of the lungs; a record is made using a peak flow meter; normal 300–500 l/min

Summary of common illnesses

Asthma

  - patient distressed, tachypnoeic, unable to talk easily
  - wheeze on expiration audible or by auscultation
  - overinflated chest with hyperresonance
  - if central cyanosis: critically ill, artificial ventilation?
  - pulsus paradoxus (may be normal between attacks)
  - often due to atopy
  - enquire about exposure to antigens:
    - house dust mite
    - cats or dogs

Obstructive airways disease (chronic)

  - barrel chest
  - accessory muscles of respiration in use

- hyperresonance
- depressed diaphragm – indrawing lower costal margin on inspiration
- diminished breath sounds:
  - **blue bloater:**
    central cyanosis
    signs of carbon dioxide retention
    obese
    not dyspnoeic
    ankle oedema: may or may not have right heart failure
  - **pink puffer:**
    not cyanosed
    no carbon dioxide retention
    thin
    dyspnoeic
    no oedema

Bronchiectasis

- clubbing
- constant green/yellow phlegm
- coarse crackles over affected area

Allergic alveolitis

- clubbing
- fine, unexplained crackles, widespread over bases

System-oriented examination

Examination of the respiratory system

Use the techniques of inspection, palpation, percussion and auscultation in each phase of the examination whilst examining the anterior, posterior and lateral thorax.

- hands: clubbing, signs of increased carbon dioxide (warm hands, bounding pulse, coarse tremor)
- face: nasal flaring
- tongue: central cyanosis
- trachea: right or left shift
- supraclavicular, infraclavicular and parasternal nodes
- inspection
  - shape of chest contour
  - chest movements
  - respiration rate/rhythm/depth/distress
  - colour and condition of the skin

- palpation
  - interspaces for abnormalities
  - sternum, ribs, clavicles and scapulae for abnormalities
  - excursion
  - vocal fremitus
- percussion: in 5 cm intervals from apex to base – upper segments (L, R), middle (L, R) and lower segments (L, R)
  - diaphragmatic excursion
- auscultation
  - breath sounds
  - added sounds (adventitious sounds)
- if COPD
  - expiration time

References

Barkauskas, V., Baumann, L. & Darling-Fisher, C. (2002) *Health and Physical Assessment*, 3rd edn. Mosby, London.

Bickley, L. & Szilagyi P. (2007) *Bates' Guide to Physical Examination*, 5th edn. Lippincott, Philadelphia.

Epstein, O., Perkin, G., de Bono, D. & Cookson, J. (2008) *Clinical Examination*, 4th edn. Mosby, London.

Hatton, C. & Blackwood, R. (2003) *Lecture Notes on Clinical Skills*, 4th edn. Blackwell Science, Oxford.

Jarvis, C. (2008) *Physical Examination and Health Assessment*, 5th edn. Saunders, St Louis.

Seidel, H., Ball, J., Dains, J. & Benedict, G. (2006) *Mosby's Guide to Physical Examination*, 6th edn. Mosby, St Louis.

Swartz, M. (2006) *Physical Diagnosis, History and Examination*, 5th edn. Saunders, London.

Talley, N. & O'Connor, S. (2006) *Clinical Examination: A Systematic Guide to Physical Diagnosis*, 5th edn. Churchill Livingstone, London.

CHAPTER 5

Examination of the Abdomen

General examination
Introduction

To facilitate examination of the abdomen, the patient needs to be as relaxed as possible. Allow the patient to lie flat with his head resting on one pillow. His arms should lie loosely at his sides and his knees should be slightly bent (to relax abdominal muscles). You may want to prop a pillow under the patient's knees to make him more comfortable. Do not allow the patient to place his hands above his head as this stretches and tightens the abdominal wall. Ensure you maintain privacy and the patient's dignity by screening the examination couch/table/bed by closing the curtains and/or the door.

It is important that the patient can be inspected fully. You should ensure that the patient can be assessed in good light and that you can observe the abdomen from above the xiphoid process to the symphysis pubis, thus exposing the patient's groin.

Introduce yourself to the patient and inform him about what you will be doing. Begin your inspection at the foot of the bed. Note the shape of the abdomen. The normal abdomen is concave and symmetrical. It will rise and fall in line with respiration. Look for signs of peristalsis. Now move to the right side and bend down so that you can view the abdomen tangentially. In this position you can more easily pick out subtle changes of contour.

- **Note the presence of any:**
  - surgical scars
  - striae, which may be silver if the patient has previously lost weight, or stretch marks resulting from pregnancy; striae are purplish/pink in *Cushing's syndrome*
  - body hair
  - dilated veins – flow of blood in vein (Fig. 5.1) is:
    - superior: due to inferior vena cava obstruction
    - inferior: due to superior vena cava obstruction
    - radiating from navel: due to portal vein hypertension
  - jaundice
  - rashes or lesions

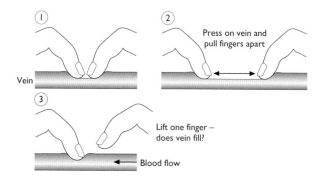

Vein

① ②   Press on vein and pull fingers apart

③   Lift one finger – does vein fill?

← Blood flow

Fig. 5.1   William Harvey's method of checking vein filling.

- distension/swellings
- central or flank
- symmetrical or asymmetrical. May be due to one of the 5 Fs:
  - flatus
  - faeces
  - fetus
  - fat
  - fluid (ascites, ovarian cyst) (Fig. 5.2)

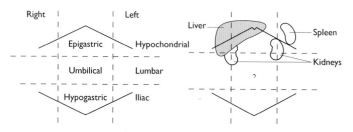

Right | Left

Epigastric | Hypochondrial

Umbilical | Lumbar

Hypogastric | Iliac

Liver — Spleen

Kidneys

Fig. 5.2   Nine abdominal quadrants and location of organs in epigastric, hypochondrial and lumbar regions.

- discolouration in the flanks or around the umbilicus
- nodules
- movement of abdomen on respiration
- peristalsis: may be visible in thin normal person
- pulsation
- hernia
- **Look for signs of:**
  - **liver disease:**
    - *clubbing*
    - *pallor*

- *leuconychia*
- *palmar erythema*
- *xanthelasmata* (*chronic cholestasis*)
- *jaundice*
- *ascites*
- *right-sided pleural effusion*
- *telangiectasia* on face
- *icterus*
- *spider naevi* (Fig. 5.3)

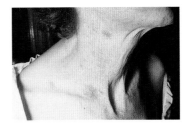

Fig. 5.3 Spider naevi in cirrhosis – telangiectasia radiating from central arteriole.

- *gynaecomastia*
- *female distribution of body hair*
- *alcohol abuse*
    - *Dupuytren's contracture* (see Fig. 2.12)
    - parotid swelling
    - *testicular atrophy*
- **liver failure:**
    - *liver flap*
    - *foetor hepaticus*
    - *Wernicke's or Korsakoff's psychosis*
    - *inability to copy a five-pointed star*

        Signs of chronic liver disease are usually obvious, but we are all allowed up to six spider naevi (particularly if pregnant) (Fig. 5.4).

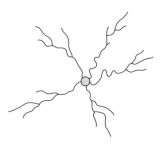

Fig. 5.4 Spider naevus: a small collection of capillaries fed by a central arteriole.

- **anaemia** – inspect palpebral conjunctiva by gently everting lower eyelid; in anaemia it appears pale pink
- **iron deficiency:**
  - *koilonychia* (see Fig. 2.4)
  - *smooth tongue*
  - *angular stomatitis* – can be from ill-fitting dentures or edentulous state
- **B$_{12}$ or folate deficiency**
  - *glossitis* – 'beef steak' or smooth shiny tongue
  - *megablastic, macrocytic anaemia*
- **Look at lips:**
  - if pale, examine conjunctivae for anaemia
    Brown freckles 1–5 mm in diameter on lips or buccal mucosa may indicate *Peutz–Jeghers syndrome*; can also be seen on fingers; another feature of this syndrome is polyps in the small bowel that can cause abdominal pain, bleed, intussuscept or become malignant.
- **Look at mouth:**
  - **dry tongue** – 'dehydration' or mouth breathing
    If the patient seems dehydrated, check for Maxwell's sign (lift fold of skin on forehead above the nose and between the eyebrows). Skin remains raised with dehydration.
  - central cyanosis in chronic liver disease from pulmonary arteriovenous shunting
  - *Candida* – red tongue, white patches on palate
  - *gingivitis*
  - ulcers
  - Crohn's disease (ulceration may be noted at the corners of the mouth)
  - aphthous with coeliac disease
  - ill-fitting dentures
  - breath – *ketosis, ethanol, foetor hepaticus* and *uraemia*
- **Palpate for nodes** (behind the left sternoclavicular joint):
  A hard node felt behind the left sternoclavicular joint may be a **Virchow's node** (Fig. 5.5) and suggests an abdominal neoplasm spread by lymphatics via the thoracic duct.

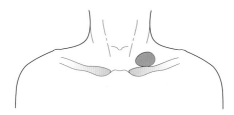

Fig. 5.5   Virchow's node.

Auscultation

Auscultation provides important information about bowel motility and it is important to listen to the bowel before performing palpation or percussion as they can alter the frequency of bowel sounds.

Bowel sounds are caused by intestinal peristalsis moving gas and fluid through the bowel.

Bowel sounds

- Listen over the abdomen with the diaphragm of the stethoscope for about 10–15 seconds. If sounds are difficult to hear, listen for up to 7 minutes.
  In progressive bowel obstruction, large amounts of fluid and gas accumulate and hyperactive 'tinkling' bowel sounds can be heard. This is an ominous sign of impending bowel paralysis.
  Paralytic ileus or *generalized peritonitis* presents with complete absence of bowel sounds.
- Listen for *hepatic bruits* in patients with liver disease.
  A soft and distant bruit heard over an enlarged liver is always abnormal and may indicate:
  - *primary liver cell cancer*
  - *alcoholic hepatitis*
  - *acquired arteriovenous shunts* from biopsy or trauma

Arterial bruits (Fig. 5.6)

If suggested by the history or examination (e.g. patient has high blood pressure), listen for bruits over the renal, iliac and femoral arteries. Renal arteries are generally best heard over the back.

> *Renal artery stenosis* may be the cause of hypertension.
> Patients with *intermittent claudication* may have flow bruits over the femoral arteries from narrowing, e.g. *atheroma*.

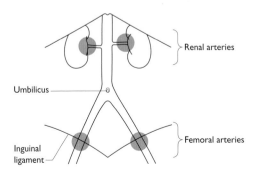

Fig. 5.6 Auscultation sites for arterial bruits.

Palpation of the abdomen

- Before you feel the patient's abdomen:
  - allow him to empty his bladder.
  - ask 'is your abdomen painful anywhere? Tell me if I hurt you.'
  - warm your hands; get the patient to lie flat with arms by his sides.
  - Lightly palpate each quadrant first, starting away from the site of pain or tenderness. Your hand should be flat on the patient's abdomen. Feel by flexing your fingers at the metacarpophalangeal joints. Be gentle.
  - Look at the patient's face to see if palpation is hurting him.

    Tenderness may be superficial, deep or rebound.

    Rebound tenderness from movement of inflamed viscera of peritonitis against parietal peritoneum. First palpate the abdomen lightly 1–2 cm in depth. If no pain, proceed to deep palpation 4–6 cm in depth.

    Guarding may be noted during palpation. This is a voluntary muscle spasm to protect from pain.

    Rigidity. Fixed, tense abdominal muscles from reflex involuntary spasm. Occurs in generalized *peritonitis*.

Liver

- **Examine from the patient's right**. Start about 10 cm below the costal margin and work up towards the ribs. Ask the patient to take a deep breath. Try and feel for the liver edge as it comes down towards your finger tips.
- **Describe position of liver edge** in centimetres below the costal margin of the midclavicular line. Liver enlargement is described as mild, moderate or massive. If enlarged, trace the shape of the liver edge and decide if it is. Feel the surface of the enlarged liver and edge for:
  - firm or hard
  - regular/irregular
  - tender
  - pulsatile (in tricuspid incompetence) (Fig. 5.7)

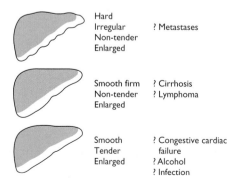

Fig. 5.7 Examination of the liver.

- **Percuss the upper and lower borders of the liver** after palpation to confirm findings.

  If the liver is not felt and the right hypochondrium is dull, the liver may extend to the hypogastrium. Palpate lower down.

If large, remember to feel for the spleen as the presence of a palpable spleen suggests cirrhosis with portal hypertension.

Spleen

- **The normal spleen** cannot be felt and only becomes palpable when it has doubled in size. Begin your palpation 10 cm beneath the costal margin in the hypochondrium, working up to the ribs.
- **Ask the patient to take a deep breath**, to bring the spleen down so it can be palpated.

  If the spleen is not palpable, **percuss** the area for splenic dullness – the spleen can be enlarged to the hypogastrium.

  If a slightly enlarged spleen is suspected, lay the patient on his right side with his left arm hanging loosely in front and again feel on deep inspiration.

- **Check** characteristics of the spleen (Fig. 5.8):
  - site
  - shape (? notch)
  - cannot get above it:
    - moves on respiration
    - enlarges towards umbilicus
    - dull to percussion
- Describe as for liver.

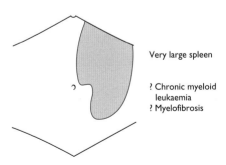

Very large spleen

? Chronic myeloid leukaemia
? Myelofibrosis

Fig. 5.8   Splenic enlargement.

Kidneys

The kidneys are difficult to feel and deep bimanual palpation is required to explore them.

- **Push up with left hand in renal angle** and feel kidney anteriorly with right hand.

- **Ask the patient to take a deep breath** to bring kidneys between hands. Tenderness is common over the kidneys if there is infection. A large kidney may indicate a tumour, *polycystic disease* or *hydronephrosis.*
- **Assess for kidney tenderness** (costal-vertebral angle tenderness). Sit the patient forward – place the palm of your hand over the renal angle. Then using the ulnar surface of your other hand, make a fist and strike your hand placed on the patient's renal angle with moderate force. Perform on each kidney in turn and assess the patient's reaction.

Masses
- **Carefully palpate the whole of the abdomen**. If a mass is found, describe:
  - site
  - size
  - shape
  - consistency – faeces may be indented by pressure
  - fixation or mobility – does it move on respiration?
  - tender
  - pulsatile – transmitted pulsation from aorta or pulsatile swelling
  - dull to percussion – particularly important to determine if bowel is in front of mass
  - does it alter after defaecation or micturition?

Aorta
- Palpate in the midline above the umbilicus for a pulsatile mass. If easily palpated, suspect aortic aneurysm and proceed to ultrasonography in men over 50 and women over 60 years.
  - may be normal aorta in a thin person
  - unfolded aorta
  - aneurysm
  - Musset's sign (bobbing of the patient's head with each pulsation of the aorta)

Percussion

- Dullness on percussion:
  - ascites – free fluid
  - an organ, e.g. liver, spleen
  - tumour, e.g. *large ovarian cyst*
- **Percuss liver, spleen and kidneys after palpation of each organ.**
- **Percuss any suspected mass.**
  The midline of the abdomen should be resonant – if not, think of *gastric neoplasm, omental secondaries, enlarged bladder, ovarian cyst, pregnancy.*

- **If there is generalized swelling of the** abdomen, lie the patient on one side and mark the upper level of dullness. Roll the patient flat and see if the level shifts. This is called **shifting dullness** (Fig. 5.9).

  Note that in ascites there is central tympani and lateral dullness. In ovarian tumour there is central dullness and lateral tympani as the gas-filled bowel is pushed laterally.

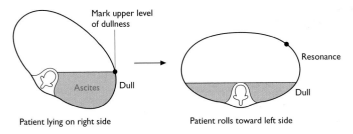

Fig. 5.9 Shifting dullness.

Summary of common illnesses

Cirrhosis

- leuconychia
- clubbing
- palmar erythema
- spider naevi
- jaundice
- firm liver

Portal hypertension

- splenomegaly
- ascites
- caput medusa

Hepatic encephalopathy

- liver flap
- drowsy
- constructional apraxia (cannot draw five-pointed star)
- musty foetor

'Dehydration' (water and salt loss)

- dry skin
- veins collapsed
- diminished skin turgor – pinched fold of skin on forehead remains raised (Maxwell's sign)
- tongue dry
- eyes sunken
- blood pressure low with postural drop

Intestinal obstruction

- patient 'dehydrated' if he has been vomiting
- abdomen swelling centrally
- visible peristalsis
- not tender (unless inflammation or some other pathology)
- resonant to percussion
- high-pitched 'tinkling' bowel sounds

Pyloric stenosis

- upper abdomen swelling
- may have 'succussion splash' on shaking abdomen
- otherwise like intestinal obstruction

Appendicitis

- slight fever
- deep tenderness in right iliac fossa or per rectum
- otherwise little to find unless has spread to peritonitis

Peritonitis

- lies still
- abdomen:
  - does not move on respiration
  - rigid on palpation (guarding)
  - tender, particularly on removing fingers rapidly (rebound tenderness)
  - absent bowel sounds

Cholecystitis

- tender right hypochondrium, particularly on breathing in (Murphy's sign – tender gallbladder descends on inspiration to touch your palpating hand)

Jaundice and palpable gallbladder

- obstruction is not due to gallstones, but from another obstruction such as neoplasm of the pancreas (Courvoisier's law); gallstones have usually caused a fibrosed gallbladder which cannot dilate due to back-pressure from gallstones in common bile duct

Enlarged spleen

- infective, e.g. septicaemia or subacute bacterial endocarditis
- portal hypertension, e.g. cirrhosis
- lymphoma
- leukaemia and other haematological diseases
- autoimmune, e.g. systemic lupus, Felty's syndrome

Per rectum examination

- Tell the patient at each stage what you are going to do.
- Lie the patient on the left side with knees flexed to the chest.
- Say: 'I am going to put a finger into your back passage'.
- Inspect anus for lumps, haemorrhoids, fissures, ulcers, inflammation, excoriation and discolouration – a bluish discolouration of perineal skin may be indicative of Crohn's disease.
- With lubricant on glove, press your fingertip against the anal verge, then gently slip the forefinger into the anal canal and then into the rectum. Feel the tone of the sphincter by asking the patient to squeeze your finger with his anal muscles, then check the size and character of the prostate and any lateral masses. If appropriate, proceed to proctoscopy.
- Test stool on your glove for occult blood.

Per vaginam examination

The per vaginam examination is discussed in Chapter 7. If you are a male nurse, do not perform a vaginal examination without a chaperone, who should be female if possible. Note that most women will prefer to be examined by a woman.

System-oriented examination

Examine the abdomen

- Inspect abdomen asymmetry: movement, pulsation, swelling
- Hands: clubbing, spider naevi, palmar erythema, liver flap, Dupuytren's contracture

- Nails: leuconychia, koilonychia in iron deficiency
- Eyes: jaundice, anaemia
- Mouth: ulceration
- Tongue: foetor, smooth
- Lips: *Peutz–Jeghers syndrome*
- Neck: Virchow's lymph node
- Chest: spider naevi, gynaecomastia
- Auscultate: bowel sounds, arterial and liver or spleen bruits/rubs
- Enquire: whether pain or tenderness
- Palpate: inguinal lymph nodes briefly
- Palpate: four quadrants for masses: note abdominal tenderness, guarding, rigidity
- Palpate: liver, kidneys, spleen, aorta (? aneurysm)
- Ascites: test for shifting dullness
- Examine for hernia: ask patient to cough; stand patient up if a hernia is a possibility
- Enquire whether appropriate:
  - to examine vulva/testes
  - to do rectal examination

CHAPTER 6

Examination of the Male Genitalia

General examination
Introduction

Patients may become embarrassed when discussing their genitals so it is important to try and put them at ease. Therefore it is important that the sexual history and examination should be undertaken in a sensitive manner. Reassure the patient that the information shared will remain confidential. This will help encourage him to be more open and honest with you. The questions asked may be perceived by the patient as intrusive and he may feel that your questioning has no bearing on the symptoms or problem that he has presented with. Take time and give clear explanations as to why you are asking certain questions. By utilizing careful questioning and tact, you are more likely to encourage patients to open up and provide you with the answers that will assist you in reaching a diagnosis.

It is useful to begin by stating something like 'I am now going to ask you some questions about your sexual health and practices'. Try and determine the patient's risk of acquiring a sexually transmitted infection (STI). Depending on the problem, you may wish to begin by asking general questions about sexual function, sexual history, and duration of relationships, timing of the last sexual encounter, whether it was with a regular or casual partner, the contraceptive methods used, the number of sexual partners that he has had and his sexual orientation. Ask about having sex with men and women or both. Ask if his partner has any symptoms. You can then ask about any previous STIs and any previous treatments that he may have had. If he has previously had a STI, ask him about the symptoms he had. Ask about any previous sexual health check-ups. Ask about the use of injected drugs. Ask if the patient has been vaccinated against hepatitis A or B and whether he has been tested for HIV, hepatitis or syphilis.

Important symptoms to consider

- Urethral discharge
- Warts

- Ulceration
- Testicular pain
- Swelling
- Ulceration
- Rashes
- Inflammation
- Frequency and urgency
- Hesitancy
- Haematuria
- Nocturia
- Impotence
- Loss of sexual desire
- Infertility
- Incontinence
- Oliguria
- Dysuria

Erectile function

If the presenting problem is erectile dysfunction, ask the following questions.
- Are you suffering from stress, in work or relationships?
- Are you afraid that sexual intercourse may cause cardiac problems?
- Do you drink alcohol? How many units?
- What medications do you take, over the counter, prescription and illicit drugs?

Note the distribution and amount of body hair, and the size of testes as testosterone levels may be reduced.

Possible sexually transmitted infection

- To assess the possibility of a STI, ask questions about any discharge or dripping from the penis.
- If the patient has a penile discharge try and ascertain the amount, colour and consistency.
- Ask if he has any other symptoms such as a temperature, rash or pain.
- Tell the patient that an STI can affect any opening that comes into contact with sexual organs.
- Ask the patient about oral and anal sex and if he answers positively, ask about the presence of sore throats, rectal bleeding, pain, itching or diarrhoea.
- Ask about the presence of any sores, warts, swelling on the penis or swelling in the scrotum/testicles.
- Ask if the patient has any concerns about HIV infection.

Examination of the male genitalia

The patient may lie down or stand whilst you carry out your inspection. If the patient is standing, it is helpful to have him lean over an examination table.

Ask permission in a sensitive way before you proceed, e.g. 'I should briefly examine you down below. Is that all right?'. Then begin your examination by inspecting the penis and groin area. Some examiners recommend that the patient hold his penis during inspection rather than the examiner holding it.

Inspection

- Note the size, colour, shape and the presence or absence of a prepuce (foreskin). The size of the penis is usually dependent on the patient's age and overall development.
- Note any abnormal curvatures.
- Examine the penis. Retract the prepuce (foreskin) to expose the glans; it may be useful to get the patient to do this for you. Note the presence of any chancres, ulceration or erythema and the presence of smegma which is a cheesy white substance that accumulates normally under the foreskin.
- Examine and inspect the glans. Look for the presence of warts, ulcers, nodules or the signs of any inflammation. Examine the external urethral meatus – ask the patient to squeeze it open gently to inspect for discharge (normally you will find none). *Balanitis* (inflamed glans of penis) should remind the examiner to check for diabetes.
  If any discharge is noted, take a swab and send for microbiology examination.
- Inspect the skin around the groin for any excoriation or inflammation. Note the presence of any nits or lice – these can usually be found at the base of the pubic hairs.
- Lift up the scrotum to inspect the posterior surface.
- Note any obvious hernia.
- Examine scrotal swellings – transilluminate.
  A poorly developed scrotum on one or both sides may suggest cryptorchidism.

Abnormalities of the penis

- Priapism (persistent, usually painful, erection of the penis).
- Hypospadias (birth defect where the urethra and urethral groove are malformed).
- Phimosis (tight prepuce that cannot be retracted over the glans).
- Paraphimosis (a tight prepuce that once retracted cannot be returned and oedema may occur). This is common following the insertion of a catheter when the healthcare professional does not return the prepuce over the glans.

Abnormalities of the scrotum

- Cryptorchidism (undescended testis).
- Inguinal hernia.
- Cystic swelling.
- Variocoele (occurs in about 8% of male population and feels like a bag of worms). Due to varicosity of the veins of the pampiniform plexus.
- Epididymal cyst.
- Hydrocoele.
- Scrotal swelling (common scrotal swellings include inguinal hernias, scrotal oedema and hydrocoeles). Tender painful swellings may indicate acute orchitis, acute epididymitis or torsion of the spermatic cord. Swelling in the scrotum can be evaluated by transillumination.

Look for signs of syphilis – primary, secondary and tertiary

- Chancre (painless hard ulcer) seen in primary syphilis.
  Skin rash, with brown sores about the size of a penny; the rash may cover the whole body or appear only in a few areas, almost always on the palms of the hands and soles of the feet. May be seen in secondary syphilis.
- Mild pyrexia, fatigue, headache, sore throat, patchy hair loss, and swollen lymph glands throughout the body. These symptoms may be very mild and, like the chancre of primary syphilis, will disappear without treatment.
- In tertiary syphilis, the brain, nervous system heart, eyes, bones and joints can be affected. This stage can last for years and may result in mental illness, blindness, other neurological problems, heart disease, and death.

Look for signs of gonorrhoea

- Painful urination.
- Yellowish urethral discharge.
- Painful discharge of bloody pus from the rectum (rectal gonorrhoea).
- Throat infection can occur as a result of oral sex with infected partner.

Look for signs of herpes

- Painful blisters or bumps in the genital or rectal area that crust over to form a scab and heal.
- Patient complains of itching, burning or tingling sensation in the genitals.
- Swollen lymph glands.
- Headache.
- Muscle ache.
- Pyrexia.
- Penile discharge.
- Infection of the urethra causing a burning sensation during urination.

Look for signs of HPV infection

- Genital warts (condylomata acuminata) usually appear as small bumps or groups of bumps. They can be raised or flat, single or multiple, small or large, and sometimes cauliflower shaped.

Look for signs of chlamydia

- No symptoms in 70–80% of cases.
- Lower abdominal pain and burning pain during urination.
- Mucopurulent discharge from the penis.
- Tenderness or pain in the testicles.
- Burning and itching around the meatus.
- Rectal pain, discharge or bleeding in patients who engage in anal sex.

Palpation

Groin

The spermatic cord, lymph nodes and arteries occupy the groin. Swellings here are usually caused by hernias or enlarged lymph nodes.
- Palpate the groin to detect enlarged lymph nodes.
- Most people have small, shotty nodes. Most enlarged tender nodes arise from infection in the legs or feet. However, in some Afro-Caribbean men this is a normal finding.
- If large nodes, palpate spleen carefully (*reticulosis* or *leukaemia*).

Hernia

When checking for the presence of hernia, examine the patient standing and ask him to cough – enlargement of a groin swelling suggests a hernia (Fig. 6.1).

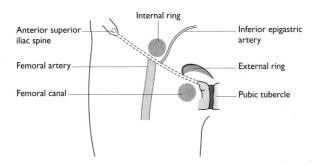

Fig. 6.1　Checking for hernia.

- **Indirect (oblique) inguinal hernia**: the swelling is reduced to the internal inguinal ring by pressure on the contents of the hernial sac and then controlled by pressure over the internal ring when the patient is asked to cough; if your hand is then removed, the impulse passes medially towards the external ring and is palpable above the pubic tubercle.
- **Direct inguinal hernia**: the impulse moves in a forward direction mainly above the groin crease **medial to the femoral artery** and swelling is not controlled by pressure over the internal ring.
- **Femoral hernia**: swelling fills out the groin crease medial to the femoral artery.

Penis

- Palpate the whole length of the penis to the perineum, and note the state of the dorsal vein. Note any hardened or tender areas. Hardness may indicate a urethral stricture or cancer whereas tenderness may indicate an infection.

Scrotum

- Ask 'Is your scrotum painful anywhere? Tell me if I hurt you'.
- Warm your hands, and remember to use gentle pressure.
- Palpate the scrotum for the testes and epididymes.
- Palpate each testis and epididymis with your thumb and first two fingers.
- Observe the patient's face.
- *Note the size, shape and consistency of each testis. Note any tenderness.*
  - Tender and enlarged testes may occur with *orchitis* or *torsion of the testis. Multiple tortuous veins may indicate a variocoele.*
  - **A large, soft swelling which transilluminates** suggests *hydrocoele* or an *epididymal cyst.* A hydrocoele surrounds the testis; an epididymal cyst lies behind the testis.
  - **A large, hard, painless testis** suggests *testicular cancer*, a potentially curable cancer with a peak incidence between the ages of 15 and 35 years.

Prostate gland

- Lie the patient on the left side with knees flexed to the chest or ask the patient to bend over the examination table.
- Inspect the anus for lumps, haemorrhoids, fissures, ulcers, inflammation, excoriation and warts.
- *Explain to the patient that you will need to place your finger into his rectum to examine the prostate. This procedure may be uncomfortable but should not be painful. Say: 'I am going to put a finger into your back passage'.*

With lubricant on the glove, press your finger tip against the anal verge, then gently slip your forefinger into the anal canal and then into the rectum. Inform the patient that he may feel the urge to pass urine but he will not. Palpate the prostate gland on the anterior rectal wall. Check the size and character of the prostate. It should feel smooth and rubbery and be approximately the size of a walnut. Note any nodules or tenderness. A swollen, tender prostate may indicate acute prostitis whereas an enlarged, smooth but firm prostate may indicate benign prostatic hypertrophy. Hard roughened areas are suggestive of cancer.

CHAPTER 7

Examination of the Female Reproductive System

General examination

Introduction

Examination of a woman's reproductive system includes an abdominal examination (discussed in Chapter 5), examination of the external genitalia, a speculum examination and bimanual examination. A rectal examination may also be needed in some circumstances (Arulkamaran *et al.*, 2007). This chapter considers the pelvic examination of a non-pregnant woman. This procedure is very intimate but is one that most women will experience at some point in their lives. It is the nurse's role to make it as bearable as possible. Most, but not all women, will prefer a woman to carry out the examination, and all women should be offered a chaperone, regardless of the gender of the person carrying out the examination. Some women may want to have a friend or relative present. It is important for the nurse undertaking the procedure to establish a rapport with the woman prior to examination. It is also important that the nurse explains fully the procedure, and why it is necessary, prior to the woman getting undressed. A diagram or model may help here. However, it is equally important to be aware that some women do not want to have a detailed explanation, and would rather the nurse 'just got on with it'.

Preparation

Ask the woman if she needs to empty her bladder prior to examination. Make sure everything is ready before asking the woman to get undressed: there is nothing worse than having to leave the bedside to search for a swab that is in another room. Make sure there is a good lighting source that can be positioned to give the best view of the genitalia. Secure the door to the consultation room and let the women know that the door is closed and no one else will come in. Explain exactly what you want the woman to do: it may seem evident to you that you need the woman to remove her underwear, but it may not be evident to the woman. Leave the woman to undress in private, having given her a gown or blanket to put over herself so she is not sitting exposed waiting for you.

In most primary care settings, the woman will be asked to lie on a couch in the dorsal position, with the soles of her feet together and knees apart. In secondary care, the lithotomy position, using leg supports, is more common. The lithotomy position gives a better view of the genitalia, but seems to be a more exposing and 'medicalized' position to ask a woman to adopt. A left lateral position may also be used, which is useful in examining women who have uterovaginal prolapse or vesicovaginal fistulae (Arulkamaran *et al.*, 2007). This position is also more comfortable for older women, particularly if they have kyphosis or arthritis/bone/joint disease. Once the woman is in the correct position, covered over her abdomen and legs with a gown or sheet, check again that there is everything to hand (Box 7.1), wash your hands and then put on gloves.

Box 7.1   Materials needed for a pelvic examination

Gloves
Warm water for lubrication
KY jelly or similar
Specula (it may be necessary to use different sizes to ensure comfort
   and facilitate visualization of the cervix)
Cervical broom/liquid-based cytology container (if cervical cytology is
   being undertaken)
Swabs (if samples are being taken for microbiology/virology)
Tissues

Adapted from O'Connor & Kovacs (2003).

Inspection of the external genitalia

Tell the woman that you are beginning the examination. Look at the perineum. Note hygiene and distribution of pubic hair. Look at the labia majora which should be generally symmetrical, but may be open or closed, full or thin. Note any lesions. Open the labia majora to inspect the labia minora, which should be darker coloured and soft. Inspect the clitoris, urethral opening and vaginal opening. Check for any inflammation, redness or discharge. Palpate the Bartholin glands and the lateral tissue of the perineum between thumb and forefinger. Check for swelling, tenderness and masses.

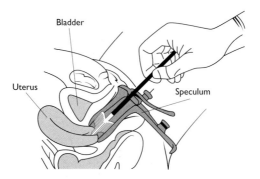

Bladder

Uterus

Speculum

Fig. 7.1 Speculum examination.

Speculum examination (Fig. 7.1)

The Cusco's (disposable) speculum is the most commonly used. Ensure you are familiar with how to open and close the blades.

Warm and lubricate the speculum using warm water. Extra lubrication can be used if no samples (for cytology or microbiology/virology) are being taken. Tell the woman what you are going to do and then gently part the labia to insert the speculum. In the dorsal position, the speculum should be inserted with the handle superior, while in the lithotomy position the handle is usually inferior (Arulkamaran *et al.*, 2007). If the handle is superior, make sure that it does not touch the clitoris, which is very sensitive. Open the speculum when it is fully inserted. Inspect the vaginal walls which should be pink and moist. The cervix should be visible between the tips of the blades. If you cannot see it, try withdrawing the speculum slightly – the cervix may 'drop' into view or you may need to close the speculum, withdraw further and change direction of the speculum slightly. If necessary a digital examination can be used to establish the position of the cervix. Putting a pillow under the woman's buttocks may also help to adequately position the woman for the examination.

Inspect the cervix. It should be symmetrical, pink and about 3 cm in diameter. The surface should be smooth. The os should be round in a nulliparous woman and slit-like in a parous woman. Note any ectropion at the transformation zone. There may be some clear or creamy odourless discharge from the os. Obtain cervical cytological samples and/or swabs at this point as needed. Remove the speculum, keeping the blades open until they are clear of the cervix. Close the blades and withdraw the instrument slowly from the vagina.

Bimanual examination (Fig. 7.2)

The purpose of the bimanual examination is to bring the pelvic organs closer to the abdominal wall, where they can be felt by the hand on the abdomen

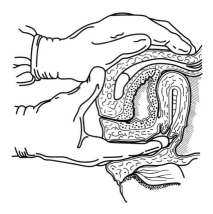

Fig. 7.2 Bimanual examination.

(Arulkamaran *et al.*, 2007). Explain again to the woman what you are going to do. Using lubrication on gloved fingers, place the index and middle fingers of the right hand into the vagina, palm upwards. Locate the cervix. Grasp the cervix between the two fingers and move it gently from side to side, watching the woman's face. The cervix should move 1–2 cm in either direction without pain. If this procedure is painful for the woman, she has 'cervical excitation' or 'cervical motion tenderness'.

Place the left hand over the lower abdomen. Feel the uterus between the hands. An anteverted uterus should be easy to feel, a retroverted one may not be. However, the body of the uterus may be palpable by the fingers in the vagina, by moving them to above and below the cervix and exerting pressure inwards. The uterus should be pear shaped, about 5.5–8 cm long in nulliparous women, larger in multiparous women (Seidel *et al.*, 2006). The contour should be round, firm and smooth. The uterus should be slightly mobile in the anterior–posterior plane and non-tender on movement. Note the presence of fibroids. The adnexae can be palpated with the fingers of the vaginal hand in the lateral fornices and with the abdominal hand over the respective iliac fossa. Try to locate the ovaries: with the fingers of the vaginal hand in the lateral fornix, the abdominal fingers should be pressing deeply over the iliac fossa towards the symphysis pubis. The ovaries, if palpable, should be smooth and firm and slightly tender. The fallopian tubes should not be palpable. Ovaries in postmenopausal women should not be palpable. If any masses are found in the uterus or adnexae, note size, contour, consistency and mobility. Finally, the pouch of Douglas and uterosacral ligaments should be examined. Note any tenderness and nodularity of the ligaments.

Having finished the examination, offer the woman some tissues and leave her to dress in private. Allow her to wash her hands afterwards.

Differential diagnosis

See Tables 7.1 and 7.2 for differential diagnosis of acute and chronic pelvic pain.

Table 7.1   Differential diagnosis of acute pelvic pain

Category	Diagnosis
Gynaecological	
Pregnancy related	Ectopic
	Miscarriage
	Fibroid degeneration (rare)
Ovarian	Mittelschmerz
	Torsion/rupture/haemorrhage of an ovarian cyst
	Ovarian hyperstimulation syndrome
Tubal	Pelvic inflammatory disease
Uterine	Dysmenorrhoea
Pelvic	Endometriosis
Non-gynaecological	
Gastrointestinal	Appendicitis
	Inflammatory bowel disease
	Diverticulitis
	Constipation
	Adhesions
	Strangulated hernia
Urinary tract	Infection
	Calculus
	Retention

Adapted from O'Connor & Kovacs (2003).

Table 7.2   Differential diagnosis of chronic pelvic pain

Category	Diagnosis
Gynaecological	
Ovarian	Mittelschmerz
	Ovarian cysts
	Ovarian cancer
Tubal	Pelvic inflammatory disease
Uterine	Dysmenorrhoea
	Fibroids
	Uterine cancer
Pelvic	Endometriosis
	Pelvic congestion syndrome

Table 7.2   (*continued*)

Category	Diagnosis
Non-gynaecological	
Gastrointestinal	Inflammatory bowel disease
	Irritable bowel syndrome
	Diverticulitis
	Constipation
	Adhesions
Urinary tract	Infection
	Retention
Orthopaedic	Disorder of spine or hip
Other	Somatization

Adapted from O'Connor & Kovacs (2003).

Selected gynaecological conditions

Infections

Infections of the female reproductive system may be non-sexually transmitted (candida and bacterial vaginosis) or sexually transmitted (gonorrhoea, chlamydia, herpes simplex virus, etc.). They may affect different parts of the reproductive tract (Table 7.3). The purely vaginal infections tend to be less severe, whereas infections that ascend the genital tract can cause pelvic inflammatory disease (PID) and infertility.

Table 7.3   Infections

	Fungal	Bacterial	Viral	Other
Vulval	Candida		HSV HPV	Syphilis
Vaginal		BV	HPV	TV
Cervical (/urethral)	Actinomyces	GC Chlamydia	HPV HSV	
Pelvic	(actinomyces)			

BV, bacterial vaginosis; GC, gonorrhoea; HSV, herpes simplex virus;
HPV, human papilloma virus; TV, *Trichomonas vaginalis*.
Reproduced from Centres for Excellence in Teaching and Learning (2008).

Pelvic inflammatory disease

Pelvic inflammatory disease is a syndrome resulting from the spread of micro-organisms to the endometrium and fallopian tubes. Chlamydia is the major cause of PID in the UK (patient.co.uk, 2008). History includes high fever, acute pelvic pain and dyspareunia, abnormal vaginal bleeding and purulent vaginal discharge. On pelvic examination, there is cervical excitation and adnexal tenderness (Sadler *et al.*, 2008).

Endometriosis

Endometriosis is the presence of tissue similar to the endometrium found outside the uterine cavity, most commonly in the pelvis. History includes pelvic pain, dyspareunia, dysmenorrhoea, menorrhagia and infertility. On examination, there may be pelvic tenderness, pelvic mass and fixation of the uterus (Sadler *et al.*, 2008).

Fibroids (uterine leiomyoma)

Fibroids are benign tumours of the myometrium. Usually they are asymp-tomatic, but they may cause menorrhagia, pain, pelvic discomfort and back-ache as well as urinary symptoms. On examination, the uterus will feel bulky and there may be a pelvic mass (Sadler *et al.*, 2008).

Prolapse

The history may be a dragging sensation or lump when standing upright. Urinary symptoms, recurrent cystitis and dyspareunia may be associated. Examination for prolapse should be carried out in the left lateral position, using a Sims speculum. For a woman who has delivered five or more babies, a large Sims speculum will be needed.

Gynaecological cancers

The National Institute for Health and Clinical Excellence (NICE, 2005) recommends urgent referral with the following findings:
- clinical features suggestive of cervical cancer
- postmenopausal bleeding (not on HRT) or continuation of bleeding 6 weeks after cessation of HRT
- unexplained vulval lump
- vulval bleeding due to ulceration.

Consider also for women with persistent intermenstrual bleeding with no identifiable cause.

The guidelines also recommend urgent referral of the woman for ultra-sound in suspected abdominal or pelvic mass that is not obviously a fibroid.

References

Arulkamaran, S., Symonds, I. & Fowlie, A. (2007) *Oxford Handbook of Obstetrics and Gynaecology*. Oxford University Press, New York.

Centres for Excellence in Teaching and Learning (2008) *Gynae Skills*. Available at: www.cetl.org.uk/learning/skills_sheets/GynaeSkills.pdf.

National Institute for Health and Clinical Excellence (NICE) (2005) *Referral Guidelines for Suspected Cancer*. National Institute for Health and Clinical Excellence, London.

O'Connor, V. & Kovacs, G. (2003) *Obstetrics, Gynaecology and Women's Health*. Cambridge University Press, Cambridge.

Patient.co.uk (2008) *Pelvic Inflammatory Disease*. Available at: www.patient.co.uk/showdoc/23069029/

Sadler, C., White, J., Everitt, H. & Simon, C. (2008) *Women's Health*. Oxford General Practice Library. Oxford University Press, Oxford.

Seidel, H., Ball, J., Dains, J. & Benedict, G. (2006) *Mosby's Physical Examination Handbook*. Mosby, St Louis.

CHAPTER 8

Mental Health Assessment

General examination

Introduction

A mental health assessment can be carried out to identify a person's needs, to assist in developing and using appropriate interventions, to contribute to diagnostic accuracy and to define a problem that needs solving. Assessing the mental state of people involves judging their psychological health and this requires experience, a degree of intelligence, self-knowledge, social skills, objectivity and the ability to deal with cognitive complexities.

A mental health assessment is usually done during an assessment interview. Motivational interviewing may lead to a more accurate assessment and involves exploring the pros and cons of the person's current state, their general life satisfaction and what help they need in making decisions about care.

Motivational interviewing (Andrews & Jenkins, 1999; Attenborough, 2006)

Working with ambivalence: ambivalence is not seen as unwillingness to seek help; rather, it may reflect the conflict the person feels between wanting help and wanting to remain the same.

Empathic listening: not making value judgements but displaying an attitude of acceptance, for example by reflecting comments back to the person to allow them to explore the possibility of help.

Self-motivational statements: eliciting comments from the person that indicate a willingness to accept help.

Counselling skills: for example, the use of open-ended questions, reflective listening, affirmations and summarizing.

Resistance: roll with the resistance by using non-confrontational methods. For example, if the person indicates that they do not want to accept treatment, you reply that they cannot see a reason to accept treatment.

Assessment of mental health status

An increasing number of people with mental health problems will be seen in general health settings. Assessment of mental health status may be necessary in all patients, not just those seen in mental health settings. An assessment of mental health status is not something you do to patients but activity undertaken in partnership with patients and during which you elicit their views of their needs. Barker (2004) suggests different levels of assessment.

- The physiological self – assessment of basic physiological needs
- The biological self – needs in relation to any symptoms a person may be experiencing, e.g. pain
- The behavioural self – the effects of our thoughts, feelings, attitudes and values on our behaviour
- The social self – how we relate to others
- The spiritual self – our values, hopes and experiences of the world

Gamble & Brennan (2006) suggest the following elements of a comprehensive mental health assessment:

- Risk
- Physical and mental health status
- Social need and functioning
- Symptomatology and coping skills
- Quality of life and its effects on others
- Housing and money
- Social support
- Medication and its effects
- Work skills and meaningful daily activity.

An assessment of mental health status may also focus on the following:

- **appearance and behaviour** – physical appearance, reaction to situation
- **mood** – mood, affect
- **speech** – rate, form, volume and quantity of information, content
- **form of thought** – amount and rate of thought, continuity of ideas
- **thought content** – delusions, suicidal thoughts, other
- **perception** – hallucinations, other perceptual disturbances
- **sensorium and cognition** – level of consciousness, memory, orientation, concentration, abstract thoughts
- **insight** – understanding of condition
- **sexual health** – sexual activity, contraceptive use, substance use, cervical screening, testicular examination, HIV status
- **patient's perception of need** – ask patients about their views of their mental health needs

Rating scales may be used with interviews as part of a mental health assessment. Some commonly used rating scales in mental health assessment are as follows.

- The Short Form-12 (SF-12_ (Ware *et al.*, 1996): a measure of general mental and physical health
- The Health of the Nation Outcome Scale (HoNOS) (Wing, 1994): a measure of 12 categories of behaviour and mental state linked to mental health status
- Brief Psychiatric Rating Scale (BPRS) (Ventura *et al.*, 1993): a measure of psychiatric symptoms
- Edinburgh Post Natal Depression Scale (EPNDS) (Cox *et al.*, 1987): a measure of depressive symptoms associated with childbirth
- Beck Depression Inventory (BDI) (Beck *et al.*, 1961): a measure of depressive symptoms
- Side Effects Checklist (SEC) (Andrews & Jenkins, 1999): a measure of side effects of drugs commonly used in psychiatry
- Suicide Assessment and Management (SAM) (Fremouw *et al.*, 1990): a measure of suicidal intent and previous self-harming behaviour
- Risk Assessment and Management – Clinical Risk Management Tool (CRMT) (Morgan, 2000): a measure of the likelihood of a potentially harmful incident happening, or that has possible beneficial outcomes for the person and others

General rules in assessing mental health status

- Be non-judgemental.
- Be alert to phenomena that are observed.
- Do not jump to conclusions about what the person is saying.
- Clarify with gentle enquiry:
  - **'Can you tell me more about that?'**
  - **'Can you give me a recent example?'**
  - **'When did that last happen?'**
  - **'What did you do about it?'**
  - **'How often/how long have you experienced that?'**

Appearance and behaviour (observation)

- Describe in simple terms:
  - unkempt appearance
  - bewildered, agitated, restless, aggressive, tearful, sullen:
    - appropriate to setting?
    - reduced activity in *depression*
    - overactive and intrusive in *mania*
    - tense and reassurance seeking with *anxiety*
  - able to respond to questions
  - evidence of responding to hallucinations
  - smell of alcohol
  - evidence of drug misuse (e.g. needle marks)

Mood (part observation, part enquiry)

Mood is a subjective state and is mainly judged by the impression conveyed during the history, although examination gives further clues.

- Ask:
    - **'How have your spirits been recently?'**
    - **'Have you been feeling your normal self?'**
    - **'Is this how you normally feel?'**
        > Depressed – depression disorder or an adjustment reaction (see questions under 'Mental Health' in Chapter 1).
        > Elevated – manic disorder or intoxication, e.g. ethanol, drugs, delirium.
        > Anxious – anxiety disorder or reaction to situation.
        > Angry – delirium or reaction to situation.
        > Flat – depressed or no emotional rapport, i.e. *schizophrenia*.
- If evidence for depression, worry, agitation, irritability – record current nature and severity. If depressed, ask:
    - 'How bad has it been?'
    - 'Have you ever thought of suicide?'
    - 'Have you seriously considered taking your life?'
- Also ask for nurses' and relatives' comments.

Speech (observation)

Describe speech in simple terms and record typical remarks verbatim.

- **Rate:**
    - fast in *mania*
    - slow in *depression*
- **Form:**
    - are there abnormalities of grammar or flow? (record examples)
        > Disordered thought processes can occur in *schizophrenia, mania, acute organic states, dementia.*
    - are there abnormal sequences of words?
    - non sequiturs with disordered logic in *schizophrenia* – 'word jumble'
    - loosely connected topics in *mania* – 'flight of ideas'
- **Content** (observations, elaborate with enquiry):
    - 'You said you . . . Tell me more about that.'
    - 'When you feel sad, what goes through your mind?'

Form of thought (form and content – largely inferred from speech)

- Record patient's main thoughts or preoccupations:
    - negative pessimistic in *depression* – ask about suicidal intentions
    - grandiose in *mania*
    - catastrophizing in *anxiety*

Obsessions – intrusive thoughts or repetitious behaviours that the patient cannot resist although he knows they are not sensible.
- perseveration – repetition of a word or phrase; can occur in *anxiety, depression, mania, delirium* or *dementia*

Thought content (odd ideas, thoughts, beliefs, delusions)

- Ask patient to describe; be non-judgemental.
- Ask why he thinks that – may reveal psychotic thoughts or hallucinations.

Delusions are fixed, false beliefs without reasonable evidence, e.g. I've got AIDS/cancer.
- 'Did it ever seem to you that people were talking about you?'
- 'Have you ever received special messages from the television, radio or newspaper?'
- 'Do people seem to be going out of their way to get at you?'
- 'Have you ever felt that you were especially important in some way or that you had special powers?'
- 'Do you ever feel you have committed a crime or done something terrible for which you should be punished?'

Perception (hallucinations and illusions – usually apparent from history)

- Ask:
  - 'Have you had any unusual experiences recently?'
  - 'Do they seem as if they are in the real world or as if they are "inside" your head?'

Hallucinations are false perceptions without a stimulus (e.g. pink elephants – experienced as real).
- They can occur in any sensory modality.
- Visual hallucinations are suggestive of an organic state.
- Third-person ('he' or 'she') auditory hallucinations are suggestive of *schizophrenia*.
- 'Do you ever hear things that other people can't hear such as the voices of people talking?'
- 'Do you ever have visions or see things that other people can't see?'
- 'Do you ever have strange sensations in your body or skin?'

Illusions are misinterpreted perceptions (e.g. he thinks you are a policeman). They are common in acute organic states (*psychosis*).

Sensorium and cognition (observations supplemented by specific enquiry)

- **Impairment of concentration** can occur in:
  - *depression*
  - *anxiety states*
  - *dementia*
  - *confusional state*
- **Orientation, thought processes, memory and logic.** These aspects must be tested as part of mental health assessment.

Insight (understanding of condition)

- 'What do you think is wrong with you?'
  - 'Is there any illness that you are particularly worried about?'
  - 'What treatment do you feel is appropriate?'
  - 'Are there any treatments you are frightened of?'
      It is important to ask all patients these questions. If the patient lacks insight into abnormal beliefs or behaviour, this suggests a psychotic illness.
  - Client's perception of his or her needs and problems

General history and examination

Mental illness can be the presentation of a physical illness and a full history and examination should be carried out for all patients.

Physical illnesses that may masquerade as mental illnesses include:
- *hypothyroid, hyperthyroid*
- *hypercalcaemia* or *hypokalaemia*
- *cerebral tumour*
- *other causes of increased intracranial pressure*
- *chronic, occult infection*
- *drugs*
- *porphyria*

There is some evidence that mental illnesses may be linked to physical imbalance of transmitters/receptor function in the brain, and the division of illness into physical and mental is often spurious. In any case, all patients, whatever the nature of their illness, should be treated non-judgementally and with respect.

Challenging behaviour

Anger and hostility

- Inordinate anger is often symptomatic of another problem.
- Assess whether the grievance is justified and whether it can be resolved.
- 'Is there anything else that is upsetting you?'
- If the antagonism is directed against you, enquire whether the patient would prefer to see somebody else.

Violence and aggression

- Do not take unnecessary risks (have help nearby).
- Attempt to defuse the situation.
- Ensure patient does not have a weapon.
- Determine orientation and whether intoxicated or deluded.
- Fear often underlies aggression – what is the fear?

Self-harming behaviour

- Assess intent and history of previous attempts (if any):
  - planning and likelihood of discovery
  - perceived dangerousness of method
  - intention at time
- Assess current intent:
  - how likely to attempt suicide?
  - what does the client want to happen?
  - what would increase/decrease risk?

Sexual disinhibition

- Often associated with manic disorders.
- Protect client's privacy and dignity.
- Work with client to agree boundaries of acceptable behaviour.
- Agree with client to operate within terms of contract.
- Take client into private space.
- Minimize others' ridiculing of client.

Summary of common mental disorders

Depression

- low mood, tearfulness (not always present)
- lack of interest and self-care
- poor concentration

- negative thought content
- low self-esteem
- wakes up early
- depressed facies
- slow movements and speech
- weight loss
- negative speech content

Anxiety

- generally worried
- thought focuses on catastrophes
- cannot get to sleep
- tense lined face, furrowed brow
- sweaty palms
- shaky
- hyperventilation
- tachycardia

Anorexia nervosa

- thin, little body fat
- increased, fine body hair
- sees self as fat even if thin
- thoughts dominated by food

Bulimia nervosa

- often normal weight
- binges followed by self-induced vomiting
- thoughts dominated by food
- erosion of teeth from vomiting

Schizophrenia

- hallucinations
- delusions
- thought disturbances
- disordered thinking
- negative symptoms

Bipolar disorder – mania

- rapid speech with 'flight of ideas'
- overactive, cannot keep still

- normal activities disrupted
- overly cheerful or irritable
- stands close and is argumentative

Bipolar disorder – depression

- depressed affect
- slow movements and speech
- negative thoughts and delusions, e.g. that brain is rotting
- suicidal thoughts
- loss of interest or pleasure in usual activities
- poor concentration

References

Andrews, G. & Jenkins, R. (eds) (1999) *Management of Mental Disorders*, UK edn. WHO Collaborating Centre for Mental Health and Substance Misuse, Sydney.

Attenborough, J. (2006) Motivational interviewing. In: Callaghan, P. & Waldock, H. (eds) *The Oxford Handbook of Mental Health Nursing.* Oxford University Press, Oxford: p98.

Barker, P. (2004) *Assessment in Psychiatric and Mental Health Nursing. In Search of the Whole Person.* Nelson Thornes, Surrey.

Beck, A., Ward, C., Mendelson, M., Mock, J. & Erbaugh, J. (1961) Inventory for measuring depression. *Archives of General Psychiatry*, **4**: 561–571.

Cox, J., Holden, J. & Sagovsky, R. (1987) Detection of postnatal depression: development of the 10-item Edinburgh Post Natal Depression Scale. *British Journal of Psychiatry*, **150**: 782–786.

Fremouw, W., de Perczel, M. & Ellis, T. (1990) *Suicide Risk Assessment and Response Guidelines.* Pergamon Press, New York.

Gamble, C. & Brennan, G. (2006) *Working with Serious Mental Illness. A Manual for Clinical Practice*, 2nd edn. Baillière Tindall, London.

Morgan, S. (2000) *Clinical Risk Assessment and Management Policy.* Lincolnshire Partnership NHS Foundation Trust. Available at: www.lpt.nhs.uk/Documents/ Policies/OPR/OPR20.pdf.

Ventura, M., Green, M., Shaner, A. & Liberman, R. (1993) Training and quality assurance with the brief psychiatric rating scale: 'the drift buster'. *International Journal of Methods in Psychiatric Research*, **3**: 221–244.

Ware, J., Kosinski, M. & Keller, S. (1996) A 12-item short-form health survey: construction of scales and preliminary tests of reliability and validity. *Medical Care*, **34**: 220–233.

Wing, J. (1994) *Health of the Nation Outcome Scales: HoNOS Field Trials.* Royal College of Psychiatrists Research Unit, London.

CHAPTER 9

Examination of the Nervous System

Introduction

The history is of prime importance in assessing the nature of the pathology, whereas the examination reveals the location and extent of the lesion. The history may also guide the order of the examination. The examination should address three questions: (1) Does the patient have a neurological illness? (2) Where in the nervous system is the pathology located? (3) What is the pathology? (Hatton & Blackwood, 2003).

The following features in the history can be informative:

- **speed of onset**
  - rapid, abrupt – *vascular, oedema* or *infective*
  - seconds – *seizure*
  - minutes – *migraine*
  - hours – *infective, inflammatory*
  - slow, progressive – *neoplasm* or *degenerative disorder*
- **duration**
  - brief episodes with recovery, e.g. *TIA, epilepsy, migraine, syncope*
  - longer episodes with recovery – *mechanical, obstruction* or *pressure*
  - demyelination, e.g. *multiple sclerosis*
- **frequency**
- **witness description** – particularly if the patient has episodic loss of consciousness or is confused.

The minute examination of the nervous system can be elaborated almost indefinitely. Of far greater importance is acquiring the ability to conduct a thorough but comparatively rapid examination with confidence in the findings. As with other examinations, it is best to develop your own basic system and perform it consistently because this will help avoid omissions.

- Adapt your examination to the situation. The order in which functions are examined may be varied according to the symptoms, but the routine examination must be mastered.

From the history, usually it will be obvious whether it is necessary to examine the mental functions in detail. A patient with sciatica would rightly be dismayed by an examination that began by asking him to name the parts of a watch.

The examination of the nervous system is approached under the following headings.

- **Mental function:**
  - appearance and behaviour
  - mood
  - orientation
  - geographical orientation
  - memory
  - intelligence
  - speech and comprehension
- **Cranial nerves**
- **Motor and sensory function**

The motor examination should be carried out in a systematic way. You should begin by assessing the upper limbs, then the neck and trunk and finally the lower extremities of the patient. When examining the limbs and trunk, you will need to observe the patient's posture, muscle tone, presence or absence of involuntary movements and muscular wasting and/or fasciculation. Your limb evaluation and examination should proceed from proximal to distal. Assess the major muscle groups first and if you note problems in any particular area then carry out a more detailed examination.

The assessment will examine the patient's proprioception, balance, gait, sensory stimuli, cortical sensory function and reflex activity.

The nervous system cannot effectively be examined in isolation. Other points of relevance may include:

- configuration of the skull and spine
- neck stiffness
- ear drums for otitis media
- blood pressure
- heart, e.g. arrhythmia, mitral stenosis
- carotid arteries – palpation and bruit
- neoplasms – breast, lung, abdominal
- jaundice

Mental function

General observation

- appearance, e.g. unkempt
- behaviour, e.g. bewildered, restless, agitated
- emotional state, e.g. depressed, euphoric, hostile

Observe, and ask for comments from nurses, other healthcare practitioners and relatives.

Consciousness level

If the patient is not fully conscious shake him gently and/or speak to him loudly but clearly. Record:
- drowsy but able to rouse to normal level
- drowsy but not able to rouse

Glasgow Coma Scale (GCS)

The GCS provides a rapid, widely used assessment of a patient's level of consciousness. It is an indirect measure of consciousness because it measures behaviours that are associated with conscious activity. Patterns of change in these behaviours, when linked with alterations to pupil size, temperature, pulse, respirations and blood pressure, provide an effective guide to the extent of damage within the central nervous system.

Monitor responses to verbal command or, if no response, to painful stimulus, e.g. nailbed pressure (with smooth round object such as a torch), earlobe pressure and trapezoid pinch. Supraorbital pressure (with thumb in supraorbital groove) carries a risk of damaging the eye and should only be used if earlobe pressure or trapezoid pinch do not elicit a response. Sternal rub (with knuckles over sternum) will damage the patient's skin and should only be used *in extremis*.

Table 9.1 Glasgow Coma Score

		Score
A	Eye opening	4 Spontaneous with normal blinking 3 Eyes open to command 2 Eyes open to pain 1 Eyes remain closed
B	Verbal response	5 Normal speech – able to hold a reasonable and relevant conversation 4 Confused speech – language is in a reasonable structure for the conversation but the meaning is inappropriate 3 Inappropriate words – single words spoken (expressing cerebral irritation) but no conversational structure 2 Incomprehensible sounds – moaning sounds only 1 No response
C	Motor response	6 Voluntary – responds normally to commands 5 Localizing – attempts to protect site of pain 4 Flexion response – normal withdrawal of limb to pain

Table 9.1   *(continued)*

	Score
	3 Abnormal flexion – exaggerated withdrawal of limb to pain with shoulder and elbow moving to the midline 2 Extension response to pain – adduction and internal rotation at shoulder, extension at elbows, pronation of forearms 1 No response

Add up total score for the patient's response, which provides the GCS, but when communicating the GCS also provide the breakdown of scores as this ensures greater clarity for other healthcare professionals.

Confusion

If a patient appears confused, move on to assess cognitive state, including disorientation.

Language/speech

Assess from conversation.
- **Is there difficulty in articulation?**
  > If necessary, ask patient to say 'British Constitution', 'West Register Street'.
  - **dysarthria**
    - cerebellar – scanning or staccato
    - lower motor neurone
    - palatal palsy – nasal
    - upper motor neurone – slow, 'spastic', seen in pseudo-bulbar palsy
    - acute alcohol poisoning
- **Is there altered voice tone?**
  - extrapyramidal (monotonous and slow)
  - lower motor neurone (slurred)
  - upper motor neurone (slurred)
  - acute alcohol poisoning (slurred)
  - **dysphonia**
    - cord lesion – hoarse
    - hysterical
- **Is there difficulty in finding the right word?**
  - **dysphasia** or **aphasia** – disorder of use of words as symbols in speech, writing and understanding; nearly always the result of left hemisphere lesion

N.B. The centres for language are in people's dominant hemisphere. In right-handed and 75% of left-handed people, the dominant hemisphere is the left.

- **expressive dysphasia or slight dysphasia** – difficult to detect; look for mispronounced words and circumlocutions in spontaneous speech; test for **nominal aphasia** by asking patient to name objects you point to, e.g. wristwatch, pen, chair, etc.; understanding should be intact

- **receptive dysphasia** – speech fluent but comprehension poor; patient may seem 'confused'; test by asking patient to follow commands – a three-step command is a good screening test (e.g. 'please pick up the glass, but first point to the curtain and then the door'); due to a lesion in Wernicke's area

- **gross dysphasia or missed dysphasia** – most common; usually obvious; the patient's spontaneous speech will be scanty, with small vocabulary, often with the wrong words used; there are also other dysphasias produced by interruption of the connecting pathways between the speech centres

- **aphasia or mutism** – no speech at all, just grunts; this may be due to aphasia, anarthria, psychiatric disease or occasionally diffuse cerebral pathology

Other defects occurring in the absence of motor or sensory dysfunction

- **dyslexia** – inappropriate difficulty with reading; ask the patient to read a few lines from a newspaper (having established that comprehension and expressive speech are intact)
- **dysgraphia** – inappropriate difficulty with writing
- **agraphia** – loss of ability to write
- **acalculia** – loss of ability to do mental and written sums
- **apraxia** – inability to perform a learned purposeful task when there is no paralysis, e.g. opening matchbox, waving goodbye; apraxia for dressing is common in *diffuse brain disease*
- **visual agnosia** – inability to visually recognize familiar objects
- **auditory agnosia** – inability to recognize familiar sounds
- **astereognosis** – tactile agnosia – the inability to recognize common objects, e.g. a key or coin, when placed in the hand
- **parietal lobe lesions** – can cause neglect of the opposite side of the body; there are no perceived sensations and so half of the body is not recognized by the conscious brain; right parietal lobe lesions cause particular problems with spatial awareness: getting lost in familiar places, inability to lay table, to draw or make patterns and neglect of left side of space

Cognitive function

Take account of any evidence you have about the patient's intelligence, education and interests.

'Cognitive' is a term that covers orientation, thought processes and logic (impaired cognitive function is also covered in Chapter 8 and Hodkinson's mental test score is in Appendix 3).

Orientation

In the process of normal conversation, you can check the patient's awareness of time, place and person. The ability to respond and contribute appropriately to a 'normal' conversation with the normal changes of parameters would indicate that understanding (Wernicke's area) and speech (Broca's area) are functioning. Issues of time, place and person provide some details that you may find easier to check but which require less use of the patient's language centres. Questions that require one-word answers should be avoided on the whole.

Disorientation indicates disruption of the pathways between language understanding and expression. *Depressed patients* may be unwilling to reply although they know the answers.

Attention and calculation

- Test the concentration of a patient by asking him to take away 7 from 100, 7 from 93, etc. or by asking him to say the months of the year backwards.

Concentration may be impaired with many cerebral abnormalities, depression and anxiety.

Memory

Immediate recall – digit span

- Ask the patient to repeat a random series of numbers. Speak slowly and start with an easy short sequence and then increase the numbers. Most people manage seven digits forwards, five backwards.

Short-term memory

- **Ask patient to tell you:**
  - what he had for breakfast
  - what he did the night before
  - what he has read in today's paper
    Demented patients will be unable to do this. They may **confabulate** (make up impressive stories) to cover their ignorance.

New memory

- **In the early part of your assessment, ask the patient to remember four or five common objects** such as orange, apple, pen, book and teddy bear; make sure the patient has learnt it. After 10 minutes or so, ask the patient to recall your objects. It is a good idea to note the objects and order.

Longer term memory
- **Ask the patient and if necessary check with relatives, etc.**
  - events before illness, e.g. last year or during last week
  - 'What is your address?'

General knowledge
- **Assess in relation to anticipated performance from history.**
  - What is the name of the Queen/President/Prime Minister?
  - Name six capital cities.
  - What were the dates of a major event relevant to the patient's societal grouping, i.e. to a Western European the Second World War may be appropriate, to a Royalist the death of Princess Diana, etc. Depending upon the questions, an inability to answer may just reflect a lack of interest or an inability to recall.

    In *acute organic states* and *dementia*, new learning, recent memory and reasoning are usually more impaired than remote memory. Vocabulary is usually well preserved in *dementia*. In *depression*, patients may be unwilling to reply, and appear demented.
  - A history from a relative or employer is very important in early dementia.

Reasoning (abstract thought)
- What does this proverb mean: 'Let sleeping dogs lie?'

Skull and spine

- **Inspect and palpate skull** if there is any possibility of a head injury.
- **Check neck stiffness** – meningeal irritation.
- **Inspect spine** – usually when examining back of chest.
- If there is any possibility of pathology, stand patient and check all movements of spine; if there is possible trauma then X-ray first.

Cranial nerves

- **Examine cranial nerves and upper limbs with patient sitting up**, preferably on side of bed or on a chair.

I Olfactory nerve

Not normally tested unless there are other neurological deficits, including papilloedema, undiagnosed headache (especially frontal) or head injury. Ask the patient to close his eyes, then close one nostril by palpation. Then present a smell such as oil of cloves, peppermint, coffee, etc. to the open nostril. Test

each nostril in turn. It is normal not to be able to name all smells, but one smell should be distinguished from another. Pungent or noxious smells such as ammonia should not be used, as they are perceived by the fifth cranial nerve and confuse results. A loss of the sensation of smell indicates possible:
– *base of skull fracture*
– *olfactory groove meningioma* } especially if loss of smell is one-sided
– *rhinitis*
– *smoking* } more likely if loss of smell is bilateral

II Optic nerve

Visual acuity
- **Test each eye separately.**
- Check that the patient can read a language you understand and then ask them to read small text such as newspaper print with each eye separately, with reading glasses if used.
- **If sight poor, test formally:**
  – **near vision** – newsprint or Jaeger type (each eye in turn) (see Appendix 1)
  – **distant vision** – Snellen type (more precise method) (see Appendix 2)
    Stand patient at 6 m from Snellen's card (each eye in turn). Results expressed as a ratio:
    – 6 – distance of person from card
    – x – distance at which patient should be able to read type
    i.e. 6/6 is good vision, 6/60 means the smallest type the patient can read is large enough to be normally read at 60 m.
    If the patient cannot read 6/6, try after correction with glasses or pinhole. Looking through a pinhole in a card obviates refractive errors, analogous to a pinhole camera. If vision remains poor, suspect a neurological or ophthalmic cause.
    A 3 m Snellen chart is shown in Appendix 2.
    A pinhole is not effective for correcting near vision for reading.

Visual fields
- Quick method for **temporal peripheral patient fields** by confrontation of patient and examiner with both eyes open. Always test fields – patients are often unaware of visual loss, the most dramatic of which is Anton's syndrome (blindness with lack of awareness of the blindness).
  – Sit opposite the patient and ask him to look at your nose with both eyes open.
  – Examine each eye in turn. (Do not examine both eyes simultaneously).
  – Bring a waggling finger forwards from behind the patient's ear in upper and lower lateral quadrants and ask when it can be seen (Fig. 9.1).
  – Normal vision is approximately 100° from axis of eye.

Patient

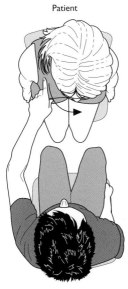

Examiner

Fig. 9.1   Testing temporal peripheral patient fields of vision.

The patient must fully understand the test. The extreme of peripheral vision can be tested with both eyes open, since the nose obstructs vision from the other eye. **If peripheral field seems restricted**, re-test with the other eye covered to ensure each eye is being tested separately.

– A peripheral defect in the visual field of one eye would indicate a nasal defect in the other eye. To test this, the patient covers the eye with the peripheral defect and then the examiner moves the waggling finger from the expected defect towards the area of better vision.

– Normal vision is approximately 50° from each axis of eye.

● **Standard method**

Hold a small red pinhead in the plane midway between the patient and examiner. With the patient's eye and the examiner's opposite eye covered, compare the visual fields of the patient with that of the examiner, with a pin brought in from temporal or nasal fields.

Defects in the central field can be assessed by the standard method with a small red pin held in the plane midway between the patient and examiner:

– **scotoma** – defects in the central field (*retinal or optic nerve lesion*)
– **enlarged blind spot** (*papilloedema*)

Map by moving the pin from inside the scotoma or blind spot outwards until the red pinhead reappears (Fig. 9.2). This is a crude test and small areas of loss

Patient

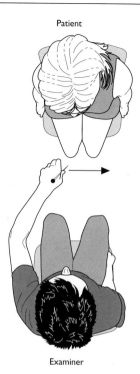

Examiner

Fig. 9.2 Visual field assessment method and testing central field vision.

of vision may need to be formally tested with a **perimetry**. (Note that the examiner must have good peripheral vision in order to perform this test).

- **Test for sensory inattention** when fields are full with both eyes open.
  - Hold your hands between you and the patient, one opposite each ear, and waggle forefingers simultaneously. Ask which moves. With a parietal defect, the patient may not recognize movement on one side, although fields are full to formal testing (Fig. 9.3).

The patterns of visual field deficit will indicate where the lesion is on the optic pathway from the optic disc to the occipital cortex. The changes in the visual field deficit occur because at the optic chiasma, half of the optic nerve crosses over to enable stereoptic vision. All light from the right reaches the left-hand side of both optic discs and then travels to the left occipital cortex (dark) and vice versa. Deficits at the optic chiasma are usually central (bitemporal hemianopia) and caused by an enlarged pituitary (such as pituitary adenoma). Deficits before the optic chiasma cause problems in one eye only, at the optic chiasma the problems are mirrored in both visual fields whereas after the optic chiasma, the deficits affect one side of the visual field in both eyes. Partial

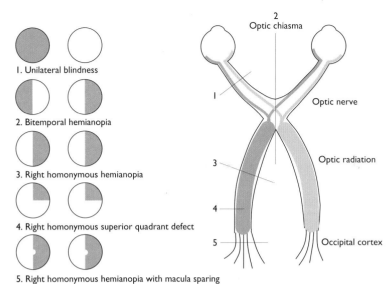

1. Unilateral blindness

2. Bitemporal hemianopia

3. Right homonymous hemianopia

4. Right homonymous superior quadrant defect

5. Right homonymous hemianopia with macula sparing

2
Optic chiasma

Optic nerve

Optic radiation

Occipital cortex

Fig. 9.3   Visual field defects.

damage to the optic radiation will produce a partial deficit (4), with a top-quadrant defect being caused by temporal damage or an occipital lesion and a lower-quadrant defect being caused by parietal damage or an occipital lesion.

Examine the fundi
- Lesions particularly relevant to neurological system:
  - *optic atrophy* – pale disc and demyelination, e.g. *multiple sclerosis: pressure on nerve*
  - *papilloedema* – caused by a raised intracranial pressure (RICP); RICP pushes cerebral tissue through the superior orbital fissure, which squashes the back of the eye; this is more likely with conditions that cause acute changes in intracranial pressure such as *tumours, trauma* and *obstructive hydrocephalus*
- **Nystagmus** – a sensitive test for nystagmus is to ask the patient to cover the other eye during fundoscopy. This removes fixation and can help to elicit nystagmus.

II Optic nerve and III oculomotor nerve

Assessment of the cranial nerves related to the eye and eye function will have a degree of overlap; constriction of a pupil to light involves the optic nerve transmitting the light stimuli and the oculomotor nerve telling the pupils to constrict.

- **Look at pupils**. Are they round and equal? (Normal pupils are between 2 and 6 mm in diameter) (Barkauskas *et al.*, 2002).
  - **Symmetrical small pupils: (<2 mm)**
    - *old age*
    - *opiates*
    - *Argyll Robertson pupils (syphilis)* are small, irregular, eccentric pupils, reacting to convergence but not light
    - pilocarpine eye drops for *narrow-angle glaucoma*
  - **Symmetrical large pupils: (>6 mm)**
    - *youth*
    - *alcohol*
    - *sympathomimetics, anxiety*
    - *atropine-like substances*
  - **Asymmetrical pupils (anisocoria):**
    - *third-nerve palsy* – affected pupil dilated, often with ptosis and diplopia
    - *Horner's syndrome* (sympathetic defect) – affected pupil constricted (miosis – smaller pupil), often with partial ptosis (drooping eyelid), enophthalmos (backward displacement of the eyeball into the orbit) and anhidrosis (abnormal deficiency of sweat)
    - *iris trauma*
    - *drugs* (see above), e.g. tropicamide 1.0% or cyclopentolate 1.0% will be used in the treatment of anterior uveitis
- **Light reflex:** shine bright light from torch into each pupil in turn in a dimly lit room. Do pupils contract equally?
  - *Holmes–Adie pupil*: large, slowly reacting to light
  - *afferent defect, ocular or optic nerve blindness*: neither pupil responds to light in blind eye; both conditions respond to light in normal eye (consensual response in blind eye)
  - *relative afferent defect* – direct response appears normal but when light moves from normal to deficient eye, paradoxical dilation of pupil occurs
  - *efferent defect – third nerve lesion*, pupil does not respond to light in either eye
- **Accommodation reflex (Fig. 9.4):** ask patient to look at distant object, and then at your finger 10–15 cm from his nose – do pupils contract?
  - Response to accommodation but not light:
    - *Argyll Robertson*
    - *Holmes–Adie*
    - *ocular blindness*
    - *midbrain lesion*
    - some recovering *third nerve lesions*

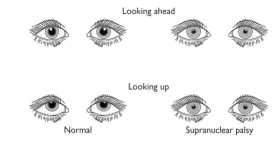

Looking ahead

Looking up

Normal   Supranuclear palsy

Fig. 9.4 Accommodation reflex.

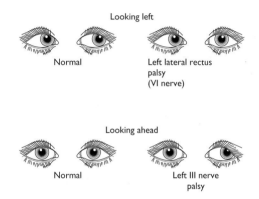

Looking left

Normal   Left lateral rectus
               palsy
               (VI nerve)

Looking ahead

Normal   Left III nerve
               palsy

Fig. 9.5 Testing external ocular movements (EOM).

III Oculomotor nerve, IV trochlear nerve and VI abducens nerve

External ocular movements (Fig. 9.5)

- **Test the eye movements in the four cardinal directions** (left, right, up and down as though you were printing a large H in the air) and convergence using your finger at 1 m distance. Look for abnormal eye movements (Fig. 9.6).

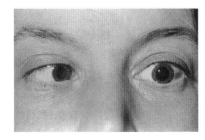

Fig. 9.6 Left sixth nerve lesion – the patient is looking to the left, but there is no lateral movement of the left eye.

● **Ask: 'Tell me if you see double.'** Upward gaze and convergence are often reduced in unco-operative patients.
● To detect minor lesions:
  – **Find direction of gaze with maximum separation of images.**
  – **Cover one eye and ask which image has gone.**
        Peripheral image is seen by the eye that is not moving fully.
        Peripheral image is displaced in the direction of action of the weak muscle, e.g. maximum diplopia on gaze to left. Left eye sees peripheral image, which is displaced laterally. Therefore left lateral rectus is weak.
● **Diplopia** may be due to a single muscle or nerve lesion (N.B. monocular diplopia usually implies ocular pathology):
  – paralytic strabismus (squint)
    – **III palsy:** ptosis, large fixed pupil, eye can be abducted only; eye is often 'down and out'
    – **IV palsy:** diplopia when eye looks down or inwards
    – **VI palsy:** abduction paralysed, diplopia when looking to side of lesion
  – **concomitant non-paralytic strabismus,** e.g. *childhood ocular lesion* – constant angle between eyes. Usually no double vision as one eye ignored (amblyopic) (Fig. 9.7)

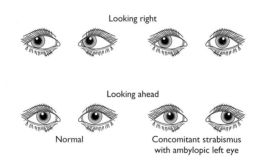

Fig. 9.7   Concomitant non-paralytic strabismus.

  – **conjugate ocular palsy**
    – *supranuclear palsies* affecting co-ordination rather than muscle weakness; inability to look in a particular direction, usually upwards
    – *intranuclear lesion*: convergence normal but cannot adduct eyes on lateral gaze (Fig. 9.8)
  – if patient sees double in all directions
    – may be *third nerve palsy*
    – *thyroid muscle disease* – worse in morning

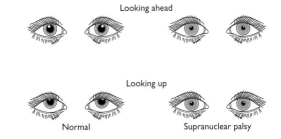

Fig. 9.8   Supranuclear palsies.

- *myasthenia gravis* – worse in evening
- manifest strabismus

Ptosis
Drooping of upper eyelid can be:
- complete – *third nerve palsy*
- incomplete
- *partial third nerve palsy*
- muscular weakness, e.g. *myasthenia gravis* (from anti-acetylcholine receptor antibodies)
- sympathetic tone decreased – *Horner's syndrome* (also small pupils – miosis and enophthalmos and decreased sweating on face)
- partial Horner's syndrome (small irregular pupils with ptosis) in *autonomic neuropathy* of *diabetes* and *syphilis*
- lid swelling
- *levator dysinsertion syndrome* (from chronic contact lens use)

Nystagmus
This is an involuntary oscillating movement of the eye in a horizontal or vertical direction or a combination of directions. The oscillating movement is labelled by the direction of fast movement. A small amount of end-position (at the extremes of gaze) lateral nystagmus is normal. However, in any other position (e.g. when present at 30° from the midline) it is abnormal (Barkauskas *et al.*, 2002).
- **Test first in the neutral position and then with the eyes deviated to right, left and upwards.** Keep object within binocular field as nystagmus is often normal in extremes of gaze. Keep your movements smooth.
  - **cerebellar nystagmus (Fig. 9.9)**
    - fast movement to side of gaze (on both sides)
    - increased when looking to lesion
    - *cerebellar* or *brainstem lesion* or *drugs* (*ethanol*, *phenytoin*)

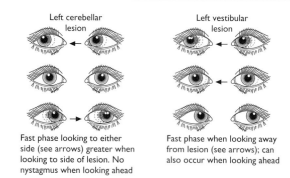

Fig. 9.9   Cerebellar nystagmus.

- **vestibular nystagmus**
  - fast movement only in one direction – away from lesion
  - reduced by fixation if peripheral in origin
  - more marked when looking away from lesion
  - *inner ear, vestibular disease* or *brainstem lesion*
    Labyrinthine nystagmus may be positional, particularly in benign positional vertigo, and can be induced by hyperextension and rotation of the neck (Hallpike manoeuvre) which after a latency of a few seconds will produce a vertical/torsional type of nystagmus for about 10–15 seconds, along with symptoms of vertigo.
- **congenital nystagmus** – constant horizontal wobbling
  - downbeat nystagmus – foramen magnum lesion or Wernicke's disease
  - retraction nystagmus – midbrain lesion
  - complex nystagmus – brainstem disease, usually multiple sclerosis

Saccades

This is the rapid eye movement used to change eye position. It is tested in the horizontal and vertical planes by asking the patient to switch fixation between two targets (e.g. the examiner's fingers). Slow saccades may be seen in a variety of disorders including degenerative disorders such as progressive supranuclear palsy.

V Trigeminal nerve

Sensory V

- Test light touch in all three divisions with cotton wool (Fig. 9.10). Ask the patient to close his eyes and to tell you when and where he is being touched. Pinprick is usually used only if needed to delineate anaesthetic area.

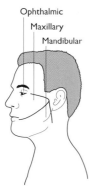

Ophthalmic
Maxillary
Mandibular

Fig. 9.10 Assessment areas for trigeminal nerve sensation.

Corneal reflex–sensory V (trigeminal) and motor VII (facial)
- **Ask the patient to look up and away from you and then touch the cornea** from the opposite side to the gaze, with a wisp of cotton wool. Both eyes should blink. The corneal reflex (Fig. 9.11) is easily prompted incorrectly by eliciting the 'eyelash' or 'menace' reflex.

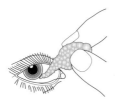

Fig. 9.11 The corneal reflex.

Motor V – muscles of jaw
- **Ask the patient to open his mouth against resistance**, and look to see if his jaw descends in the midline. Palsy of the nerve causes deviation of the jaw to the side of the lesion. Fifth nerve palsies are very rare in isolation (Fig. 9.12).

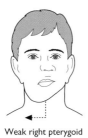

Weak right pterygoid

Fig. 9.12 Fifth nerve palsy.

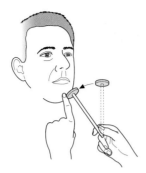

Fig. 9.13   Jaw jerk test.

- **Jaw jerk (Fig. 9.13)** – only if other neurological findings, e.g. upper motor neurone lesion. Increased jaw jerk is only present if there is a bilateral upper motor neurone fifth nerve lesion, e.g. *bilateral strokes* or *pseudo-bulbar palsy*.
  - Put your forefinger gently on the patient's loosely opened jaw. Tap your finger gently with a tendon hammer. Explain the test to the patient or relaxation of his jaw will be impossible. A brisk jerk is a positive finding.

VII Facial nerve

- **Ask the patient to:**
  - raise his eyebrows
  - close his eyes tightly
  - smile
  - frown
  - show you his teeth
  - puff out his cheeks
    Demonstrate these to the patient yourself if necessary.
    Lower motor neurone lesion: all muscles on the side of the lesion are affected, e.g. *Bell's palsy*: widened palpebral fissure, weak blink, drooped mouth.
    Upper motor neurone lesion: only the lower muscles are affected, i.e. mouth drops to one side but eyebrows raise normally. This is because the upper half of the face is bilaterally innervated. This abnormality is very common in a hemiparesis (Fig. 9.14).
- **Taste** – can only be tested easily on anterior two-thirds of tongue.
  Ask patient to close his eyes and stick his tongue out; small amounts of sugar, tartaric acid or salt can be placed on the appropriate part of the tongue.

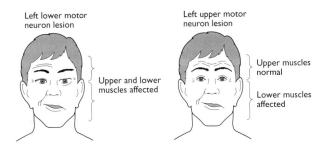

Left lower motor
neuron lesion

Upper and lower
muscles affected

Left upper motor
neuron lesion

Upper muscles
normal

Lower muscles
affected

Fig. 9.14 Upper and lower motor neurone lesions.

VIII Vestibulo-auditory nerve

Vestibular

There is no easy bedside test for this nerve except looking for nystagmus.

Acoustic

- **Block one ear by pressing the tragus. Whisper numbers increasingly loudly until the patient can repeat them. A ticking watch may be more useful.**

More accurate tests are as follows:

Rinne's test. Place a high-pitched vibrating tuning fork on the mastoid (1 in figure). When the patient says the sound stops, hold the fork at the meatus (2 in figure).

- If still heard: air conduction > bone conduction (normal or nerve deafness).
- If not heard: air conduction < bone conduction (middle ear conduction defect).

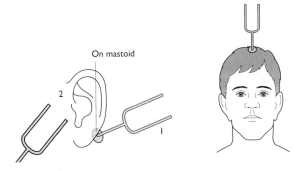

On mastoid

2

1

Fig. 9.15 Rinne's and Weber's tests.

Weber's test. Hold a lightly vibrating tuning fork firmly on the top of the patient's head or on the forehead. If the sound is heard to one side, middle ear deafness exists on that side or the opposing ear has nerve deafness.

IX Glossopharyngeal

- **Ask patient to say 'Ahh'** and watch for symmetrical upwards movement of uvula – pulled away from weak side.
- **Touch the back of the pharynx with an orange-stick or spatula gently.** If the patient gags the nerve is intact (Fig. 9.16).

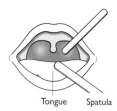

Tongue   Spatula

Fig. 9.16   Stimulating the gag reflex.

This gag reflex depends on the IX and X nerves, the former being the sensory side and the latter the motor aspect. It is frequently absent with ageing and abuse of tobacco.

X Vagus nerve

- **Ask if the patient can swallow normally.**
  There are so many branches of the vagus nerve that it is impossible to be sure it is all functioning normally. If the vagus nerve is seriously damaged, swallowing is a problem; spillage into the lungs may occur. Swallowing can be assessed by initially ensuring that cranial nerves V, VII, IX and XII are working correctly (oral stage) and then asking the patient to swallow (without food or fluid). The pharyngeal stage lasts one second. Observe that the throat muscles (pharyngeal constrictor muscles) move evenly and effectively. If the dry swallow is effective then ask the patient to take a small drink of water. Coughing on attempted swallow indicates a high risk of aspiration. Check speech afterwards. A change of voice quality ('wet' speech) indicates pooling of fluids on the vocal cords, and indicates a high risk of aspiration. Check for a voluntary cough as this can become quiet and ineffective. Check speech for dysarthria. Whenever patients have been intubated and had an endotracheal tube *in situ*, a swallowing assessment should be undertaken before fluids or food are given by mouth to ensure aspiration is prevented.

XI Spinal accessory nerve

- **Ask the patient to flex his neck**, pressing his chin against your resisting hand. Check that both sternomastoids contract normally.
- **Ask the patient to raise both shoulders.** If he cannot, the trapezius muscle is not functioning.

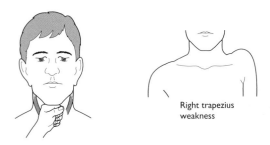

Right trapezius weakness

Fig. 9.17   Flexing the neck and raising both shoulders.

Failure of the trapezius muscle on one side is often associated with a *hemiplegia* (particularly anterior cerebral artery infarctions).

- **Ask the patient to turn his head against your resisting hand.** This tests the contralateral sternomastoid, and can help to demonstrate normal motor functioning in a *hysterical hemiplegia*.

XII Hypoglossal nerve

- **Ask the patient to put out his tongue.** If it protrudes to one side, this is the side of the weakness, e.g. deviating to left on protrusion from left hypoglossal lesion (Fig. 9.18).
- **Look for fasciculation or wasting** with mouth open.

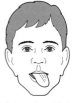

Left hypoglossal lesion

Fig. 9.18   Left hypoglossal lesion.

Limbs and trunk

General inspection

- **Look at the patient's resting and standing posture:**
  - flexed upper limb, extended lower limb – *hemiplegia*
  - wrist drop – *radial nerve palsy*
- **Look for abnormal movements:**
  - tremor
  - *Parkinson's* – coarse rhythmical tremor at rest, lessens on movement
  - *essential tremor (thyrotoxicosis)* – tremor present on action; look at outstretched hands
  - *chorea* – abrupt, involuntary repetitive semi-purposeful movement
  - *athetosis* – slow, continuous writhing movement of limb
  - *spasm* – exaggerated, involuntary muscular contraction
- **Look for muscle wasting.** Check distribution:
  - symmetrical, e.g. *Duchenne muscular dystrophy*
  - asymmetrical, e.g. *poliomyelitis*
  - proximal, e.g. *limb girdle muscular dystrophy*
  - distal, e.g. *peripheral neuropathy*
  - generalized, e.g. *motor neurone disease*
  - localized, e.g. with *joint disease*
- **Look for fasciculation.** This is irregular involuntary contractions of small bundles of muscle fibres, not perceived by the patient.

  > This is typical of denervation, e.g. *motor neurone disease*, when it is widespread. It is caused by the death of anterior horn cells.

Arms

Inspection

In addition to the general inspection it is important to make an initial assessment.

- **Ask the patient to hold both his arms straight out in front him with his palms up and eyes shut.** Observe gross weakness, posture and whether the arms remain stationary:
  - hypotonic posture – wrist flexed and fingers extended
  - drift
    - gradually upwards with sensory loss, may be *cerebellar damage*
    - gradually downwards, may be *pyramidal weakness*
    - downward without pronation can be seen in *hysteria* or in profound *proximal muscle weakness*
  - athetoid tremors – *sensory loss* (peripheral nerve) or *cerebellar disease*
- **Tap both arms downwards.** They should by reflex return to their former position.

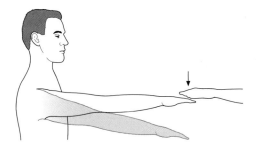

Fig. 9.19 Tapping both arms downwards.

If the arm overswings in its return to its position, weakness or *cerebellar dys-function* may be present (Fig. 9.19).

● **Ask the patient to do fast finger movements.** Quickly touch each finger tip on one hand to the thumb and repeat several times, or ask them to pretend they are playing a fast tune on the piano. You may have to demonstrate this yourself. Clumsy movements can be a sensitive index of a slight *pyramidal lesion*. The dominant side should always be quicker than the non-dominant side.

Co-ordination
● **Ask the patient to touch his nose with his index finger (Fig. 9.20).**

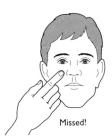

Missed!

Fig. 9.20 Testing co-ordination – index finger to nose.

● **With the patient's eyes open, ask him to touch his nose, then your finger, which is held up in front of him.** This can be repeated rapidly with your finger moving from place to place in front of him, but your finger must be in position before the patient's finger leaves his nose (Fig. 9.21). Past pointing and marked intention tremor in the absence of muscular weakness suggest *cerebellar dysfunction*. If you suspect a cerebellar abnormality, check rapid alternating movements (*dysdiadochokinesia*):

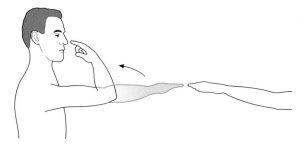

Fig. 9.21 Cerebellar function – index finger to nose to examiner's moving finger.

- **fast rotation of the hands on the patient's lap** (supination and pronation)
- **tapping back of other hand as quickly as possible**
  Damage to the cerebellum results in a loss of proprioception, the brain's unconsciousness awareness of the position of the joints, muscles and limbs. Proprioception enables normal movement to be a smoothly co-ordinated process. Any disruption creates clumsiness, especially at night when vision is less able to compensate (Barkauskas *et al.*, 2002; Epstein *et al.*, 2008; Swartz, 2006).

Tone

Always check tone before you assess strength. This is a difficult test to perform as patients often do not relax. Try to distract the patient with conversation.

- **Ask the patient to relax his arm and then you flex and extend his wrist or elbow.** Move through a wide arc moderately slowly, at irregular intervals to prevent patient co-operation.
- **Ask the patient to let his leg go loose, lift it up and move at the knee joint** (hip and ankle if required). It can be difficult to assess this in the legs because patients often cannot relax. Ankle clonus can be assessed at the same time (refer to examination technique below).

Hypertonia (increased tone):
- pyramidal: more obvious in flexion of upper limbs and extension of lower limbs, Occasionally 'clasp knife', i.e. diminution of tone during movement
- extrapyramidal: uniform, 'lead pipe' rigidity. If associated with tremor, the movement feels like a 'cog wheel'
- hysterical: increases with increased movement

Hypotonia (decreased tone):
  lower motor neurone lesion
  recent upper motor neurone lesion
  cerebellar lesion
  unconsciousness

Muscle power

For screening purposes, examine two distal muscles, one flexor and one extensor (e.g. finger flexion and extension), and two proximal muscles in each limb. Compare each side. Confirm the weakness suspected by palpation of the muscle.

Strength/power is usually graded:

0 No active contraction
1 Visible as palpable contraction with *no* active movement
2 Movement with gravity eliminated, i.e. in horizontal direction
3 Movement against gravity
4 Movement against gravity plus resistance
5 Normal power.

- **Look for patterns of weakness:**
  - *hemiplegia* – muscles weak all down one side
  - *monoplegia* – weakness of one limb
  - *paraplegia* – weakness of both lower limbs
  - *tetraplegia* – weakness of all four limbs
  - *myasthenia* – weakness developing after repeated contractions – most obvious in smaller muscles, e.g. repeated blinking
  - proximal muscles, e.g. *myopathy*
  - nerve root distribution, e.g. *disc prolapse*
  - nerve distribution, e.g. wrist drop from *radial nerve palsy*

Upper limbs

- As indicated previously, compare each side and confirm the weakness suspected by palpation of the muscle. For example:

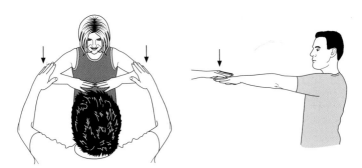

Fig. 9.22   Testing muscle power.

- 'Squeeze my fingers'. Present the two forefingers of each hand. The patient may hurt you if he squeezes your whole hand.
- Ask the patient to extend his arms (show him) and then say, 'Stop me pressing them down'.

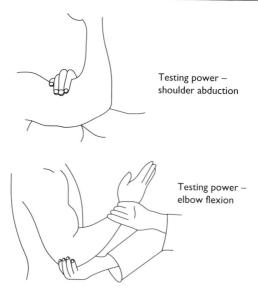

Testing power –
shoulder abduction

Testing power –
elbow flexion

Fig. 9.23 Testing power: shoulder abduction and elbow flexion.

- Ask the patient to bend his arm and as you hold his wrist, ask him to force his arm down against resistance to check extension (Fig. 9.23).
- Resistance to extension:
  - Ask patient to bend his arm and as you hold his wrist, ask him to pull his arm up against resistance to check flexion.
    Gross power loss will have been noted on inspection of extended arm position or on walking.
- If the patient is in bed, start the examination by asking him to:
  - raise both arms
  - raise one leg off the bed
- Test power at joints against your own strength – shoulder, elbow, wrist.
  - power at main joints cannot normally be overcome by permissible force.
- **If there is weakness or other neurological signs in a limb, test the individual muscle groups:**
  - shoulder – abduction, extension, flexion
  - elbow – flexion, extension
  - wrist – flexion, extension: 'Hold wrists up, don't let me push them down'
  - finger – flexion, grasp, extension, adduction (put a piece of paper between straight fingers held in extension and ask the patient to hold it, as you remove it), abduction (with fingers in extension, ask patient to spread them apart against your force)

Tendon reflexes

Arms

● Place arms comfortably by side with elbows flexed and hands on upper abdomen. Tell the patient to relax because reflexes are easier to see; continuing to talk with the patient during this part of the examination may provide distraction and help accuracy. Compare sides.

– **supinator reflex:** tap the distal end of the radius with a tendon hammer
– **biceps reflex:** tap your forefinger or thumb over the biceps tendon
– **triceps reflex:** hold arm across chest to tap your thumb over the triceps tendon (Fig. 9.24)

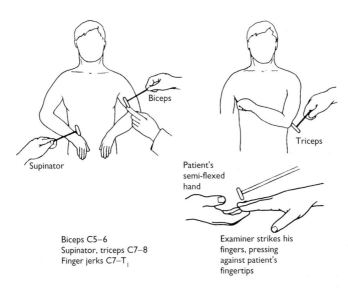

Biceps

Triceps

Supinator

Patient's semi-flexed hand

Biceps C5–6
Supinator, triceps C7–8
Finger jerks C7–T₁

Examiner strikes his fingers, pressing against patient's fingertips

Fig. 9.24 Tendon reflexes.

Increased jerks – *upper motor neurone lesion* (e.g. hemiparesis).
Decreased jerks – *lower motor neurone lesion* or acute *upper motor neurone lesion.*
Clonus – pressure stretching a muscle group causes rhythmical involuntary contraction. If a brisk reflex is obtained, test for clonus. Found in *marked hypertonia* from stretching tendon. No need to strike tendon with tendon hammer. Clonus confirms an increased tendon jerk and suggests an upper motor neurone lesion. A few symmetrical beats may be normal.

Trunk
- **The superficial abdominal reflexes rarely need to be tested.**
  - Lightly stroke each quadrant with an orange-stick or the back of your fingernail. Note the contractions of the muscles and movement of the umbilicus towards the stimulus. These reflexes are absent or decreased in an upper or lower motor neurone lesion (Fig. 9.25).

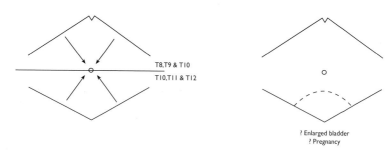

Fig. 9.25   Trunk reflexes.

- **Cremasteric reflex T12–L1**
  - Stroke inside of leg – induces testis to rise from cremaster muscle contraction.
- Palpate the bladder.

  The patient with a distended bladder will feel very uncomfortable as you palpate it.

  Many neurological lesions, sensory or motor, will lead to a distended bladder, giving the patient *retention with overflow incontinence.*
- Examine the strength of the abdominal muscles by asking the patient to attempt to sit up without using his hands.

Lower limbs

Inspection
As for arms.

Co-ordination
- Ask the patient to run the heel of one leg up and down the shin of the other leg. Lack of coordination will be apparent (Fig. 9.26).

  Gait may become broad based, and the patient may be unable to perform a tandem gait (heel–toe walking).

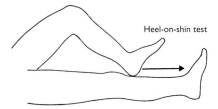

Heel-on-shin test

Fig. 9.26   Lower limb co-ordination.

Tone
- Ask the patient to let the limb go loose, lift it up and move at the knee joint (hip and ankle if required).

  Tone may be difficult to assess in the legs because patients may have difficulty relaxing. Ankle clonus can be assessed at the same time (see below).

Muscle power
Bending and straightening the knee as well as dorsiflexion and plantarflexion of the ankle against resistance will demonstrate the muscle power in the legs. Lifting the straight leg off the bed against resistance will demonstrate hip flexion (Fig. 9.27).

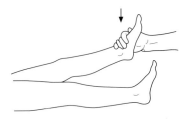

Fig. 9.27   Muscle power in the legs. Hip flexion.

- Hip flexion: ask the patient to lift the leg, and say, 'Don't let me push it down'.
- Hip extension: ask the patient to keep the leg straight on the couch or bed surface, and try to lift at the ankle; you can test for abduction and adduction against resistance as well; refer to Chapter 11 for further information on performing these tests (Fig. 9.28)
- Knee – flexion and extension
- Ankle – plantarflexion, dorsiflexion, eversion and inversion

  Only severe weakness will be detected because the legs are stronger than the arms. If no weakness is detected and the patient is complaining of weakness, then more sensitive tests can

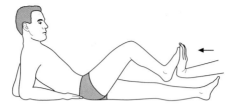

Fig. 9.28   Knee flexion.

be helpful, e.g. walking on tiptoes, heels, arising from a squat position, hopping on either leg.

Hip weakness is easily overlooked. If a weakness is suspected, test the patient's ability to lift his own weight, i.e. rising from a chair or climbing stairs.

Occasionally patients will have hysterical weakness. A useful test is Hoover's sign. This is tested by placing your hand under the ankle of the patient's paralysed leg. The patient is first asked to extend the paralysed leg (which should produce no effort), and then by asking for hip flexion of the non–paralysed leg, resulting in contraction of the 'paralysed' hip extensor (a reflex fixation that we all do). Unlike other tests for non-organic illness, this test demonstrates normalcy in the paralysed limb (Hatton & Blackwood, 2003).

Tendon reflexes

- **Test knee reflexes** by passing left forearm behind both knees, supporting them partly flexed. Ask the patient to let the leg go loose and tap the tendons below patella (Fig. 9.29). Compare both sides. Reflexes can be normal, brisk (can occur in normal subjects or *upper motor* neurone lesion), decreased or absent (always abnormal).

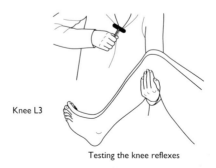

Knee L3

Testing the knee reflexes

Fig. 9.29   Testing knee reflexes.

- **Test ankle reflex** by flexing the knee and abducting the leg. Apply gentle pressure to the ball of the foot, with it at a right angle, and tap the tendon. Ankle jerks are often absent in the elderly.
- **Compare sides** – right versus left and arms versus legs. It is essential that the patient is relaxed when reflexes are tested. This is not always easy for the patient, particularly the elderly. You can elicit **reinforcement** (an apparently absent reflex may become present) by asking the patient to clasp his hands together and pull one hand against the other just as you strike with the hammer (Fig. 9.30).

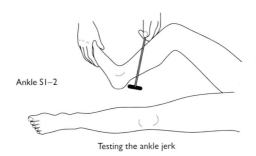

Ankle S1–2

Testing the ankle jerk

Fig. 9.30 Testing the ankle jerk.

Increased jerks – *upper motor neurone lesion* (e.g. hemiparesis).
Decreased jerks – *lower motor neurone lesion* or *acute upper motor neurone lesion.*
Clonus – if a brisk reflex is obtained, test for clonus. A sharp, then sustained dorsiflexion of the foot, by pressure on ball of the foot, may result in the foot 'beating' for many seconds. Clonus confirms an increased tendon jerk and suggests an *upper motor neurone lesion.* A few symmetrical beats may be normal.

Plantar reflexes

- Tell patient what you are doing, and scratch the side of the sole with a firm but not painful implement (orange-stick or rounded spike on tendon hammer). Watch for flexion or extension of the toes (Fig. 9.31).

  Normal plantar responses = flexion of all toes.

  Extensor (Babinski) response = slow extension of the big toe with spreading of the other toes. Withdrawal from pain or tickle is rapid and not abnormal. In individuals with sensitive feet, the reflex can be elicited by noxious stimuli elsewhere in the leg; stroking the lateral aspect of the foot can be very useful or testing for sharp sensation on the dorsum of the great toe. (Do not use needles or pins to test for 'pinprick' sensation. Use a disposable

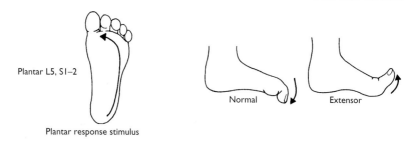

Plantar L5, S1–2

Plantar response stimulus

Fig. 9.31 Plantar response stimulus.

'neurostick', 'neuropin' or paper clip and ask the patient to tell you whether the sensation is sharp or dull.)

An extensor reflex is normal up to 6 months of age.

Sensation

If there are no grounds to expect sensory loss, sensation can rapidly examined.

Briefly examine each extremity. Success depends on making the patient understand what you are doing and co-operating effectively with you. This examination is very subjective. As in the motor examination, you are looking for patterns of loss, e.g. nerve root (dermatome), nerve, sensory level (spinal cord), glove/stocking (peripheral neuropathy), dissociation (i.e. pain and temperature versus vibration and proprioception, e.g. syringomyelia).

Vibration sense

- **Test vibration sense using a 128 Hz tuning fork**. Place the fork on the sternum first, so that the patient appreciates what vibration is. Ask the patient to close his eyes, then place the vibrating fork on the lateral malleoli and wrists. Ask the patient to tell you when it stops vibrating. You stop the vibrating fork and if vibration sense is normal, the patient will tell you the vibration has stopped. If the periphery is normal, proximal sensation need not be examined. Occasionally a patient will claim to feel vibration when it is absent. If this is suspected, try a non-vibrating fork or surreptitiously stop the fork vibrating and see if the patient notices. If the patient says he can feel it vibrate, testing is not valid. Vibration sense often diminishes with age and may be absent in the legs of the elderly patient.

Position sense – proprioception

- Show the patient what you are doing. 'I am going to move your finger/toe up or down' (doing so). 'I want you to tell me up or down each time I move it. Now close your eyes.'

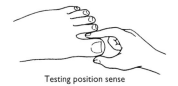

Testing position sense

Fig. 9.32 Testing position sense.

- Hold distal to the joint and either side with your forefinger and thumb so that pressure does not also indicate the direction of movement. Make small movements in an irregular, not alternate, sequence. e.g. up, up, down, up, down, down, down (Fig. 9.32).

  Normal threshold is very low – the smallest, slowest passive movement you can produce in the terminal phalanges should always be correctly detected.

Pain, touch and temperature
Pain and touch

- Take a new clean neurostick/neuropin (do not reuse the same neurostick/neuropin on another patient). Also take a tongue depressor.
- With the patient's eyes open, touch the sharp end of the neurostick/neuropin on the skin. Do not draw blood. Ask, 'Does this feel sharp?'.
- Also touch the skin with the tongue depressor. 'Does this feel blunt?'

    Ask the patient to close his eyes and to tell you where you touch his skin and whether it is sharp or blunt. Then randomly assess the patient's sensory function. If you find sensory loss, map out that area by proceeding from the abnormal to normal area of skin.

Temperature

- This process can be repeated with test tubes of hot (but not burning) and cold water to test perception of temperature. Ask the patient to close his eyes and then tell you if he feels 'hot' or 'cold' as you touch his skin with the test tubes.

Light touch

- Ask the patient to close his eyes.
- Ask him to tell you when and where you touch him with a wisp of cotton wool. Touch at irregular intervals.
- Compare both sides of body.

    Two-point discrimination. Normal threshold on fingertip is 2 mm. If sensory impairment is peripheral or in cord, a raised threshold is found, e.g. 5 mm. If cortical, no threshold is found.

    Stereognosis is tested by placing coins, keys, pen top, etc. in the patient's hand and, with eyes closed, the patient attempts to identify by feeling.

Sensory exclusion is assessed by bilateral simultaneous, e.g. touch; sensations are felt only on the normal side, while each is felt if applied separately. Indicates a parietal lobe lesion as brain is unable to process all stimuli.

Dermatomes

Most are easily detected with a neurostick/neuropin. Map out from area of impaired sensation.

Note in arms: **middle finger – C7** and dermatomes either side symmetrical up to mid upper arm.

Note in legs: **lateral border of foot and heel (S1)**, back of legs and anal region have sacral supply.

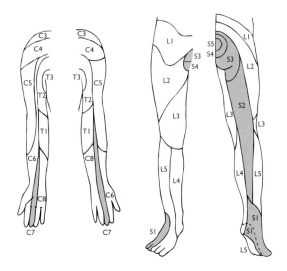

Fig. 9.33 Dermatomes.

Gait

● Observe the patient as he walks in. If ataxia is suspected but not seen on ordinary walking, ask the patient to do heel-to-toe walking. (Demonstrate it yourself.)

There are many examples of abnormal gait.

– **Parkinson's disease**. Patient has stooped posture with most joints flexed and walks with small shuffling steps without swinging arms; tremor of hands (Fig. 9.34).

– **Spastic gait**. Patient scrapes his toe on one or both sides as he walks; to prevent this, he moves his foot in a lateral arc (Fig. 9.35).

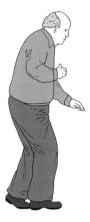

Fig. 9.34 Parkinson's disease gait.

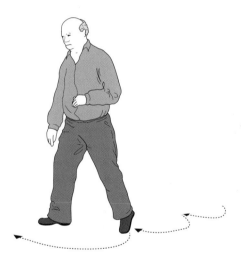

Fig. 9.35 Spastic gait.

- **Sensory ataxia**. Patient has a high stepping gait, with a slapping down of his feet. Seen with peripheral neuropathy (Fig. 9.36).
- **Cerebellar gait**. Patient has his feet wide apart as he walks (Fig. 9.37).
- **Foot drop**. Patient's toe scrapes on the ground in spite of excessive lifting up of leg on affected side.
- **Shuffling gait**. Patient takes multiple little steps – typical of diffuse cerebrovascular disease.
- **Hysterical gait**. Patient usually lurches wildly but without falling over, with the pattern marked by inconsistency.

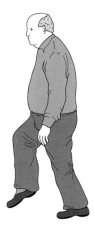

Fig. 9.36   Sensory ataxia gait.

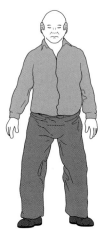

Fig. 9.37   Cerebellar gait.

Romberg's test is often performed at this time but is mainly a test of position sense. Ask the patient to stand upright with his feet together and close his eyes. If there is any falling noted, the test is positive. Be sure you stand to the side of the patient with one arm held out in front and one arm held out to the patient's back in case the patient begins to fall so that you can steady him (Fig. 9.38).

Elderly patients may fail this test and may begin to fall sideways but stop just before they topple over due to reduced proprioceptive awareness. Test positive with posterior column loss of tabes dorsalis of syphilis. Anxious patients may sway excessively; try distracting them by testing stereognosis at the same time – the excess swaying may disappear (Hatton & Blackwood, 2003).

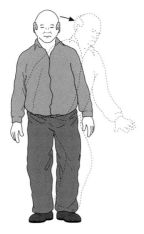

Fig. 9.38 Romberg's test.

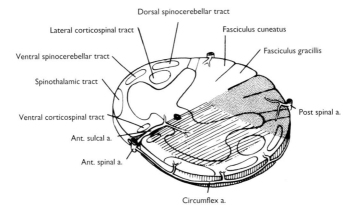

Fig. 9.39 Anatomy and vascular supply of the spinal cord. Note: Anterior spinal artery occlusion spares posterior column function. Reproduced from Talley & O'Connor (2006).

Dorsal column loss of sensation
– decreased position, vibration and deep pain sensation (squeeze Achilles tendon)
– touch often not lost, as half carried in anterior column

Cortical loss of sensation
Defect shown by deficient function:
– position sense
– tactile discrimination
– sensory inattention

Signs of meningeal irritation
  - neck rigidity – try to flex neck, is there resistance or pain?
  - Kernig's sign – not as sensitive as neck rigidity (Fig. 9.40)

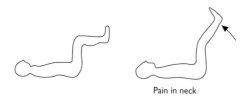

Pain in neck

Fig. 9.40   Signs of meningeal irritation.

Straight-leg-raising for sciatica
  - Lift straight leg until there is pain in back. Then slightly lower leg until there is no pain and then dorsiflex the foot to 'stretch' the sciatic nerve until the patient says there is pain present down the back of the leg (Fig. 9.41).

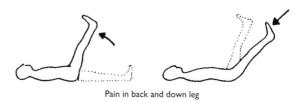

Pain in back and down leg

Fig. 9.41   Straight-leg raising for sciatica.

Summary of common illnesses
Lower motor neurone lesion

  - wasting
  - fasciculation
  - hypotonia
  - power diminished
  - absent reflexes
  - + or – sensory loss
  - **T1 palsy**
    - weakness of the intrinsic muscles of the hand: finger adduction and abduction, thumb abduction (cf. median nerve palsy and ulnar nerve palsy)
    - sensory loss: medial forearm

- **median nerve palsy**
  - abductor pollicis brevis weakness (other thenar muscles may be weak), wrist drop
  - sensory loss: thumb, first two fingers and palmar surface
- **ulnar nerve palsy**
  - interversion, hypothenar muscles wasted (Fig. 9.42), weakness of finger abduction and adduction; clawhand, cannot extend fingers
  - sensory loss: half fourth, all fifth fingers, palmar surface

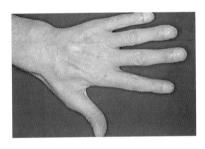

Fig. 9.42 Wasted interossei and hypothenar eminence from an ulnar nerve or T$_1$ lesion.

- **radial nerve palsy**
  - wrist drop
  - sensory loss: small area/dorsal web of thumb (Fig. 9.43)

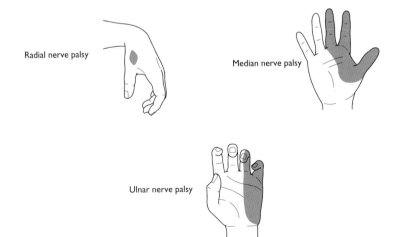

Radial nerve palsy

Median nerve palsy

Ulnar nerve palsy

Fig. 9.43 Radial, median and ulnar nerve palsies.

- **L5 palsy** – foot drop and weak inversion; sensory loss on medial aspect of foot
- **peroneal nerve palsy** – foot drop and weak eversion; minor sensory loss of dorsum of foot
- **S1 palsy** – cannot stand on toes, sensory loss of lateral aspect of foot, absent ankle reflex

Upper motor neurone lesion

- no wasting
- extended arms – hand drifts down
- overswing when hands are tapped
- hypertonia
  - spastic flexion of upper limbs, extension of lower limbs
  - clasp knife
- power diminished
- increased tendon reflexes (+ or – clonus)
- extensor plantar response
- + or – sphincter disturbance
- spastic gait
- extended stiff leg with foot drop
- arm does not swing, held flexed

N.B. Check 'level' first, then pathology.

Cerebellar dysfunction

- no wasting
- hypotonia with overswing; irregularity of movements
- intention tremor
- inability to execute rapid alternating movement smoothly (dysdiado-chokinesia)
- ataxic gait
- nystagmus
- scanning or staccato speech
- inco-ordination not improved by sight (whereas it is with a defect of proprioception)

Extrapyramidal dysfunction – Parkinson's disease

- flexed posture of body, neck, arms and legs
- expressionless, impassive face, staring eyes
- 'pill-rolling' tremor of hands at rest
- delay in initiating movements

- tone – 'lead pipe' rigidity, possibly with 'cog-wheeling'
- normal power and sensation
- speech quiet and monotonal
- gait – shuffling small steps, possibly with difficulty starting or stopping
- postural instability: test by having the patient standing comfortably; stand behind the patient and give a sharp tug backwards; normal patients should show a slight sway; taking steps backwards, particularly multiple steps, is abnormal

Muitiple sclerosis

- **evidence of 'different lesions in space and time' from history and examination; usually affects cerebral white matter;** common sites:
  - optic atrophy – optic neuritis
  - nystagmus – vestibular or cerebellar tracts
  - brisk jaw jerk – pyramidal lesion above fifth nerve
- cerebellar signs in arms or gait – cerebellar tracts
- upper motor neurone signs in arms or legs – pyramidal, right or left (absent superficial abdominal reflexes)
- transverse myelitis with sensory level – indicates level of lesion
- urine retention – usually sensory tract
- sensory perception loss – sensory tract

System-oriented examination
Examine the higher cerebral functions

- general appearance
- consciousness level
- mood
- speech
- cognitive
- confusion
- orientation
- attention/calculation
- memory – short-term, long-term
- reasoning – understanding of proverb

Examine the cranial nerves

Table 9.2   Cranial nerves

Number	Name	Function
I	Olfactory	Smell
II	Optic	Visual acuity Visual field Fundi
III, IV and VI	Oculomotor, trochlear and abducens	Ptosis Nystagmus Eye movements Pupils
V	Trigeminal	Facial sensation Corneal reflex Jaw muscles/jerk Tongue taste
VII	Facial	Face muscles
VIII	Vestibulo-auditory	Hearing Rinne's/Weber's tests Nystagmus/gait
IX, X	Glossopharyngeal, vagus	Palate Swallowing Taste – posterior third of tongue
XI	Spinal accessory	Trapezius
XII	Hypoglossal	Tongue wasting

Examine the arms neurologically

- **Inspect:**
  - abnormal position
  - wasting
  - fasciculation
  - tremor/athetosis
- Ask patient to extend arms in front, keep them there with eyes closed, then check:
  - posture/drift
  - tap back of wrists to assess whether position is stable
  - fast finger movements (pyramidal)
  - touch nose (co-ordination) – finger-to-nose test
  - 'Hold my fingers'; push and pull against resistance

- Tone
- Muscle power – each group if indicated
- Reflexes
- Sensation:
  - light touch
  - pinprick
  - vibration
  - proprioception

Examine the legs neurologically

- **Inspect**:
  - abnormal positions
  - wasting
  - fasciculation
- 'Lift one leg off the bed'
- 'Lift other leg off the bed'
- Co-ordination – heel–toe
- Tone
- Power – 'Pull up toes. Push down toes' against resistance
- Reflexes
- Plantar reflexes
- Sensation (as hands)
- Romberg's test
- Gait and tandem gait

Examine the arms or legs

- **Inspect:**
  - colour
  - skin/nail changes
  - ulcers
  - wasting (are both arms and legs involved?)
  - joints
- **Palpate:**
  - temperature, pulses
  - lumps (see above)
  - joints
  - active movements
  - feel for crepitus, e.g. hand over knee during flexion
  - passive movements (do not hurt patient)
  - reflexes
  - sensation

References

Barkauskas, V., Baumann, L. & Darling-Fisher, C. (2002) *Health and Physical Assessment*, 3rd edn. Mosby, London.

Epstein, O., Perkin, G., de Bono, D. & Cookson, J. (2008) *Clinical Examination*, 4th edn. Mosby, London.

Hatton, C. & Blackwood, R. (2003) *Lecture Notes on Clinical Skills*, 4th edn. Blackwell Science, Oxford.

Swartz, M. (2006) *Physical Diagnosis, History and Examination*, 5th edn. Saunders, London.

Talley, N. & O'Connor, S. (2006) *Clinical Examination: A Systematic Guide to Physical Diagnosis*, 5th edn. Churchill Livingstone, London.

CHAPTER 10

Ophthalmic Examination

Introduction

The purpose of examining the eye is to assess the function of the eye, check its anatomy and discern pathology that affects vision. Until recently, patients with ophthalmic conditions were seen in specialist eye centres. However, today more and more nurses are assessing ophthalmic conditions in outreach centres, accident and emergency, walk-in centres and general practice settings. Assessment of the eye is important because, for example, primary open angle glaucoma (POAG) is a major cause of visual impairment and blindness in the United Kingdom (Kroese & Burton, 2003). Many patients that you will see will be unaware that they have POAG or other pathological conditions of the eye; therefore your assessment and intervention are essential.

This chapter begins by reviewing the anatomy and physiology of the eye and then presents examination techniques.

Anatomy and physiology of the eye (Fig. 10.1)

The eyeball is approximately 25 mm in diameter.

Orbit

The eye sits within the orbit; the optic nerve leaves the eye at the optic disc and transports the entire visual image to the brain. The ophthalmic artery also leaves here, running underneath the optic nerve.

Eyelids

- Provide protection to the eye itself (blinking action)
- Secrete oily part of the tear film
- Help the tear film to spread over the eye
- Prevent the eye drying out
- Contain the puncta whereby tears drain into the lacrimal system

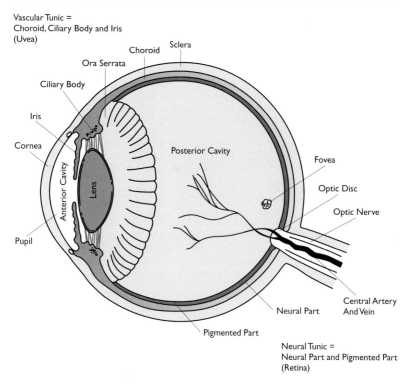

Vascular Tunic =
Choroid, Ciliary Body and Iris
(Uvea)

Fig. 10.1   The eye.

- Eyelid opening performed by the levator muscle
- Eyelid closed by orbicularis muscle

Cornea

A transparent structure, convex shaped (like a watch glass cover), the cornea is 0.5 mm thick. This allows light rays through and the shape allows light rays to bend. It is highly sensitive and protects the front of the eyeball.

It has five layers, with the epithelium being the only layer able to regenerate. The layers are:
- Epithelium
- Bowman's membrane
- Stroma
- Descemet's membrane
- Endothelium (damage to these cells results in a hazy cornea).
The cornea is avascular.

Anterior chamber

The area between the posterior surface of the cornea and the anterior surface of the iris.

When the eye is inflamed, cells may be visible here.

Posterior chamber

The area between the posterior surface of the iris and the anterior surface of the lens and suspensory ligaments.

Both the anterior and posterior chambers are filled with aqueous; this nourishes the lens and maintains intraocular eye pressure. Aqueous is made up of 99% water and 1% nutrients.

Ciliary body

A triangular structure lying between the choroid and iris. It consists of the cilary processes and the ciliary muscle.

Iris

- The coloured circular diaphragm which lies behind the cornea and in front of the lens, and forms the pupil at its centre. It is attached at the periphery to the ciliary body.
- The sphincter muscle constricts the iris, restricting the amount of light allowed into the eye.
  The dilator muscle dilates the pupil.
- The sphincter muscle is more powerful than the dilator muscle so if inflammation in the eye affects both muscles, the sphincter muscle will be dominant and constrict the pupil.

Lens

- The focusing mechanism of the eye.
- It is held in place by zonules (supensory ligaments).

Vitreous

- The vitreous is transparent and fills the posterior segment of the eye (between the lens and the retina).
- It is composed of 98–99% water, 1–2% hyaluronic acid and collagen fibres.
- It maintains the shape of the eye, if taken out and not replaced with an artificial replacement, the eye would collapse.
- It helps with refraction of light.

Sclera

- The sclera extends from the cornea (limbal area) to the optic nerve.
- It is often described as the hard protective coating of the eye.
- It is composed of dense, white, non-uniform collagen fibres.

Choroid

- The choroid lies between the sclera and the retina.
- Its function is to provide nourishment to the underlying retina.
- It contains blood vessels to supply the underlying retina.

Retina

- The retina has ten layers:
  - Layer 1 pigmented epithelium
  - Layers 2–10 neural layers
- The retina is transparent; it gets its colour from the choroid's blood supply.
- The retina is responsible for converting light into electrical signals.
- It contains rods and cones.
  - Rods are important for night vision; they are sensitive to light and do not signal colour information.
  - Cones are responsible for daytime vision. Some of the cones are responsible for red, green and blue colour vision. Cones are concentrated at the fovea which is responsible for reading vision and fine print.

Optic disc

The area where the retinal fibres leave the eyeball as the optic nerve.

Macula

- The region of the retina where precise central vision occurs.
- Not fully developed in the child until 6 months of age.

Fovea centralis

Found in the centre of the macula and responsible for detailed vision, e.g. fine print.

History Taking

It is fundamentally important when examining a patient with an ophthalmic condition to have a logical and systematic approach to history taking, visual assessment, examination and diagnosis. If this approach is not adopted then vital signs and symptoms may be missed during the examination.

Walsh (2006) suggests that patients with ocular symptoms often have high levels of anxiety and therefore need tact and understanding during their examination. It is therefore import to appear calm and confident in your approach. Goldblum (2004) suggests that if patients are not treated in a friendly and professional manner then often they will not express all their concerns to the examiner.

In the first two years of life the eyeball grows rapidly. By the age of between ten and thirteen years of age the eyeball will have reached its adult size. The scleral thickness and rigidity also increases from around 0.5 mm in childhood to 1 mm by adulthood (Wright 2003).

Children need to be treated with special care when being examined as they will often remember negative experiences which then make re examination more traumatic; especially if they need regular follow up. There are local anaesthetics on the market which don't smart and can be instilled before other drops that do smart to make the child's experience more comfortable.

As noted previously, it is essential to use a systematic approach in your examination and treatment of ophthalmic patients, it is suggested that it is good practice to:

> Take a history
> Perform visual assessment using a snellen visual acuity chart, near vision chart and colour vision or Amsler grid as required.
> Carry out a detailed examination using a good quality torch, magnifying light and preferably a slit-lamp.

The following features in the history are a requirement:

Presenting complaint

> Why has the patient attended
> Which eye is the problem (*If both, did it start in one eye and transfer to the other?*)

Duration and description of symptoms

- Identify:
  - How long the symptoms have been present.
  - Whether the symptoms are there all the time or whether they come and go.
  - Whether the pain occurred suddenly or gradually.
  - What the patient was doing at the time (*be very suspicious of penetrating injury if the patient has been drilling, chiselling, hammering or carrying out a task that could have caused a high-speed injury*).

- If it was a chemical injury, what type of chemical? (*these patients need immediate irrigation with at least 1 litre of normal saline, ensuring the eyelids are everted*). Establish whether the PH of the chemical is alkaline or acid and contact the local ophthalmology unit for advice.
- If the eye has a foreign body sensation, ask the patient wearing eye protection and whether the protection chosen was a good fit.
- If there is a discharge, it is relevant to ask whether the patient has had a recent cough or cold as a high proportion of conjunctivitis comes from viral aetiology. Establish colour and consistency of discharge.
- Whether the patient has tried any over-the-counter treatments themselves at home; if yes, whether the treatments had any effect.
- If the patient has a photophobic red eye with a foreign body sensation that came on gradually, does he suffer with cold sores on his face or lip? (*It could be a herpes simplex keratitis*).
- If the complaint is of a headache, in what region of the patient's head is the headache positioned? Does he suffer with migraine? If the headache is temporal, is the patient well? Has he suffered weight loss; is there pain on touching the temporal area or jaw claudication? (*If yes to these questions and the patient has visual symptoms, this could be temporal arteritis. Thus the patient needs an urgent blood test for C-reactive protein (CRP) and erythrocyte sedimentation rate (ESR) and urgent referral to the ophthalmologists. Listen for bruits over the temporal artery as on occasion this may be heard*). If temporal pain and no visual symptoms, refer to general practitioner urgently.
- Whether he has any nausea and/or headache. If yes, is the eye red, with a hazy cornea and a fixed dilated pupil? *This could indicate an attack of acute glaucoma. These patients need urgent referral to an ophthalmologist for immediate treatment.*
- Whether the patient complains of vision loss. Ask whether the vision is blurred. Did it worsen rapidly or over a course of weeks or months? Was it like a camera shutter closing over the eye with complete loss of vision or can he make out blurred images? Is his vision distorted when he is reading? *In sudden onset of loss of vision, check blood pressure and blood sugar to exclude underlying medical conditions.*
- Whether the patient is experiencing flashing lights +/− floaters; is he experiencing a cobweb or net curtain-like appearance in their vision? Is he a high myope? *These patients are at higher risk of retinal detachment (James et al., 2003) and require prompt referral to an ophthalmologist.*

Past ocular history

- Identify:
  - Whether the patient has ever had anything similar before? If yes, does he know what eye condition he had and what treatment was required?

– Whether he has a history of:
Iritis/uveitis
Episcleritis/scleritis
Previous eye trauma
Diabetic eye disease
Previous corneal abrasion/recurrent erosion syndrome
– Whether he wears glasses for distance or reading
If he wears contact lenses, what type are they? How does he clean them? What is the average length of time that lenses are worn? (Overwear of contact lenses is a common cause of red eye.)

Family ocular history

● Does he have a history of familiar eye problems?
Glaucoma
Diabetic eye disease
Retinal detachment
Diabetic eye disease
Squints/glasses/lazy eye

General medical health

● Ask whether the patient has:
Hypertension
Diabetes (how is it controlled, type and duration of symptoms)
Heart disease
Thyroid disorders
Joint complaints, e.g. rheumatoid arthritis
Bowel problems such as Crohn's disease
Chest problems such as asthma or sarcoidosis
Any other relevant problems

Questions relevant to child's history taking

● Who is accompanying the child?
Parent
Carer
Sibling
Other relative
● What source has the referral come from?
School
Accident and Emergency
Parent

Child's birth and developmental information

- Was the child full term or premature?
- Was it a normal delivery, C-section or assisted, e.g. forceps?
- Does the parent have any concerns over developmental issues?
- Did the mother experience any problems during pregnancy, e.g. infections, amniocentesis?

Other questions relevant to child's history

For the young child, ask the parent. For a child who is able to verbalize, direct the question to the child.

- When do you notice the problem?
  - All the time
  - When tired
  - When unwell
- Is the problem getting worse?
- Does your child complain of headaches?
- Does your child bump into things?
- Have you noticed your child sitting close to the television?
- Do you sit near the board where your teacher writes?
- Can you see what your teacher is writing on the board?
- When your teacher uses different colours on the board, are some colours missing?
- Is the child frightened of the dark?
- Is the child scared when you cover one eye?

Allergies

What allergies does the patient have? What reaction occurs when he uses this medicine, food or product (e.g. swelling/rash)?

Occupation

- Consider what the patient's occupation is.
- Consider whether a child is at school or nursery as this may have implications for him. For example, a patient with acute bacterial or viral conjunctivitis working in a school environment or attending a nursery school needs to be advised that his condition is highly contagious and he should refrain from work or attending school until symptoms resolve (can be anything from 24 hours to 1 week).

Examination

Visual acuity assessment

Preceding formal ocular examination, it is an essential requirement to check and fully document a formal visual acuity assessment. The standard tool for measuring distance visual acuity is a Snellen chart, with acuity measured at a distance of 6 metres from the chart. (*Some charts are designed for use at shorter distances; for example, if using a reverse Snellen chart in a mirror, the vision can be measured at 3 metres but still be recorded as 6 metres.*) The main advantage of Snellen charts is that they are relatively straightforward to use.

Snellen chart

A Snellen chart is a commonly used method of measuring visual acuity. It consists of nine rows of letters that get progressively smaller. The letters are heavy block letters, numbers or symbols printed in black on a white background. The top letter can be read by a normal eye at a distance of 60 metres, the smallest line at a distance of 4 metres. The vision recorded is expressed as a fraction; for example, if the patient is seated 6 metres away from the chart and he can read the top line only, then his vision in the eye being tested is 6/60. It is essential that you record whether the patient had his glasses or contact lenses *in situ*. It is not acceptable practice to record 'vision normal' or 'not affected'. If the patient is reassessed at a later date, there will not be any recordings to compare the results with, and if the patient requires referral to an eye clinic, visual acuity will be one of the first questions that will be asked.

Procedure

- Ensure the patient is seated comfortably with his feet firmly on the floor or foot rest of the chair.
- Ask the patient to use distance glasses if needed. Test each eye individually, starting with the right eye and then the left. Cover the untested eye with an occluder or a fresh tissue. (The occluder needs to be cleaned in between patients according to local policy.)
- Ask the patient to read down the chart from left to right as far as he can read. Encourage him to try another couple of letters and reassure him that it doesn't matter if he gets a letter wrong.
- If the patient's visual acuity is anything less than 6/9 with or without glasses, it is advisable to use a pinhole to establish whether the decreased vision is correctable or not, as in some cases reduced vision is due to a refractive error and nothing more serious.
- If the patient cannot read any letters on the chart, move him 1 metre closer to the chart and try the test again. If he is still unable to read the top letter, continue to move him forward 1 metre at a time. If at 1 metre from the chart he is still unable to read the top letter, stand about 1 metre

away and ask the patient to count the number of fingers held up and record as CF (counting fingers). If he cannot recognize the number of fingers held up, wave your hand 30 cm in front of his eye and ask if he can see your hand moving. If he can see your hand moving, record this as HM (hand movements). If the patient is unable to see hand movements, using your bright torch shine the light from different directions whilst asking the patient if he can see the light and which direction it is coming from. If he can see the light, it can be recorded as PL (perception to light). If unable to see the light in any direction, record as NPL (no perception to light).

The Sheridan–Gardiner method

This test can be used in illiterate patients or in young children to obtain a Snellen vision. The examiner holds a card at 6 metres from the patient and asks him to match the letter on the corresponding card which he is holding. This gives a Snellen recording.

LogMAR vision testing

Although more complex, LogMAR vision testing is well documented as being more accurate in its measurement of visual acuity (Rosser *et al.*, 2001). The main advantage of a LogMAR chart is that there are five letters on each line, each of which is scored and therefore gives the patient a fairer chance of being able to read the letters. The main disadvantage to the tester is that it takes longer in the early stages and people are put off by having to work out the scores for each individual patient. However, most departments have a conversion chart which can be used to easily record the score (Elliott, 2007). The LogMAR vision chart is primarily used in low vision, glaucoma and macular degeneration clinics.

Near vision testing

Near vision is assessed with a specifically designed reading card using different sizes of ordinary printer's type; each size is numbered. As in testing distance vision, the patient's eyes are tested individually and using reading glasses if applicable. The chart should be used in good light, preferably with a reading light positioned over the patient's shoulder. The chart should be positioned at approximately 25 cm from the patient (Stollery, 1997). Record the number of the lowest line read (e.g. N8).

Colour vision assessment

Colour vision assessment should be carried out in any patient who presents with painful loss of vision and whom you suspect may have an optic nerve condition, or in the patient who requests a colour vision assessment for work purposes. The standard method for colour vision assessment is performed using pseudo-isochromatic plates such as Ishihara colour plates, which test for red/green colour blindness. The plates appear as a circle of dots and within the circle a number is placed. The patient covers one eye and reads the number. If a plate cannot be distinguished, a number is taken away from the total score (e.g. 16/17 read).

Contrast sensitivity testing

This test is designed to test subtle levels of vision changes not accounted for in the normal visual acuity testing, for example in patients with cataracts. It measures real-life vision compared to black on white (Yannoff & Duker, 1998). It is not routinely assessed in ophthalmology clinics but more often in research clinics. The standard chart used is a Pelli–Robson which has six letters per line, all the same size on all eight lines. The letters fade in blackness until on the eighth row, they are barely visible. Like the LogMAR test, each letter is given a score. A printed conversion sheet is provided with the Pelli–Robson chart to ensure correct interpretation of results is recorded.

Testing central vision with the Amsler grid

This test uses an A5 sheet of paper with a grid of black lines. In the centre of the grid is a black spot.

Each eye is tested individually. The patient needs to wear his reading glasses and holds the test at a distance of approximately 25 cm and looks at the centre spot. He informs the examiner of any distortion, blurring, wavy or missing parts on the grid and this is recorded on the chart. This test is of great importance in patients with suspected macular degeneration. In these cases the patient would see wavy or distorted lines.

Testing eye movements

This test must be done in all patients who complain of double vision.
- The examiner sits in front of the patient at the same height. Explain to the patient that he must follow the pen torch with his eyes.
- Using a light from a pen torch, ask the patient to cover his left eye and then move the light slowly up and down, left and right, asking the patient to report any double vision or any pain on eye movement. Observe for full eye movement in all directions in both eyes.

Recording visual fields

Confrontational field testing
- Make sure your patient is seated comfortably with his feet on the floor or foot rest. You should adjust his chair to ensure that he is seated at arm's length distance from you and at eye level. You face the patient.

- Using a large red hat pin, ask the patient to close or cover his left eye (you do the same to your opposite, right eye), bring the pin into vision and ask the patient to state when he can see the pin in his visual field – upper right, middle and lower right.
- Repeat on the left eye.
  Use your own observation of the pin as a guide to when the pin should come into view for the patient. Note that you must have good visual fields to perform this assessment.

Perimetry visual field testing

- These tests are carried out in optometry practices and ophthalmic clinics. They measure the degree of peripheral and central visual field loss.
- They are used most frequently in glaucoma clinics to detect progression of the disease.
- The most common machine is a Humphrey field analyser. This provides an electronic record of the patient's visual field. Each eye is tested individually with the patient's refractive error corrected.
- The patient is given a buzzer to press when he sees a light being shone. These lights are shone in all $360°$. Recordings will show any changes from that of a normal visual field.
- The test not only records the spots correctly identified but can tell when the patient has pressed the buzzer incorrectly, and whether there was any loss of fixation.

Testing the child's vision

There are several different methods for checking a child's visual acuity, and the choice greatly depends on the child's age and ability. Testing of a young child's visual acuity is best performed by orthoptists in an ophthalmic unit as they are best equipped and experienced to obtain the best vision assessment from a young child.

Vision in the child varies. At birth, visual acuity is very poor and newborn babies are unable to fix on an object. By the age of 2–4 months, babies are able to fix and their vision starts to develop and will continue to do so until its peak of development at around age 7–9 years (Wright, 2003).

Non-verbal children

Young babies should be able to fix on a bright toy or object, even if only for a few moments. By the age of 6 months and over, the infant will try and reach out for the toy or object, or pick up small sweets (small cake decorations are a useful tool for this test).

Verbal children

From the age of 1 year, there are tests specifically designed to test children's vision and some are outlined below.

Cardiff acuity test

- This is a preferential test based on the perspective that children like to look at complex rather than plain targets (James *et al.*, 2003).
- It is aimed at young children from about 12 months to 3 years of age.
- The examiner observes eye movements and responses from the child to establish whether or not the child can see the target on a card.
- The cards have a grey background with a white picture. If the picture is too small for the child to see, the card will just appear grey and the child will lose interest.
- The test is carried out at a distance of 1 metre and covers vision down to 6/3.75.

Kay pictures

- This test is aimed at children as young as 2 years of age and requires the examiner to hold a series of pictures at 3 or 6 metres distance.
- Each card has a picture or, if using a LogMAR equivalent, five pictures, getting smaller as each new card is presented. The child is asked to say what picture is on each card. If the child is shy or not communicating, he can be asked to match the pictures on a corresponding card that he holds. Once the child reaches school age he can try matching the letters on a Snellen or LogMAR chart until he is able to read the letters for himself (Fig. 10.2).

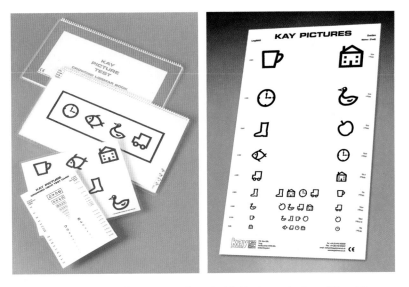

Fig. 10.2 Kay picture charts. Reproduced with kind permission of Hazel Kay (www.kaypictures.co.uk).

Visual electrophysiology testing

In some children, it is impossible to obtain a visual acuity or colour vision measurement and therefore electrophysiology in the form of an electroretinogram (ERG), visual evoked potential (VEP) and electro-oculogram (EOG) tests may be performed. These are non-invasive tests and serve as integrated parts of the ophthalmology examination. They determine how the retina and the visual cortex are functioning. These tests provide important and objective information for eye disease diagnosis, prognosis and treatment and are carried out in specialist units.

Ocular examination of the adult

The eye should always be examined from the outside in. When examining the patient's eye, first look at his face as a whole to ensure facial symmetry and note any obvious palsy, ptosis, proptosis or allergic reaction. Always consider the patient's age and psychological state. Patients with Parkinson's disease may, for example, find it very difficult to position themselves when a slit-lamp is used to carry out the examination (Stollery, 1997).

At the beginning of the examination, ask the patient to open both eyes as this is easier to do than opening one alone. Use of a good pen torch or magnifying light is essential (if a slit-lamp is unavailable) to examine the eye and check pupil reactions. If the patient is in pain, local anaesthetic drops may be required prior to the examination. In the case of a glass foreign body or if the history indicates a possible penetrating injury or perforation, local anaesthetic should **NOT** be instilled. These patients need immediate referral to an eye unit or ophthalmic A&E department day or night. **DO NOT PAD THE EYE OR PUT ANY PRESSURE ON IT.** A cartella eye shield should be used to cover the entire eye to prevent further accidental injury.

It is essential to look under the patient's top eyelid by everting it, if he is complaining of a foreign body sensation and a corneal foreign body cannot be seen. Use fluorescein eye drops to highlight any scratches or abrasions to the eye.

Ocular examination of the child

When a child attends with an eye problem requiring examination, it is essential that he feels at ease as much as possible. Encourage young children to bring in their favourite comforter and to sit on their parent's lap if they wish. Offer the child lots of patience and reassurance. If, however, you are unsure of a diagnosis or you find a corneal foreign body, for example, contact your local eye unit for advice.

Table 10.1 gives clear guidance on what to look for when examining eyes in both adults and children.

Table 10.1 Eye examination in adults and children

Face	Evaluate	Facial symmetry, look for drooping mouth and eyelids (common in Bell's palsy)
Eye movements	Can the patient Is there	Look upwards, downwards, left and right comfortably? Any obvious squint present?
Eyelids	Look for	Swelling of the lids *(is the swelling hard or soft? Is it hot to touch?)* Ptosis *(droopy eyelid)* Entropion *(inturning lid)* Ectropion *(out-turning lid)* Trichiasis *(ingrowing eyelashes)* Any lacerations to lids Chalazions Blepharitis *(inflammation of the eyelid margins)*
Conjunctiva	Assess	Redness *(position and degree of redness. Is it all over? Is it localized or limbal?)* Is there any haemorrhage? Any swelling? Can a foreign body be seen? Is there a laceration? Any conjunctival cysts *(look like a balloon filled with water)*? Pterygium *(wing-shaped growth that can encroach onto cornea, causing irritation)*
Cornea	Is it Is there Are there	Clear/hazy? Any scarring? Staining when fluorescein dye instilled? Any ulcers? Any foreign bodies? Any lacerations?
Anterior chamber	Is it Is there Are there	Shallow/deep? *(compare both eyes together)* A hyphaema? *(blood in the anterior chamber)* A hypopyon? *(pus in the anterior chamber)* Cells? *(seen when carrying out a slit-lamp examination)*
Iris	Are they Are there Is there	The same colour? *(some patients have different coloured irises; some medications change the iris colour)* Any naevi present? Any trauma? *(has the patient had any previous surgery?)*
Pupil	Is it Are they	Round? *(a peaked pupil could indicate posterior synechiae in uveitis; an oval pupil with a hazy cornea indicates acute glaucoma)* Equal and reactive Black in colour *(in an adult a white or grey pupil often indicates a cataract; in an infant, a cataract or more seriously retinoblastoma)*

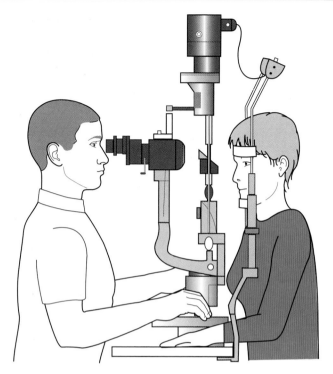

Fig. 10.3 Slit-lamp examination.

Use of a slit-lamp

It is almost impossible to obtain a definite diagnosis of an eye condition without using a slit-lamp (Fig. 10.3). The slit-lamp consists of a microscope and a light source.

Technique
- Explain to the patient that the light may be a little bright but that it will give a highly magnified view of the eye, thus aiding diagnosis.
- Patient and examiner are seated (both must be comfortable) with the chin height adjusted, to ensure the eye is aligned with the slit-lamp guide.
- The patient places his chin and forehead on the bars; the examiner looks through the eyepieces (ensuring that the eye pieces are adjusted to her own glasses prescription, if any).
- The lids, cornea, anterior chamber and iris can be easily viewed by moving the focus using the joystick, forward and backwards as required.

– Use fluorescein and the blue cobalt light to look for corneal staining and corneal abrasions.
– Use the slit beam, approximately 1 mm wide and 3 mm long, with high magnification to look for anterior chamber cells and flare.

Use of a 90 dioptre lens with a slit-lamp to view the retina

This examination is usually carried out in optometry practices and hospital clinics. Extra training should be undertaken prior to carrying out this procedure. It gives a much better view of the retina than direct ophthalmoscopy and is therefore used more in the hospital setting than a direct ophthalmoscope.

This procedure can be carried out with an undilated pupil but a better image will be seen through a dilated pupil.

– Ensure the 90 D lens is clean and smear free (only clean with a lens cloth to prevent scratching on the lens coating.)
– Ensure that the patient is comfortably and correctly positioned at the slit-lamp with his
  chin on the chin rest, forehead firmly pressed against the plastic strap, head pointing straight ahead and eye in line with the mark on the metal frame of the slit-lamp.
– Adjust the power of the light so that it is not too bright for the patient. Adjust the width of the slit so that it is 2–3 mm wide and the height of the beam to about 8 mm.
– Pull the slit-lamp joystick towards you.
– To examine the patient's right eye, hold the 90 D lens in your left hand.
– Ask the patient to look at your right ear or use the fixation light.
– Hold the 90 D lens just in front of the patient's right eye, without touching the eye with the lens. Hold the lens with the thumb and index finger.
– Using your right hand, *slowly* advance the slit-lamp towards the eye. At first, the lens will be seen with an inverted image of the eye in its centre. (The image is vertically and laterally inverted and virtual.)
– As the slit-lamp is moved closer to the patient, the vitreous and then the retina should come into view. With the patient looking at your right ear, the disc should come into view. Nasal to the disc in the image seen is the macula. Examine the retinal vessels for any signs of haemorrhages or occlusion.
  – To examine the temporal retina, ask the patient to look to his right.
  – To examine the nasal retina, ask the patient to look to his left.
  – Get the patient to look up for the superior retina, then down for the inferior retina. The patient's upper lid will need to be kept open by gently lifting it with a finger when the patient looks down.
  N.B. The image seen in all directions of gaze is vertically and laterally inverted; for example, on upgaze, the superior-most part of the retina is

in the inferior field. This must be remembered when drawing the image, but a useful tip is to turn the page upside down so you can draw what you are seeing and on turning the page round, the image will be presented correctly.
- Repeat the entire process to examine the patient's left fundus, this time using your right hand to hold the lens, with the patient looking at your left ear, to see the disc.

Measurement of intraocular pressure (IOP)

This test is carried out on most patients who attend an ophthalmology clinic, and on all patients who are over the age of 40 in optometry practices. The usual intraocular eye pressure is between 10 and 21 mmHg (Coakes & Holmes, 1995).

Goldmann tonometry
The gold standard method is Goldmann tonometry (Fig. 10.4). This provides the most accurate measurement but it is difficult to master and should only be carried out after specialist training.
- Fluorescein dye and anaesthetic are instilled in the eye.
- A clear plastic prism is advanced until it touches the cornea. Two semi-circles are seen and the two inner circles meet. The measurement can then be read on the dial at the side of the instrument.

Perkins applanation tonometry
- This is a handheld device useful for patients unable to be seen on a slit-lamp.
- Same principles as Goldmann tonometry.
- Difficult to master.
- In order to obtain this measurement, the examiner needs to get very close to the patient.

Tonopen
This is easy to use and is good for emergency departments and patients who are unable to reach a slit-lamp. It is a pen-like device which when gently tapped on an anaesthetized cornea will give an IOP reading.

Air puff
- Most commonly used in optometry practices.
- Can give abnormally high readings as it makes the patient jump or hold their breath.
- The time taken to flatten the cornea is converted into a figure to give an IOP.

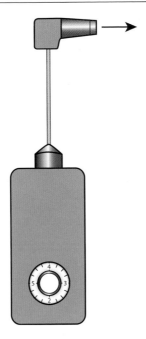

Fig. 10.4   Alignment of semi-circles in Goldmann tonometry.

Palpation of the globe
Palpation of the eye using two fingers on a closed eyelid with the patient looking downwards.

This is of no value other than to detect the hardness in an acute glaucoma (Coakes & Holmes, 1995).

Use of an ophthalmoscope

- Make sure that the ophthalmoscope is fully charged, has a bright light and the bulb is in working order before the examination commences.
- The patient should be sitting. Remove spectacles from yourself and the patient.
- Begin by setting the lens dioptre dial at 0 if you do not use spectacles. If you are myopic, you should start with the 'minus' lenses. Set the lens dioptre at −4 to begin, which is indicated as a red number. If you are hyperopic you should use the 'plus' lenses which are indicated by black numbers. Keep your index finger on the dial to permit easy focusing. Hold the ophthalmoscope about 30 cm from the patient, shine the light into the patient's pupil, identify the red reflex (from the retina)

and approach the patient at an angle of 15°. Approach on the same horizontal plane as the equator of the patient's eye. This will bring you straight to the patient's optic disc. After observing the disc, examine the peripheral retina fully by following the blood vessels to and back from the four main quadrants.

- Hold the ophthalmoscope in your right hand in front of your right eye to examine the patient's right eye, and your left eye to examine the patient's left eye. Try to hold your breath when using the ophthalmoscope. Do not breathe into the patient's face.
- If the patient's pupils are small, dilate with 1% tropicamide, one drop per eye. Tropicamide works in 15–20 minutes and lasts 2–4 hours. Warn the patient that his vision will be blurred for approximately 4 hours. Do **not** dilate if neurological observation of pupils is needed.
- The patient should be told he cannot drive for at least 4–6 hours, if his pupils have been dilated.

Look at the optic disc
- normally pink rim with white 'cup' below surface of disc
- *optic atrophy*
  - disc pale: rim no longer pink
    multiple sclerosis
    after optic neuritis
    optic nerve compression, e.g., *tumour*
- papilloedema
- disc pink, indistinct margin
- cup disappears
  - dilated retinal veins
    increased cerebral pressure, e.g., *tumour*
    accelerated hypertension
    optic neuritis, acute stage
- glaucoma – enlarged cup, diminished rim
- new vessels – new fronds of vessels coming forward from disc
  ischaemic diabetic retinopathy

Look at the arteries
- arteries narrowed in hypertension, with increased light reflex along top of vessel
  Hypertension grading:
  1 narrow arteries
  2 'nipping' (narrowing of veins by arteries)
  3 flame-shaped haemorrhages and cotton-wool spots
  4 papilloedem
- occlusion artery – pale retina
- occlusion vein – haemorrhages

Look at the retina
- hard exudates (shiny, yellow circumscribed patches of lipid)
    diabetes
- cotton-wool spots (soft, fluffy white patches)
    microinfarcts causing local swelling of nerve fibres
    diabetes
    hypertension
    vasculitis
    human immunodeficiency virus (HIV)
- small, red dots
    microaneurysms – retinal capillary expansion adjacent to capillary closure
    diabetes
- haemorrhages
    - round 'blots': haemorrhages deep in retina larger than microaneurysms
    diabetes
    - flame-shaped: superficial haemorrhages along nerve fibres
    hypertension
    gross anaemia
    hyperviscosity
    bleeding tendency
    - Roth's spots (white-centred haemorrhages)
    microembolic disorder
    subacute bacterial endocarditis
- pigmentation
    - widespread
    retinitis pigmentosa
    - localized
    choroiditis (clumping of pigment into patches)
    drug toxicity, e.g. chloroquine
    - tigroid or tabby fundus: normal variant in choroid beneath retina
- peripheral new vessels
    ischaemic diabetic retinopathy
    retinal vein occlusion
- medullated nerve fibres – normal variant, areas of white nerves radiating from optic disc

Pupil assessment for relative afferent papillary defect (RAPD)

This is an essential test to perform prior to instilling dilating drops, especially in patients whom you suspect of having optic nerve conditions.
- Assess size and shape of pupils.
- Sit the patient in a dimly lit room.
- Ask the patient to gaze into the distance.

– Shine the bright torch from one eye to the other (hold light on pupil for 2–3 seconds on each eye); if there is a pupil defect, the pupil will dilate instead of constricting when the eye is illuminated. The normal response would be for the pupil to constrict when the light is shone on it.

Documentation

It is essential to document your findings in a systematic format. An example is outlined below.

Right eye		Left eye
	Visual acuity	
	Lids	
	Conjunctiva	
	Cornea	
	Anterior chamber	
	Iris	
	Pupil	
	Intraocular pressure	
	Fundus	

References

Coakes, R. & Holmes, S. (1995) *Outline of Ophthalmology*, 2nd edn. Butterworth Heinemann, Oxford.

Elliott, D. (2007) *Clinical Procedures in Primary Eye Care*, 3rd edn. Butterworth Heinemann, Edinburgh.

James, B., Chew, C. & Bron, A. (2003) *Lecture Notes on Ophthalmology*, 9th edn. Blackwell Publishing, Oxford.

Kroese, M. & Burton, H. (2003) Primary open angle glaucoma. The need for a consensus case definition. *Journal of Epidemiology and Community Health*, **57**(9): 752–754.

Rosser, D., Laidlaw, D. & Murdoch, I. (2001) The development of a "reduced LogMAR" visual acuity chart for use in routine clinical practice. *British Journal of Ophthalmology*, **85**: 432–436.

Stollery, R. (1997) *Ophthalmic Nursing*, 2nd edn. Blackwell Publishing, Oxford.

Wright, K. (2003) *Paediatric Ophthalmology for Primary Care*, 2nd edn. Elsevier, Edinburgh.

Yannoff, M. & Duker, J. (1999) *Ophthalmology*. Mosby, London.

CHAPTER 11

Examination of the Musculoskeletal System

General examination

Introduction

For the patient presenting with a musculoskeletal problem, the primary complaint is likely to be pain or a decrease in functional ability. These are symptoms that the patient is unlikely to ignore so musculoskeletal complaints make up a large amount of the primary care or minor injury nurse practitioner's caseload. Thus, the aim of the musculoskeletal assessment is to determine the degree to which the patient's activities of daily living are affected, through a systematic assessment.

The musculoskeletal system performs several essential functions: supports and maintains body shape, supports and protects internal organs, enables movement, stores calcium and phosphate in bone and produces red blood cells. The musculoskeletal system comprises bones, muscles, ligaments, joints and cartilage.

The musculoskeletal assessment is closely linked with the neurological assessment as bone and muscle functioning are directly co-ordinated by the central nervous system. You should read the neurological assessment in Chapter 9 in conjunction with this chapter.

Frequent musculoskeletal complaints

Osteo-arthritis

A degenerative joint disease due to a progressive breakdown of the joint surfaces. Direct and indirect trauma to the articular cartilage and infection can both lead to osteo-arthritis. Osteo-arthritis primarily affects weight-bearing joints (hips, knees) with patients presenting to their GP with increased pain and a decrease in functional ability. The end result is often a joint replacement but symptoms can be managed/reduced through a range of pharmacological and non-pharmacological means.

Rheumatoid arthritis

This is the most common chronic inflammatory disease of joints. It is systemic disease affecting many different structures, unlike osteo-arthritis which invariably affects one joint in isolation. Treatment aims to control the pain associated with synovitis and maintain as much function as possible.

Osteoporosis

Due to a lack of oestrogen in postmenopausal women, a reduction in the amount of collagen in bones occurs. The bone becomes very thin and a kyphosis of the spine is often seen with pain over the spinous processes. Fractures of the femoral neck and crush fractures of the vertebrae are common after a fairly minor trip or fall.

Fractures

Fractures are usually caused by trauma, either significant, or minor and repeated. Pathological fractures occur as a result of disease, e.g. tumours, osteoporosis, Paget's disease and osteomalacia. There are many types of fracture but the principles behind their management remain the same.

General aspects

- In order that a comprehensive musculoskeletal assessment is undertaken, the patient will need to be exposed. He should be allowed to redress as the examination proceeds or be covered as appropriate to ensure privacy and dignity.
- The musculoskeletal assessment has two stages: inspection and palpation. Unlike other systems examinations, you should work through the two stages together rather than inspecting all joints and then returning to palpate.
- Always ask whether the patient has any pain and if so, assess the pain-free side first.
- Arrange your assessment by examining position for patient comfort, allowing the joint to be supported.
- Always compare each side.
- Organize your examination of the bones, muscles and joints in a head-to-toe method. This will help avoid omissions.
- Always start each part of the examination from the neutral position (Fig. 11.1).

Inspection

For a comprehensive assessment, inspection should be carried out observing from anterior, posterior and lateral views. Inspection should assess for:

- size
- contour

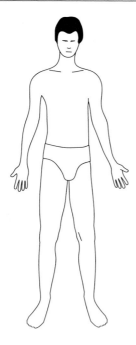

Fig. 11.1 The neutral position.

- symmetry
- involuntary movements (tremors, fasciculations)
- deformities (subluxation, dislocation, varus, valgus)
- swelling/oedema (effusions, haematoma)
- discolouration (vascular insufficiency, bruising, haematoma)
- hypertrophy/atrophy of muscles (steroid use, malnutrition, spinal cord lesion)
- posture and body alignment
- structural relationships
- scars indicating any previous surgery or trauma
- condition of skin (pressure ulcers, necrosis, scarring)

Palpation

- Palpate joints, bursal sites, bones and surrounding muscles.
- Assess the patient for both verbal and non-verbal cues of pain.
- Ask the patient, **'Does the pain radiate elsewhere from the initial region?'**
- Palpation should assess for the following:
    - increased temperature (use the back of the hand above, below and on the joint and compare with the other side)
    - swelling/oedema

- tenderness
- crepitus (loose cartilage, etc.; listen for crepitus as well as feeling)
- consistency and tone of muscle

Range of movement (ROM)

- Assess the degree of deviation away from the neutral position.
- A goniometer should be used to obtain an accurate range of movement (Jarvis, 2008).
- Active ROM involves the patient moving the joint himself.
  - Movement should be smooth and pain free.
- Passive ROM involves you providing motion in order to move the joint.
Question whether:
- Active ROM is less than passive ROM – **focus on true weakness, joint stability, pain and malignancy**.
- Active and passive ROM are limited – **determine whether there is any excess fluid or loose body in the joint (e.g. cartilage), joint surface irregularity (e.g. osteo-arthritis, contracture of muscle, ligaments or capsule)** (Barkauskas *et al.*, 2002; Bickley & Szilagyi, 2007; Epstein *et al.*, 2008; Swartz, 2006; Talley & O'Connor, 2006; Thomas & Monoghan, 2007; Walsh, 2006).

Limb measurement

- Ensure limbs are in the neutral position.
- Ensure the patient is lying straight – many discrepancies in limb length are due to inaccurate positioning.
- Full length upper limb – measure from the acromion process to the end of the middle finger.
- Upper arm only – acromion process to the olecranon process.
- Lower arm only – olecranon process to the styloid process of the ulna.
- Full length lower limb – lower edge of the ileum to tibial malleolus.
- Upper leg only – lower edge of the ileum to the medial aspect of the knee.
- Lower leg only – medial aspect of the knee to the tibial malleolus.
Establish whether shortening is due to a loss of bone length or to a deformity at the joint, e.g. a hip dislocation.

Bones

Examine for:
- Deformity
- Tumours
- Pain – is the pain focal (**fracture/trauma, infection, malignancy, Paget's disease, osteoid osteoma**) or diffuse (**malignancy, Paget's disease, osteomalacia, osteoporosis, metabolic bone disease**)?

- Consider; character, onset, site, radiation, severity, periodicity, exacerbating and relieving factors, diurnal variation.

Joints

Always compare each joint bilaterally to make a comparison. Examine for:
- Pain – causes include: **inflammatory (e.g. rheumatoid arthritis), mechanical (e.g. osteo-arthritis), infective (e.g. pyogenic tuberculosis) or traumatic (e.g. fractures)**.
- Questions to ask:
  - **Where is the site of maximum pain?**
  - **Does the pain change during the course of the day?**
  - **Has the pain been there for a short or long time?**
  - **Does the pain get better or worse as the patient moves about?**
- Tenderness
- Swelling
- Partial or complete loss of mobility
- Stiffness
- Deformity
- Weakness
- Fatigue
- Warmth
- Redness
- Lesions or ulcers

Pitting of nails is present in 50% of cases of joint disease.

Muscles

Assess:
- Size
- Contour
- Tone
- Strength/weakness
  - **Is the weakness global or focal?**
  - **Is the weakness secondary to a painful limb?**
  - **Does the weakness fluctuate in degree?**
  - **Is the weakness increasing in severity?**
  - **Is the weakness associated with sensory symptoms or signs?**
  - **Is there a family history of muscle disease?**
  - **Is the weakness symmetrical?**
  - **Is the weakness predominantly proximal or distal?**
- Pain – causes include: **inflammatory (e.g. polymyalgia rheumatica), infective (e.g. pyogenic cysticercosis), traumatic or neuropathic (e.g. Guillain–Barré syndrome)**.

The examination

When asking the patient to perform active ROM, instruct him in a way that will be understood. It may be necessary for you to perform the movement first so that the patient can then copy it.

GALS screen

The GALS (gait, arms, legs, spine) screen provides a useful rapid screen of the overall integrity of the locomotor system. It is felt that the general survey below followed by a regional joint examination is necessary for the patient presenting with a musculoskeletal complaint. However, the GALS screen may be used to make a quick 'screening' examination of the whole locomotor system in order to identify an abnormality in the absence of symptoms (Doherty *et al.*, 1992; Thomas & Monoghan, 2007).

General survey

The general survey should start as soon as you meet the patient. Call him into the examination room and watch how he moves. You can gain an accurate assessment of the patient's pattern of gait as he enters the room – once you ask the patient to walk for you, his gait may change. Watch the patient throughout the examination. Observe how he gets on and off the examination couch and up from a chair. Look at the speed of his manoeuvres and note any pain elicited.

Shake the patient's hand and gain an idea of his muscle strength.

Observe the patient's gait anteriorly and posteriorly, with and without shoes on.

- Does the patient trip?
- Is there a limp? **Look at the patient's shoes and see if one side of the heel is worn more than the other.**
- Note alignment of the pelvis and shoulders during walking.
- Does the patient stagger to one particular side?
- Does the patient, despite apparently severe ataxia, seldom sustain injury?
- If a Trendelenburg gait pattern is suspected, ask the patient to stand on one leg; if the hip abductors are weak, the pelvis will tilt towards the non-weight bearing side.

For examples of abnormal gait patterns, refer to Chapter 9.

General inspection:

- Posture
- Body alignment
- Hypertrophy/atrophy of the muscles – dominant side is usually slightly bigger than the non-dominant. Hypertrophy can be seen in young men using steroids. Atrophy of the muscles can be due to malnutrition, lack of

use of muscles due to joint disease or a spinal cord lesion due to the lack of neural input to the muscle. May need to measure the circumference of muscle bulk and document on each visit to assess any decrease. Differences of <1 cm noted at different times are not significant.

- Genu valgum/varum
- Hyperextension of the knees – will often indicate hypermobility of all joints but could could be due to ligament ruptures, intra-articular fractures or connective tissue disruption, e.g. Marfan's syndrome.
- Carrying angle – elbows should be at approximately 5–15° in an adult (see Fig. 11.1).
- Spine – scoliosis, kyphosis, lordosis, gibbus
- Symmetry
- Contour
- Size
- Involuntary movements
- Gross deformities
- Limb measurement

Regional examination

Jaw

The temporomandibular joint (TMJ) – the articulation between the temporal bone and the mandible.
- Place fingertips over the TMJ, anterior to the external meatus of the ear.
- Palpate whilst the patient goes through the range of movements:
  - open and close the mouth – **extension**
  - project the lower jaw – **flexion**
  - move the jaw from side to side – **abduction and adduction**
  - **is there any crepitus?**
- Ask the patient to bite down hard – palpate the muscle strength of the **masseter muscles**.
- Ask the patient to clench his teeth while you push lightly on the chin – **also tests the motor function of cranial nerve V**.

Spine
- Normal curvatures at the spine are **concave at the cervical region, convex at the thoracic region** and **concave at the lumbar region**.

Cervical spine
The sternoclavicular joint – the articulation between the sternum and the clavicle.
The cervical vertebrae – C1–C7, most mobile of all spinal vertebrae.
- Using thumbs, palpate all spinous processes.
- Palpate along the clavicles and manubrium of the sternum.

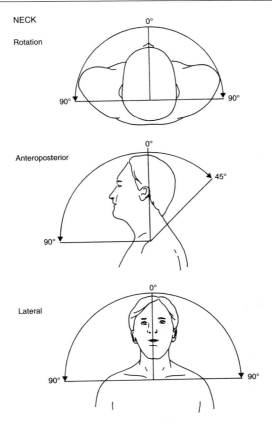

NECK

Rotation

Anteroposterior

Lateral

Fig. 11.2 Movements of the neck. Reproduced from Talley & O'Connor (1998). © 1998, Elsevier, Sydney.

- Observe patient as he goes through the range of movements (Fig. 11.2):
  - chin to chest – **flexion**
  - raise the head back to the neutral position – **extension**
  - bend the head backwards – **hyperextension**
  - turn head to each side – **lateral rotation**
  - place each ear to each shoulder – **lateral bending**
- To test the muscle strength of the trapezius and sternocleidomastoid muscles, the above range of movements should be performed to resistance.

Thoracic and lumbar spine

Thoracic vertebrae – T1–T12.
Lumbar vertebrae – L1–L5.

- Look at the equality of height at the shoulders and the iliac crests.
- Using your thumbs, palpate along all spinous processes – if no pain is elicited but **malignancy or osteoporosis is suspected**, light percussion of the spinous processes using the ulnar aspect of your fist may prove a useful technique.
- Palpate around the scapulae and assess for equality in height.
- Have the patient stand with his feet 15 cm apart and ask him to bend forward slowly as if touching his toes. Observe for any abnormal curvatures of the spine (Fig. 11.3):

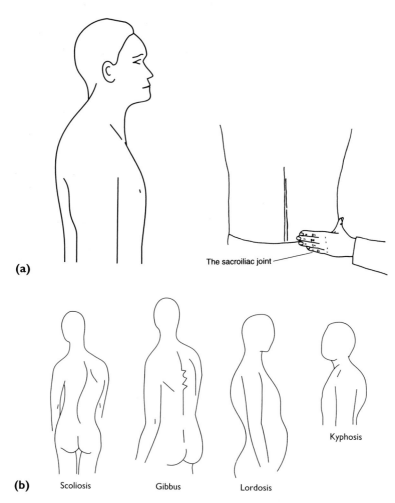

Fig. 11.3   (a) Thoracolumbar spine and sacroiliac joint. Reproduced from Talley & O'Connor (1998). © 1998, Elsevier, Sydney. (b) Changes in the thoracolumbar spine.

- **scoliosis** – a lateral curvature of the spine
- **lordosis** – an exaggerated lumbar curvature (can be normal during pregnancy, in the obese or women of Afro-Caribbean origin)
- **kyphosis** – a rounded thoracic convexity (commonly known as the 'dowagers hump'); common in osteoporotic women
- **gibbus** – when a defect is of a sharp angle, the spinous processes are seen more prominently on the back, forming an apex
- **list** – the spine is tilted to one side with no compensation

- If the patient is able to stay in a flexed position, it is useful to palpate the spinous processes. An early scoliosis may be detected through palpation, which may be missed upon inspection in the upright position.
- A spinal curvature may have an effect on the patient's respiratory function so attention may also need to be paid to a respiratory assessment.
- Observe the patient as he goes through the range of movements (Fig. 11.4).
  - Bend forward to touch toes – **flexion**.
  - Stand back up into the neutral position – **extension**.
  - Bend back as far as possible, running hands down the back of the thighs – **hyperextension**.
  - Run a hand down each leg laterally – **lateral bending**.
  - Turn to the right and left in a circular motion – **rotation**.

    It is important that you stabilize the patient's pelvis during this range of motion, or the movement will come from the pelvis and not the spine. You should have the patient sitting in a chair with his arms crossed to assess this movement.
- To assess the muscle strength of the trapezius and paravertebral muscles, the above should be performed to resistance.

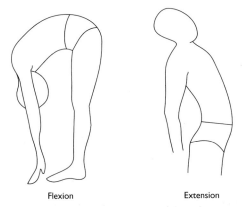

Flexion   Extension

Fig. 11.4 Flexion and extension of the spine.

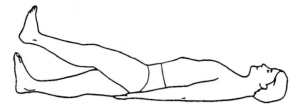

Fig. 11.5   Straight leg raise with pain increased on dorsiflexion of the foot (Bragard's test).

Stretch tests

- If a patient presents with a history of lower back pain, you should assess his ability to raise a straight leg **(Bragard's test)** (Fig. 11.5).
  - The patient should lie supine with the leg as relaxed as possible. You should slowly raise the foot, keeping the knee straight until the patient complains of pain, then dorsiflex the foot.
  - Make a note of the range of movement obtained before a complaint of pain and whether the pain intensifies upon dorsiflexion of the foot.
  - A positive test includes pain before 70° is reached in an L5 or S1 distribution, increased pain on dorsiflexion of the foot and relief of pain on flexion of the knee (Barkauskas *et al.*, 2002; Seidel *et al.*, 2006; Walsh, 2006).
  - A positive test is indicative of a herniated lumbar disc.
- If it is felt that a lumbar disc may have prolapsed higher **(L2–L4)**, a stretch test for the femoral nerve should be performed (Fig. 11.6).
  - The patient should lie prone and extend the hip with the knee in a flexed position.
  - Note the point at which the patient complains of pain.
  - Pain will be elicited in the lumbar region as the femoral nerve roots are tightened.

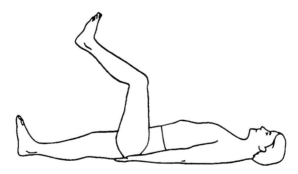

Fig.11.6   Further extension of the nerve root increases pain when the knee is extended (Lasegue's test).

- Lying prone may not be possible for all patients, so an alternative test can be performed with the patient lying laterally with his knees bent. This position produces a stretch of the femoral nerve. The stretch is enhanced as the patient bends his head toward his chest.
- Patella and Achilles reflexes should also be tested.

Upper limb
Shoulder

The acromioclavicular joint – the articulation between the acromion process of the scapula and the clavicle.

The glenohumeral joint – the articulation between the glenoid fossa and the humerus.

The sternoclavicular joint – the articulation between the sternum and the clavicle.

- Inspect the shoulder from anterior and posterior views.
- Look at the shape of the shoulders – **anterior dislocation of the shoulder can be seen as a flattening of the lateral aspect**. Check for altered sensation laterally as the axillary nerve may have been damaged by the dislocation.
- Look for swelling at the joint.
- Observe the equality of shoulder height.
- Look for muscle wasting – **may be present in arthritic joints when the patient does not use his arm**.
- Palpate each of the shoulder joints and the bursal sites **(subacromial bursa and subscapular bursa)**.
- Assess the temperature of the joint and note any colour changes in conjunction with an increased temperature.
- Palpate the clavicles, scapulae, acromion process and biceps groove.
- Palpate the associated muscles – **particularly those of the rotator cuff**.
- Observe the patient as he goes through the range of movement:
  - extend both arms forward – **flexion**
  - back to the neutral position – **extension**
  - extend both arms backwards – **hyperextension**
  - put an arm out to the side – **abduction**
  - put an arm across the body – **adduction**
  - roll arms forwards and backwards in a circular motion – **circumduction**
  - put an arm behind the back and touch the opposite shoulder blade – **internal rotation**
  - put an arm behind the head – **external rotation**
  - draw shoulders upwards – **elevation**
  - draw the shoulders downwards – **depression**
  - draw the shoulders forward – **protraction**
  - draw the shoulder back – **retraction** – gives a good view of the equality of scapula height (Figs 11.7 and 11.8)

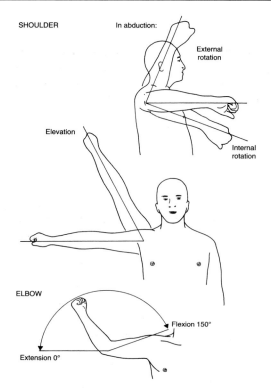

Fig. 11.7   Movements of the shoulder. Reproduced from Talley & O'Connor (1998). © 1998, Elsevier, Sydney.

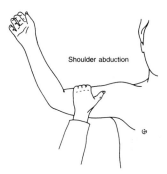

Fig. 11.8   Shoulder abduction. Reproduced from Talley & O'Connor (1998). © 1998, Elsevier, Sydney.

Elbow

The articulation between the humerus, radius and ulna.

- Inspect and palpate with the elbow in a flexed and extended position.
- Inspect for swelling, redness and increased temperature.

- Inspect for tracking marks and any associated cellulitis in the cubital fossa region – **drug misuse**.
- Palpate the olecranon bursa, the distal humerus, medial and lateral epicondyles, the olecranon process, coronoid process of the ulna and the radius.
- Assess for any pain or tenderness over the annular ligament.
- Assess for any joint swelling in the grooves either side of the olecranon process.
- Observe the patient as he goes through the range of movement:
  - bend the arm – **flexion**
  - straighten the arm – **extension**
  - turn the hand palm up – **supination**
  - turn the hand palm down – **pronation**

    Ensure that the elbow is flexed to 90° and is locked against the side of the body when testing supination and pronation, otherwise the movement will come from the glenohumeral joint and not the elbow (Figs 11.9 and 11.10).

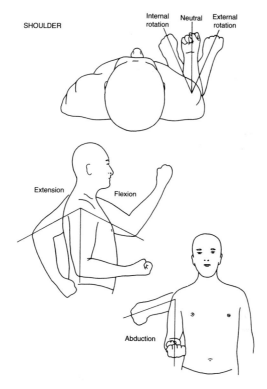

Fig. 11.9 Movements of the elbows and shoulders. Reproduced from Talley & O'Connor (1998). © 1998, Elsevier, Sydney.

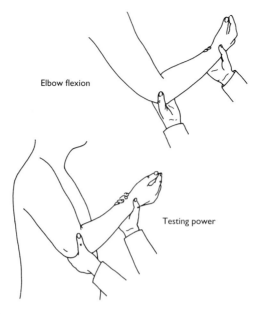

Elbow flexion

Testing power

Fig. 11.10 Flexion and testing power of the elbow. Reproduced from Talley & O'Connor (1998). © 1998, Elsevier, Sydney.

Wrist

The articulation between the distal radius and the proximal portions of the carpus.

- Inspect both wrists for symmetry, contour, swelling, atrophy and smoothness.
- As there is little tissue covering the dorsal aspect of the wrist joint, swelling is clearly visible.
- Use thumbs and index fingers to palpate the wrist and proximal portions of the carpus.
- Apply pressure in the anatomical snuffbox – **fractures of the scaphoid are not clearly visible on plain A–P and lateral X-rays and scaphoid views are needed. Pain in the anatomical snuffbox is a good indicator of a fracture. If not diagnosed and treated quickly, the patient is at risk of avascular necrosis, particularly if the fracture is through the highly vascular proximal pole**.
- Palpate the ulna tip for any pain and across the underlying bones of the carpus – **scaphoid, lunate, pisiform, trapezium, trapezoid, hamate and capitate**.
- Observe the patient as he goes through the range of movements (Fig. 11.11):

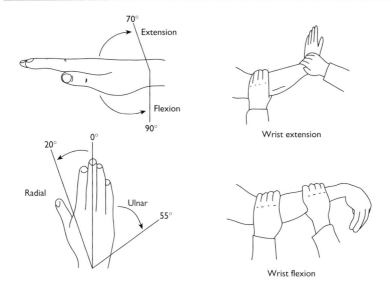

Fig. 11.11 Movements of the wrist. Reproduced from Talley & O'Connor (1998). © 1998, Elsevier, Sydney.

- – bend hand down – **flexion**
- – bend hand upwards – **extension**
- – with the hand pronated, turn it towards the right – **radial deviation**
- – with the hand pronated, turn it towards the left – **ulnar deviation**
- ● If **carpal tunnel syndrome** is suspected, one of two tests can be carried out:
  - – **Phalen's test** – ask the patient to maintain palmar flexion for 1 minute. This will produce numbness. When hands are brought back to the normal position, the numbness disappears.
  - – **Tinel's test** – lightly tap the median nerve. This will produce a tingling which will stop when tapping is ceased.

Fingers

Metacarpophalangeal joints – the articulation between the distal portions of the carpus and metacarpal bones.

Proximal interphalangeal joints – the articulation between the metacarpal and the proximal phalanges.

Distal interphalangeal joints – the articulation between the proximal and distal phalanges.

- ● Inspect each of the fingers and each of the joints – **rheumatoid arthritis is particularly evident in the joints of the fingers.**
- ● Look at the condition of the nails.

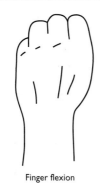

Finger flexion

Fig.11.12   Flexion of the fingers. Reproduced from Talley & O'Connor (1998). © 1998, Elsevier, Sydney.

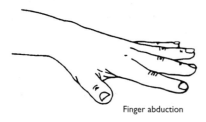

Finger abduction

Fig. 11.13   Abduction of the fingers. Reproduced from Talley & O'Connor (1998). © 1998, Elsevier, Sydney.

- Using the thumb and index finger, palpate each of the MC and IP joints.
- Observe the patient as he goes through the range of movements:
  - make a fist – **full finger flexion** (Fig. 11.12)
  - open a fist – **full finger extension**
  - spread fingers out – **abduction** (Fig. 11.13)
  - bring fingers in together from abduction – **adduction**
  - push fingers forward – **hyperflexion**
  - push fingers backwards – **hyperextension**
  - little finger to thumb – **opposition**
  - thumb to little finger – **opposition**
- **Carry out range of movement with wrist flexed as well as in neutral to test for tendon shortening.**

Lower limb
Pelvis and hips

The sacroiliac joints – the articulation between the sacrum and the ileum.
The symphysis pubis – the articulation bilaterally between the inferior and superior pubic rami.
The hip joint – the articulation between the acetabulum and the femur.
- Inspect the iliac crests for symmetry and equality of height.
- Look at the number and level of gluteal folds.
- Look at the size of the buttocks.

- Inspect the femoral area for signs of tracking and associated cellulitus – **drug misuse**.
- In supine position, inspect the body alignment, looking for external rotation of the hips and inequality of leg length – **often seen in osteo-arthritis, fractures or dislocations of the hip**.
- Gait **(refer to the general survey in this chapter and Chapters 2 and 9)**.
- Palpate bursal sites.
- In supine position, palpate hips and pelvis for tenderness, increased temperature or crepitus.
- Rock the pelvis from side to side while holding the iliac crests to test for stability at the sacroiliac joints.
- With the patient lying prone, apply slight pressure to the sacrum to test for stability at the symphysis pubis – **this joint can become lax in women carrying and/or following the birth of large babies**.
- Observe the patient as he goes through the range of movements:
  - in supine position:
    - raise the leg above the body keeping the knee in extension – **flexion**
    - raise the leg above the body and then flex the knee and bring it towards the chest – **flexion** (Fig. 11.14)

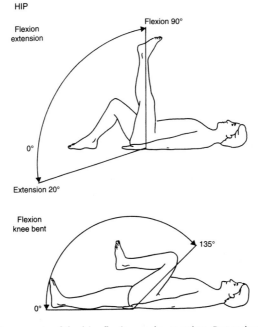

HIP

Flexion extension

Flexion 90°

0°

Extension 20°

Flexion knee bent

135°

0°

Fig. 11.14 Movements of the hip, flexion and extension. Reproduced from Talley & O'Connor (1998). © 1998, Elsevier, Sydney.

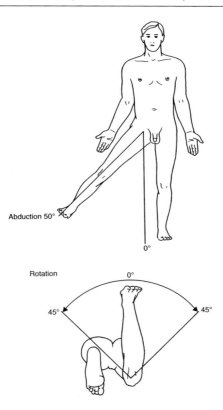

Abduction 50°

0°

Rotation   0°

45°   45°

Fig. 11.15 Movements of the hip, abduction and rotation. Reproduced from Talley & O'Connor (1998). © 1998, Elsevier, Sydney.

Hold the iliac crest as the patient goes through the movement and feel when the pelvis takes over from the hip joint. This will enable an accurate measurement of range (Fig. 11.15).

- swing the leg across the body – **adduction**
- swing the leg outwards – **abduction**
- place the side of the patient's foot on his opposite knee and move the flexed knee towards the side of the examination couch – **external rotation**
- place the side of the patient's foot on the side of the examination couch with the knee flexed and let the patient's leg fall inwards – **internal rotation**
- in prone or standing position:
  - ask the patient to swing his straightened leg behind his body – **hyperextension**

Knees

The articulation between the femur, patella and tibia.

- Inspect the knee in flexion and extension.
- Inspect for swelling, contour and symmetry.
- Inspect the popliteal region for swelling with the knee in extension.
- Inspect the patella, particularly as the knee is flexed. **Ensure that the patella tracks in a straight line and the quadriceps femoris tendon is not pulling it laterally due to the muscle being lax.**
- During walking, observe for any locking of the knee or giving way – **ligament injuries, loose bodies within the joint, meniscal tears.**
- Palpate the suprapatellar pouch and bursae of the knee – **suprapatellar, prepatellar, infrapatellar ligaments and semimembranosus.**
- Palpate the medial and lateral collateral ligaments for any pain, and the cruciate ligaments.
- Palpate the patella, holding at the apex of the patella, to ensure that it moves freely.
- Palpate the head of fibula and tibial tuberosity for any pain or tenderness.
- Palpate the medial and lateral joint surfaces.
- If swelling is present at the knee, test for an effusion – **'bulge sign'.** Milk up the medial side of the swelling so that it disappears behind the patella, lightly tap the lateral side and the bulge will reappear. A positive bulge sign may be absent in large effusions.
- Observe the patient as he goes through the range of movements:
  - bend the knee – **flexion**
  - straighten the knee – **extension** (Fig. 11.16)
  - in supine position, place your hand under the patient's knee and ask him to press down against your hand – **hyperextension; if a patient has hyperextended knees, you will not be able to place your hand between his knee and the examination couch**

Flexion to 135° ↓

Extension to 5° ↑

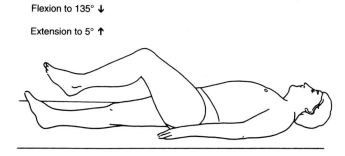

Fig. 11.16 Movements of the knee. Reproduced from Talley & O'Connor (1998). © 1998, Elsevier, Sydney.

- If ligament injury is suspected, ligament instability tests should be performed; these tests are beyond the scope of this chapter, refer to texts that address sports injury.

Ankles

The articulation between the tibia, fibula and talus.
The subtalar joint – the articulation between the calcaneum and the talus.

- Inspect the ankle during weight bearing and non-weight bearing.
- Inspect the Achilles tendon for ulcers or necrosis – **damage to the Achilles tendon can result in a *foot drop*, so the patient's foot should be inspected for plantarflexion and adduction at rest**.
- Inspect the condition of the medial and lateral malleoli.
- Inspect the condition of the calcaneum.
- Inspect the ankle for swelling and contour – **particularly over the anterior aspect of the ankle where swelling is more visible**.
- Palpate the ankle for oedema, pain or tenderness.
- Palpate the Achilles tendon for any pain – **to test if the Achilles is intact, have the patient either kneeling or with his legs hanging over the edge of an examination couch. Apply pressure just below the fullest part of the calf; if the Achilles tendon is intact the foot will plantarflex. If it does plantarflex but with pain, the gastrocnemius muscle is causing the problem rather than the Achilles tendon. If the Achilles tendon is ruptured, the foot will not plantarflex**.
- Palpate the calcaneum for any pain.
- If spinal cord compression is suspected assess for ankle clonus.
- Observe the patient as he goes through the range of movements:
  - point the foot downwards – **plantarflexion**
  - point the foot upwards – **dorsiflexion**
  - rotate the foot laterally – **abduction**
  - rotate the foot medially – **adduction**
  - point the medial side of the foot towards the floor – **eversion**
  - point the lateral side of the foot towards the floor – **inversion**

Toes

The tarsometatarsal joint – the articulation between the distal portions of the talus and the metatarsal bones.
The metatarsophalangeal joints – the articulation between the metatarsal bone and the proximal phalanx.
The interphalangeal joint – the articulation between the distal and proximal phalanx bones.

- Inspect each toe for calluses, corns, hammer toes and general condition of the skin.
- Inspect the hallux for evidence of valgus deformities (**bunions**).
- On weight bearing, inspect for the presence of an arch.
- Inspect the condition of the plantar aspect of the foot.
- Palpate each of the toes for pain or tenderness.
- Palpate for any pain on the plantar, lateral and medial aspects of the foot.
- Provide passive movement to each of the metatarsophalangeal and interphalangeal joints to assess for **flexion**, **extension** and **hypertension** using the index finger and thumb. Assess for any bogginess of the joints or pain elicited during movement.
- Observe the patient as he goes through the active range of movements:
  - curl up the toes – **full flexion**
  - straighten the toes – **full extension**
  - spread the toes out – **abduction**

Muscle strength tests

Upper limb
- With elbows flexed, ask the patient to hold his arms above his head. You should apply pressure to the palm of his hands – **deltoids**.
- With arms in extension, ask the patient to flex his elbows; you should try and hold his arms in extension – **biceps**.
- With the arms flexed, ask the patient to extend them whilst you try to hold them in a flexed position – **triceps**.
- Ask the patient to shrug his shoulders against resistance from you – **trapezius. (This test will also assess the motor function of cranial nerve XI.)**
- Ask the patient to maintain wrist flexion whilst you try to extend the wrist – **wrist flexors**.
- Ask the patient to maintain his wrist in extension as you try to flex it – **wrist extensors**.
- Ask the patient to squeeze your first two fingers bilaterally to assess his **grip strength**.
- Ask the patient to maintain a fist whilst you try to extend the fingers.
- Ask the patient to keep his fingers in extension as you try to flex them into a fist.
- Ask the patient to spread his fingers out while you try to push them together.
- Ask the patient to put his fingers together as you try to pull them apart (Fig. 11.17).

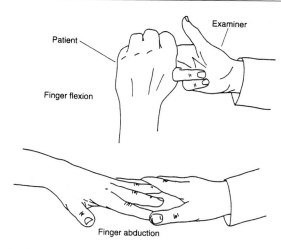

Fig. 11.17 Testing power in the hand.
Reproduced from Talley & O'Connor (1998). © 1998, Elsevier, Sydney.

Lower limb

In supine position:

- Ask the patient to raise his extended leg while you try to hold it down – **gluteals**.
- Ask the patient to push his extended knees outwards against your hands – **gluteals and tensor fascia lata**.
- Ask the patient to push his extended knees inwards against your hands – **gluteals and adductors**.
- Ask the patient to extend his knee as you try to flex it – **quadriceps**.
- Ask the patient to flex his knee you try to extend it – **hamstrings**.
- Ask the patient to dorsiflex his foot against your hand – **tibialis anterior and extensors**.
- Ask the patient to plantarflex his foot against your hand – **tibialis posterior, flexors, gastrocnemius and soleus**.
- Ask the patient to push the side of his foot against your hands.

In sitting position (with legs hanging):

- Ask the patient to cross his legs alternately – **hamstrings, gluteals, hip abductors and hip adductors**.

Terms of location

Anterior	The front of the body.
Posterior	The back of the body.
Medial	Towards the midline of the body.
Lateral	Away from the midline of the body.
Inferior	Below, or in the direction of the bottom of the body.
Superior	Above, or in the direction of the top of the body.
Proximal	Towards the midpoint of the body, or another structure.
Distal	Away from the midpoint of the body, or another structure.
Dorsal	On, or in the direction of the back of the hand, or top of the foot.
Plantar	On, or in the direction of the sole of the foot.
Palmar	On, or in the direction of the palm of the hand.

Terms used to describe ROM

Flexion	To make the inner angle of the joint smaller.
Extension	To make the inner angle of the joint larger.
Abduction	To move away from the midline of the body.
Adduction	To move towards the midline of the body.
Lateral bending	Side bending.
Internal rotation	Rotating around a long axis, inwardly.
External rotation	Rotating around a long axis, outwardly.
Circumduction	Circular movement.
Dorsiflexion	To bend the ankle with the foot moving upwards.
Plantarflexion	To bend the ankle with the foot moving downwards.
Eversion	Turning the sole of the foot out.
Inversion	Turning the sole of the foot inwards.
Pronation	To rotate the forearm with the palm turning inwards.
Supination	To rotate the forearm with the palm turning outwards.
Elevation	Draw up.
Depression	Draw down.
Protraction	Draw forwards.
Retraction	Draw backwards.
Radial deviation	With palm facing down, hand moves towards the body.
Ulnar deviation	With palm facing down, hand moves away from the body.

Reference grid for examination

Joint	Position	Flexion	Hyperflexion	Extension	Hyperextension	Internal rotation	External rotation	Lateral rotation	Adduction	Abduction	Supination	Pronation	Dorsiflexion	Plantarflexion	Eversion	Inversion	Lateral bending	Circumduction	Radial deviation	Ulnar deviation	Opposition	Depression	Elevation	Protraction	Retraction
Jaw	Sitting			■						■															
Neck	Sitting	■		■	■			■									■								
Shoulder	Standing	■		■	■	■	■		■	■								■				■	■	■	■
Elbow	Sitting	■		■							■	■													
Wrist	Sitting	■		■	■						■	■							■	■					
Fingers	Sitting	■	■	■					■	■											■				
Hips	Supine/ Prone	■		■		■	■		■	■															
Knees	Supine	■		■	■																				
Ankles	Supine/ standing												■	■	■	■									
Toes	Supine	■		■					■																
Spine (thoracic and lumbar)	Standing	■		■	■			■									■								

References

Barkauskas, V., Baumann, L. & Darling-Fisher, C. (2002) *Health and Physical Assessment*, 3rd edn. Mosby, London.

Bickley, L. & Szilagyi P. (2007) *Bates' Guide to Physical Examination*, 5th edn. Lippincott, Philadelphia.

Doherty, M., Dacre, J., Dieppe, P. & Snaith, M. (1992) The 'GALS' locomotor screen. *Annals of the Rheumatic Diseases*, **51**(10): 1165–1169.

Epstein, O., Perkin, G., de Bono, D. & Cookson, J. (2008) *Clinical Examination*, 4th edn. Mosby, London.

Jarvis, C. (2008) *Physical Examination and Health Assessment*, 5th edn. Saunders, St Louis.

Seidel, H., Ball, J., Dains, J. & Benedict, G. (2006) *Mosby's Guide to Physical Examination*, 6th edn. Mosby, St Louis.

Swartz, M. (2006) *Textbook of Physical Diagnosis, History and Examination*, 5th edn. Saunders, Philadelphia.

Talley, N. & O'Connor, S. (1998) *Pocket Clinical Examination*. Elsevier, Sydney.

Talley, N. & O'Connor, S. (2006) *Clinical Examination: A Systematic Guide to Physical Diagnosis*, 5th edn. Elsevier, Edinburgh.

Thomas, J. & Monoghan, T. (2007) *Oxford Handbook of Clinical Examination and Practical Skills*. Oxford University Press, Oxford.

Walsh, M. (2006) *Nurse Practitioner's Clinical Skills and Professional Issues*, 2nd edn. Elsevier.

CHAPTER 12

Assessment of the Child

General examination

Introduction

The child health assessment and physical examination is aimed at promoting the health of the child and preventing illness and disability through early identification of actual and potential problems. As a nurse, your anticipatory guidance can be used to help parents deal with physical and developmental issues before they become problems as well as providing early intervention for healthcare needs (Barkauskas *et al.*, 2002; DH, 2004; Epstein *et al.*, 2008; Swartz, 2006).

Approaching the patient

- **Approach the infant/child/young person from the perspective of wellness.** (The term 'young person' is used throughout this text to represent the outdated term 'adolescent' and the term 'young people' is used for 'adolescents'.)
- **Greet the parent/carer and the infant/child/young person using a gentle/normal tone of voice. It is important to use age-appropriate and developmentally appropriate language when talking to infants/ children/young people.**
- **State your name and that you are a nurse.**
- **Make sure the patient is comfortable.**
- **Explain that you wish to ask questions to find out about the health history of the infant/child/young person or what happened to the infant/child/young person.**

> Appropriate consent for this should be obtained from both the parent/carer and child/young person, remembering that different guidance pertains to a child/young person refusing to consent.
>
> Inform the parent/carer and patient how long you are likely to take and what to expect. For example, that after discussing the

infant's/child's/young person's history or what has happened to the infant/child/young person, you would like to examine the infant/child/young person.
- **Use gentle touch.**

General considerations

You will see the infant/child frequently, generally every 2–3 months during infancy when growth changes are the most rapid and dramatic.

Assess the quality of the parent/carer–infant/child/young person relationship. This along with other signs could raise issues of safeguarding children.

Give recognition and praise for parenting/caring skills.

Ask neutral questions.

The history will follow the same sequence as for the adult. Keep in mind physiological differences between infants, children, young people and adults. The format that is generally followed is:
- Biographical information
- Chief complaint
- Present illness or health status
- Past medical history
- Developmental data
- Nutritional data (e.g. breast feeding, if so when started/stopped and bottle augmentation)
- Family history
- Review of systems (physical, sociological and psychological)
- Anticipatory guidance

The physical examination will generally follow the same sequence as for the adult. For example, the physical examination of an infant less than 5 months is relatively straightforward and can proceed cephalocaudally (Barnes, 2003). In the examination you should be prepared for following.
- Infant: respect the parent/carer relationship. Stranger and separation anxiety are important in infants older than 6 months. This peaks at 9 months.
- Toddler: independence is developing. Separation and stranger anxiety makes social interaction challenging. Modify the examination.
- Preschool child: fear of bodily harm is an issue. Allow for play with the equipment on a doll or on you/parent/carer. This reduces fear.
- School-age child: willing participants and curious about what is going on around them. Encourage questions.
- Young person: a period of tremendous growth. Behaviours are not predictable. Young people have a strong orientation toward independence and peer group. They will be starting to question authority. They may be

primarily concerned about themselves and egocentric. Older young people will be goal oriented. Encourage relevant conversation, be non-judgemental. Request opinions/thoughts regarding life/health decisions. Privacy is important. Give the option of an interview with or without the parent/ carer present. Talk with the young person alone as well as with the parent/carer. Examine older young people without the parent/carer present but with a chaperone if necessary.

Usual sequence of events

1. History
2. Examination
3. Problem list
4. Differential diagnosis
5. Investigations
6. Diagnosis confirmed
7. Treatment

Approach to the assessment of the child

Well infant/child/young person visit

- **Biographical data:** DOB, address, phone, nickname, birthplace, ethnicity, primary provider, name of school, last well visit.
- **Source of data:** accompanied by whom, reliability of historian, use of translator or other special circumstances.
- **Chief complaint/reason for visit:** well child versus episodic visit.
- **Past medical history:** prenatal care/exposures, birth history, postnatal period, milestones, childhood illnesses, accidents/injuries, chronic illness, operations/hospitalizations, immunizations, allergies, medications. (In an infant assessment, consider gestational age at birth, birth weight, prenatal care, intrauterine exposures, any problems during labour, delivery and/or the neonatal period) (Barnes, 2003).
- **Interval history:** current status with regard to nutrition, growth and development, elimination and sleep.
- **Review of systems:** any special concerns or worries (systems based).

Episodic visit

- **History of present illness:** location, character/quality, quantity/severity, timing, setting, aggravating/relieving factors, associated factors, parent/ child's perception, any other people sick at home, does illness awaken from sleep, is child **playing, eating, sleeping**, what has already been done to treat illness, coping of family with illness.

Note: young people will not require as much depth with regard to prenatal, birth history and early developmental history (see Box 12.1).

Box 12.1   Approach to history taking – age-related history

Infant (birth–12 months)
- Parent's/carer's perception of infant
- Parent/carer comfort with handling/care
- Condition of parent/carer
- Parent's/carer's perception of growth and development
- Breast versus bottle feeding
- Introduction of solids
- Night waking
- Food intolerances
- Parent's/carer's plans to return to work
- Possible childcare plans
- Siblings/rivalry

Toddler (1–2 years)
- Parent's/carer's reaction to increasing independence
- Struggles/tantrums
- How discipline is managed
- Problems with negativity, autonomy and egocentrism
- Family stressors
- Parent's/carer's perception of growth and development
- Language acquisition
- Feeding/diet
- Sleeping patterns

Preschool (3–5 years)
- School readiness
- Discipline
- Childcare
- Family stressors
- Sibling relations
- Toileting/potty training
- Bladder control
- Bowel control

School age (6–11 years)

- School performance
- Friends/peers
- Extracurricular activities
- Discipline

Young person (12–18 years)

- Home environment: parents/carers, employed, with whom living, parental/carer relationship, other adult relationships
- Education or employment: school performance, favourite subjects, plans after completing school, truant or expelled, employment
- Activities: after-school activities, spare time interests, who young person spends time with

The points that follow are important to discern, if possible. It is extremely difficult to gain information on these points, especially in front of parents/carers, and even when young people are alone they may not answer these questions honestly for fear that their parents would be told. Use discretion when approaching these issues.

- Drugs/alcohol/smoking: use or sale of illicit and over-the-counter/natural drugs, use of steroids or other prescription drugs, friends using or selling drugs (it is useful to acknowledge that many young people experiment with drugs, alcohol or smoking and then proceed to ask about the young person's and friends' use)
- Sexual activity/sexuality: sexual orientation, sexually active (age of first encounter, condom use/birth control, number of partners), history of sexual or physical abuse
- Suicide/depression: unhappy, sad or tearful, tired/unmotivated, feelings of worthlessness, wish/plan for self-harm
- Safety: access to guns, seatbelt use, helmet use, risk taking/high-risk situations (joy riding/car theft, shoplifting, arrests)

Adapted from Barnes & Smart (2003). Additional information from Gill & O'Brien (2007) and Engle (2002).

Differences in anatomy and physiology (Box 12.2)

Box 12.2 Differences in anatomy and physiology

Infant

- Head and neck comprise ~45% of total body surface area
- Higher % of body composition is water (65–75% at birth)
- Infant head is 25% of body length and one-third of weight
- Rapid brain growth reflected in head circumference
- Presence of fontanelles
- Palpable sutures (newborn to 6 months)
- Skin thinner and eccrine (sweat) glands not functioning until 1–2 months
- Unstable/decreased ability to control temperature due to immature hypothalamus
- Poor protection from cold; cannot contract skin/shiver and subcutaneous layer ineffective at insulation
- Melanocytes inefficient at birth
- Well-developed system of lymphoid tissue that grows rapidly after birth
- Dramatic growth and development of nervous system during year 1 of life
- Motor activity under control of spinal cord and medulla; little cortical control
- Peripheral neurones not yet myelinated
- Movements are primarily reflexive (for the first few months)
- Development of cerebral cortex inhibits reflexes with subsequent disappearance of primitive reflexes
- Development proceeds in cephalocaudal and proximodistal directions, paralleling spinal cord myelination
- Rapidly improving visual acuity
- Nasolacrimal duct system not functioning until 3 months
- Tongue is larger in proportion to the mouth
- Ethmoid, maxillary and sphenoid sinuses present but small
- External auditory canal relatively short and straight
- Eustachian tubes shorter, wider, more horizontal

- Heart is more horizontal and higher in the thoracic cavity (apex 4th ICS)
- Smaller/narrower airways
- Supporting structures of respiratory tree not fully developed
- Respiratory efforts are largely abdominal due to reliance on the diaphragm for breathing
- Chest wall much thinner with little musculature; sounds easily transmitted
- Obligate nose breathers (up to 6–12 weeks); nasal obstruction can be dangerous
- Prominent abdomen with poor muscle tone.
- Stomach capacity is small but increases rapidly with age, while gastric emptying time is faster.
- Proportionately longer gastrointestinal tract is a source of greater fluid loss
- Liver takes up proportionately more space in the abdomen
- Bladder located higher in the abdomen (between symphysis pubis and umbilicus)
- C-shaped curvature of the spine

Toddler
- Continues to have disproportionately large head
- 40% total body surface area composed of head and trunk
- By the end of the first year of life, the brain has reached approximately two-thirds of its adult size and is 90% complete by 2 years of age
- Chest circumference surpasses head circumference by 18 months
- Myelination of the spinal cord almost complete by 2 years of age
- Ear canals narrow with upward slope
- Ethmoid and maxillary sinuses slightly more developed (no frontal and sphenoid is minute)
- Lymphoid tissue well developed with rapid growth rate
- Heart continues to be more horizontal and higher in the thoracic cavity (apex 4th ICS and S_3 may be heard)
- Thin chest wall; sounds easily transmitted
- Weak abdominal musculature gives appearance of a potbelly
- Erect posture develops anterior curve to lumbar spine
- Voluntary movement under cortical control
- Development of gross motor skills parallels distal myelination

Preschool

- Face tends to grow proportionally
- Most physiological systems mature
- Elongation of the limbs
- Total body surface area of head and trunk ~38%
- Neck with adult proportions by 4 years of age
- Hypertrophied lymph tissue (reaches adult size by 6 years of age)
- Superficial lymph nodes often palpable as normal variant
- Ethmoid and maxillary sinuses slightly more developed (no frontal and sphenoid still minute)
- Heart is more horizontal and higher in the thoracic cavity (reaches adult position at 7 years of age)
- Thin chest wall; sounds easily transmitted
- Adult proportions

School age

- Adult proportions
- Ethmoid sinus grows rapidly between 6 and 8 years of age
- Frontal sinus develops ~7 years of age; sphenoid minute until puberty
- Jaw widens for eruption of permanent teeth
- Heart reaches adult position in thoracic cavity by 7 years of age
- Under age 7 respiratory movement is primarily abdominal or diaphragmatic
- Lymph tissues hypertrophied to greater than adult size and are at the peak of their development (regression of tissue to adult size occurs during adolescence)
- Continued growth and development of nervous system

Young person

- Rapidly accelerating physical growth (reaches peak at 11–14 years of age)
- In females, an increase in total body fat content is associated with pubertal development
- Growth decelerates in females by 14–17 years of age
- Males become more muscular with a peak deceleration in the rate of fat accumulation at the time of growth spurt
- In general, females reach maturity about 1.5–2 years earlier than males

- Testosterone stimulates growth of thyroid and cricoid cartilages and laryngeal muscles, resulting in deepening of the male voice
- Major organ systems mature with orderly development of musculoskeletal system from distal to proximal parts of the body
- Increased size and strength of the heart
- Lungs increase in diameter and length with concomitant increase in respiratory volume, vital capacity and respiratory functional efficiency
- Gastrointestinal development leads to increase in size and capacity which assume adult levels at about 14 years of age
- Development of secondary sex characteristics which develop as a result of puberty
- Menarche closely related to the peak of the weight velocity curve and the deceleration phase of the height velocity curve and genetic and nutritional factors
- Neurophysiological structures and function completely developed by the end of middle adolescence
- Slight atrophy of lymph tissue to adult size

Adapted from Todd & Barnes (2003), and Barnes (1998). Additional information from Gill & O'Brien (2007) and Engle (2002).

Developmental considerations affecting the physical assessment
(Box 12.3)

Box 12.3   Developmental considerations affecting the physical assessment

Infant
- Most dramatic and rapid period of growth and development
- Attachment to and trust in parent/carer are important
- Stranger anxiety appears ~6 months of age
- Object permanence not developed until ~10–12 months of age
- Separation anxiety starts to affect social interactions at about 9 months of age
- Safety is paramount as gross and fine motor development progress rapidly

Toddler

- Separation and stranger anxiety continue to influence social interactions
- Autonomy, egocentrism and negativism are major developmental issues
- Parent/carer is home-base for explorations
- Knows 6–8 body parts by 30 months
- Fears bodily harm
- Verbal communication skills limited
- Safety continues to be paramount

Preschool

- Development of sense of initiative is important
- Able to 'help', participate and co-operate
- Knows most body parts and some internal parts
- Fears bodily harm
- Verbal communication skills more advanced
- Cognition characterized by egocentricity, literal interpretations and magical thinking

School age

- Sense of industry is important
- Articulate and active participant in care
- Increased self-control
- Understands simple scientific explanations (cause and effect) although thinking still concrete

Young person

- Increasing independence
- Time of tremendous growth and change
- Older young people have an orientation to the future
- Separates easily from parents/carers
- Peer group important
- Knows basic anatomy and physiology
- Has own opinions/ideas
- Active and articulate participant in care

Adapted from Barnes & Smart (2003). Additional information from Gill & O'Brien (2007) and Engle (2002).

Developmental approach to the physical assessment (Box 12.4)

Box 12.4   Developmental approach to the physical assessment

Infant

- Keep parent/carer in view
- Before 6 months of age examine on table; after 6 months examine in parent's/carer's lap
- Undress fully in warm room
- Careful with nappy removal
- Distract with bright objects/rattles
- Soft manner, avoid loud noises and abrupt movements
- Have bottle or dummy handy
- Vary examination sequence with activity level (if asleep/quiet, auscultate heart, lungs and abdomen first)
- Proceed in a cephalocaudal sequence
- Elicit reflexes during the examination
- Save the traumatic procedures for last (ears and temperature, for example)

Toddler

- Most difficult group to examine
- Approach gradually and minimize initial physical contact
- Leave with parent (sitting or standing if possible)
- Allow toddler to inspect equipment (demonstration usually not helpful)
- Start inspection distally through play (toes/fingers)
- Praise the toddler
- Parent removes clothes gradually as needed (toddlers do not like being undressed or touched)
- Describe examination in short phrases
- Save ears, mouth and anything lying down for last

Preschool

- Allow close proximity to parent/carer
- Usually co-operative; able to proceed head to toe
- Request self-undressing (bit by bit exposure – modesty important)
- Expect co-operation

- Allow for choice when possible
- If unco-operative, start distally with play
- Allow brief inspection of equipment with demonstration and brief explanation
- Use games/stories for co-operation
- Paper-doll technique very effective*
- Praise, reward and positive reinforcement
- Examine the genitalia last

School age

- Usually co-operative
- Child should undress self; privacy is important, provide gown if possible
- Explain purpose/function of equipment; spare equipment is useful for them to hold/look at and use on a doll, paper doll* or on you or parent/carer
- Examination can be an important teaching exercise
- Examine in a head-to-toe direction
- Examine the genitalia last
- Praise and feedback regarding normalcy is important

Young person

- Give option of parent/carer being present during the examination
- Undress in private, provide gown
- Expose one area at a time
- The examination can be an important teaching exercise
- Examine in head-to-toe sequence
- Examine genitalia last
- Feedback regarding normalcy is important
- Anticipatory guidance regarding sexual development (use Tanner staging)
- Matter-of-fact approach to history and examination
- Encourage appropriate decision-making skills

* Draw doll on examination table paper. Point out/draw where body parts are located on the doll.
Adapted from Barnes & Smart (2003). Additional information from Gill & O'Brien (2007) and Engle (2002).

The examination of infants, children and young people requires flexibility.

- **Allow the infant's/child's/young person's developmental level** to guide your history taking and physical examination.
- **The atmosphere and environment** are important. The room should be warm with appropriate decoration and the use of toys. Take into consideration the special needs of young people, including an unhurried social environment. Always limit the number of people in the room.
- **Remain organized.** Things can easily slip into chaos, particularly with children.
- **Exercise care in the use of equipment and remember safety.** Little hands can grab equipment. Do not leave the child unattended on the examination table. Maintain safety with outlets and equipment.
- **The assessment**, whether comprehensive or episodic, is always head to abdomen.
- **Incorporate health education and growth and development** anticipatory guidance into the examination.
- **Move from the easy/simple** to more distressing; use positive reinforcement and 'prizes'.
- **Use demonstration** and play to your advantage.
- **Expect an age-appropriate level of co-operation.**

Table 12.1 Physical examination of the infant and toddler

System	Normal variants	Abnormal variants
General appearance • Parent/carer/ child interaction • Posture, position, movement • Hygiene • Nutrition • Weight • Height • Head circumference	• Pink, well-nourished, well-dressed, bright-eyed and alert infant in no apparent distress, positive parent/carer/child interaction, moving all 4 extremities • 0–6 months: weight gain = 140–210 g/week (35–57 ounces); increase in length = 1.25 cm (0.5 inches/month – PLOT) • Head is ~2 cm > chest until 6–24 months when chest > head – PLOT • Birth weight regained by 7–10 days • Birth weight doubled by 4–6 months • Birth weight tripled by 1 year • Height at 2 years about half adult height • Growth can be characterized by 'spurts'	• Parent/carer displays uninterested attitude toward infant and/or lack of attachment • Dysmorphic features, facies and/or movements • Foul or unusual odour from child • Rapidly growing or non-growing head • Weight loss or failure to gain weight (after 10 days of age) • Wide discrepancy between height, weight and head percentiles

Vital signs (observations)
• Temperature
• Apical pulse
• Respiratory rate
• Blood pressure (auscultate, palpate, or flush methods)
	• Vital signs within expected range:
	  – Count apical pulse for 60 seconds – sinus arrhythmic normal (rate increases on inspiration)
	  – Respiratory pattern in infants can be erratic – count for 60 seconds and watch abdomen as breathing is more diaphragmatic than thoracic
	  – Palpation yields systolic pressure, flush yields mean B/P
		• Vital signs outside expected range

Table 12.1 *(continued)*

System	Normal variants	Abnormal variants
Skin, nails and hair	• Warm skin with pink undertones • Mongolian spots common (especially in black, Latino and Asian infants) • *Café-au-lait* spots common • Haemangiomas common (stork bite/salmon patch, cherry angioma and strawberry haemangioma) • Neonatal acne, milia, erythema toxicum, seborrhoea of the scalp are common • Mottling/reticulated pattern over extremities in response to cold room (cutis marmorata) • Jaundice in newborn (3rd–4th day of life) requires investigation (assess in natural light) • Assess turgor on abdomen • Pink nailbeds with good capillary refill • Infant hair may be patchy especially at temples and occiput • Newborn with lanugo (downy hair)	• Poor colour or cyanosis • 6 or >6 *café-au-lait* spots requires evaluation (neurofibromatosis) • Cavernous haemangioma or naevus flammeus (port wine stain) • Unfamiliar rash • Persistent mottling/cyanosis • Jaundice on 1st day of life or after 2 weeks of age • Bruising • Poor turgor/lack of subcutaneous fat • Discoloured nailbeds of clubbing • Hair tufts/dimples/break in skin on spine requires investigation

Head, neck, lymph nodes, eyes, ears, nose, mouth and throat

- Palpate suture lines in newborn: frontal, coronal, sagittal, lambdoidal
- Sutures may overlap at birth with moulded appearance to head
- Newborn: bogginess (bleeding into the periosteum) evidenced by swelling that does not cross the suture line (cephalohaematoma) or oedematous swelling of the superficial tissues of the scalp evidenced by generalized soft swelling not bounded by suture lines (caput succedaneum)
- Frontal bossing (prominence of the forehead) characteristic of premature infants
- Anterior fontanelle begins to close at ~9 months; closes ~18 months (soft but firm, slightly concave, may pulsate slightly and will tense slightly with crying)
- Posterior fontanelle closes ~1–2 months (may be closed/ absent at birth)
- Supple neck that moves easily, symmetrical alignment of head and clavicles
- Short neck
- An infant <4 months of age may show head lag when pulled to a sitting position
- Lymph glands not normally palpable in infants
- Cervical lymph nodes difficult to examine in toddlers: soft, round, slightly boggy, non-tender (diffuse cervical nodes common)

- Palpable sutures >6 months
- Marked asymmetry of the head that persists (investigate)
- Absence of or markedly enlarged (>2.5 or 2.6 cm) anterior fontanelle
- Bulging or sunken anterior fontanelle
- Resistance or pained crying with ROM of neck and/or head tilt
- Webbed neck/congenital torticollis (investigate)
- Poor head control or marked lag >4 months
- Firm/hard warm, red, tender, enlarged nodes
- Prominent supraclavicular node (investigate)
- Lack of papillary or blink reflex/response
- Lack of vestibular function reflex
- Absence of red reflex (retinal disorders) and presence of white reflex

Table 12.1 (continued)

System	Normal variants	Abnormal variants
Head, neck, lymph nodes, eyes, ears, nose, mouth and throat (continued)	• Inguinal nodes often palpable • Epitrochlear and axillary nodes usually not palpable • Pupils equal, round, reactive to light (PERRL) • Newborn blinks when bright light is introduced • Tilt to open eyes and turn head to one side whilst holding upright: assess for fixation (tests vestibular function reflex), red reflex and white reflex (cataract or retinoblastoma) • At 2 weeks fixates on bright object • At 1 month fixates on object and follows to midline • At 6 months fixates and follows 180° • Symmetry of corneal light reflex >6 months • Bright clear eyes, white sclera, no discharge • Tiny dark flecks in sclera of black and Asian children is common • Grey blue or 'muddy' colour of sclera in black children • Newborn may have residual chemical inflammation s/p eye drops (< or = 24 h); sclera may have blue tint; lacrimal glands not functioning at birth, eye colour not confirmed until 9 months of age	• Inability to fixate and follow objects • Asymmetry of corneal light reflex • Purulent discharge from eyes • Swelling of lachrymal duct with discharge • Low-set ears or deviation in alignment (mental retardation or GU problem), foul or sweet odour from canal • TM: abnormal light reflex, contour, lack of landmarks or movement; red/purple • Nasal flaring • Cleft or notched palate (hard or soft) • White non-removable plaques on tongue or buccal mucosa (thrush)

- Tip of pinna at height of outer corner of eye and 10° from vertical (posteriorly)
- Canal with some soft cerumen
- Tympanic membrane (TM) difficult to see before 1 month of age
- Pearly TM with sharp landmarks, cone of light and gentle movement
- TM will redden with crying (fades on inspiration)
- Patent nares (check for breath on stethoscope with one nare blocked)
- Ethmoid, maxillary and sphenoid sinuses present at birth, however quite small (sphenoid is minute)
- Sucking tubercle possible finding in older infants (salivation starts ~3 months)
- Newborn: fused palate, pink gingivae with raised ridge, pearls on palate/gum
- Moist pink membranes
- Eruption of lower centrals at ~6 months (to estimate dentition in children <2 years subtract '6' from the child's age in months)
- Throat is clear and pink
- Tonsils not visible in newborn
- No teeth by 12–15 months of age
- 3+ to 4+ tonsils

Table 12.1 *(continued)*

System	Normal variants	Abnormal variants
Breasts and chest	<ul><li>Toddler: 1+ to 2+ common</li><li>Rounded symmetrical thoracic cage that is smaller in circumference than head (at nipple line ~2 cm smaller than head until about 2 years of age)</li><li>2nd rib attaches at sternal angle (angle of Louis)</li><li>Anteroposterior measurement is equal to side-to-side (lateral) measurement, giving chest a circular or 'barrel' shape</li><li>Symmetrical nipples placed (slightly lateral of midclavicular line between 4th or 5th ribs) with flat nipple and slightly darker pigmentation to areola</li><li>Newborn may have a slight enlargement of breast tissue with clear or white fluid from nipple (witch's milk) – resolves within a few days/weeks</li></ul>	<ul><li>Variations in shape, symmetry or movement</li><li>Supernumerary nipple(s)</li></ul>
Pulmonary (respiratory)	<ul><li>Count rate for full minute (easiest to count when sleeping)</li><li>Common for respiratory pattern to be irregular (patterns of apnoea for 10–15 seconds not unusual)</li><li>Abdominal bulge with respiration with little chest movement</li><li>May have slight flaring of lower costal margins normal</li><li>Palpation yields no masses or lumps</li><li>Percussion is not very useful in infants</li><li>Crying can enhance auscultation of breath sounds (listen closely on expiration)</li><li>Auscultate all fields systematically and symmetrically from apices to bases</li></ul>	<ul><li>Rate not within normal limits for age</li><li>Nasal flaring, sternal/intercostal retractions or grunting</li><li>Adventitious sounds: discontinuous sounds (crackles) or continuous sounds (wheezes = high-pitched hissing or shrill quality and ronchi = low pitched and have a snoring quality)</li></ul>

- Bronchovesicular sounds throughout lung fields
- Transmission of upper airway sounds common
- Breath sounds may sound louder/harsher due to thinness of chest wall
- Upper airway sounds easily transmitted (listen at nose, sounds will be louder)
- Paediatric stethoscope makes auscultation easier (less 'noise' since diaphragm is smaller)

- Diminished or absent breath sounds, tubular sounds over lung fields/prolonged expiratory phase (indicating consolidation)

Cardiovascular		

- Inspect nailbeds (hands and feet) = pink with brisk capillary refill
- Note any extracardiac signs (pallor, cyanosis, distress)
- Palpate the precordium and locate the PMI (higher up on the thorax – 4th ISC lateral of MCL)
- Auscultate as for adult, one sound at a time; follow systematic approach
- Sinus arrhythmic normal (accelerates with inspiration)
- Heart sounds louder due to thin chest wall
- Infant – difficult to separate S_1 and S_2 (S_2 higher pitch and louder at the base)
- Soft murmurs (e.g. S_3) grade 1/6 or 2/6 systolic murmur in newborn for first 2–3 days or continuous 'machinery' murmur (PDA) within first 2–3 days in newborn
- If newborn has a murmur at birth, re-evaluate after day 3 of life

- Poor refill or absence of pink undertones
- Infant or toddler with signs and symptoms of CHF (respiratory distress, wet lungs, enlarged liver and tachycardia)
- Murmurs persisting after 3 days of life in newborn (although S_3 may remain present and is not considered pathological)
- Very loud holosystolic (pansystolic) or diastolic murmurs

Table 12.1 *(continued)*

System	Normal variants	Abnormal variants
Abdomen	• Contour of abdomen is protuberant but symmetrical • Fine superficial venous pattern • Inspect umbilical cord in newborn • + bowel sounds • Tympani over stomach with dullness at liver edge and bladder • Assess turgor over abdomen • Soft abdomen (flex knees up by holding feet frog-legged; feed or use dummy if crying) • Umbilical hernia common (increased incidence in black infants) with increased prominence when crying (can be up to 2.5 cm) • Diastasis recti common (increased incidence in black infants) – separation of rectus muscle causing a visible bulge • Caecum easily palpable in RLQ and sigmoid colon (soft sausage in left inguinal area that moves) • Infant liver fills RUQ with border ~ at right costal margin or 1–2 cm below • May feel spleen tip 1–2 cm below left costal margin (roll onto left side) • Palpate for femoral pulses (strong and equal bilaterally) • Palpate for femoral hernia (3 fingers spread medially from pulse)	• Scaphoid shape • Dilated veins • Inflammation or drainage at umbilicus or cord • Absent or diminished bowel sounds • Tethering or poor recoil of skin • Crying or obvious pain with palpation • Masses or lumps (check epigastric area for olive shaped mass = pyloric stenosis and pyloric regurgitation may be auscultated) • Umbilical hernia >2.5 cm • Diastasis recti after 3 months of age • Masses • Enlarged liver • Enlarged spleen (feels like a water balloon) • Full, bounding or absent femoral pulses • Femoral hernia

Musculoskeletal

- Observe movement, general symmetry and muscle strength/tone
- Count fingers and toes
- Slight tremulousness in hands/feet of newborn normal
- Start at feet and work up
- Toddlers: wide-based gait with arms out for balance
- Check flexibility of heel cords (angle of foot to tibia 80° or less)
- Feet often appear flat (pes planus) due to fat pads and non-weight bearing
- Palpate forefoot for mobility and positioning in relation to hindfoot (flexible metatarsus adductus – concave medial border and convex lateral border of foot – acceptable up to age 3 although position and stretching exercises may be done)
- Bow-legged (genu varum) stance of toddlers (<2.5 cm between knees when medial malleoli are together)
- Check for tibial torsion: with knees bent, place fingers on malleoli (all 4 malleoli should be parallel or less than 20° out of straight with medial malleolus anterior to lateral malleolus)
- Check hips for Galeazzi's or Allis' sign
- Unequal thigh folds
- Ortolani's sign (check every visit until 1 year of age) – With the infant supine, put your thumbs on the inner aspect of both thighs and your fingertips resting over the trochanter muscles, flex both hips and knees; abduct each knee until the lateral aspects of the knees touch the examining table; note that this test is reliable until the child is 1 year of age; in the older infant it is less reliable (use ROM of hips after 1 year)

- Hyper/hypotonia and scissoring
- Extra digits
- Marked tremors
- Abnormal gait
- Tight heel cords or foot rigidity
- Fixed adduction of forefoot with inversion (metatarsus varus – not able to be brought to neutral position with passive ROM)
- Talipes equinovarus (clubfoot) fixed metatarsus varus with downward pointing of foot (equinus)
- Tibial torsion (lateral malleolus anterior to medial malleolus)
- Click/clunk during manoeuvre = DDH (developmental dysplasia of the hip)
- Uneven knees – Galeazzi's or Allis'
- Uneven gluteal folds (investigate)
- Limited abduction (investigate)
- Lack of symmetry, simian crease or webbing of fingers/toes
- Fractured clavicle or irregularity
- Tufts, dimples, cysts, masses along spine

Table 12.1 *(continued)*

System	Normal variants	Abnormal variants
Musculoskeletal *(continued)*	• Barlow's test (this test is less reliable in the neonate) – with the infant supine, flex and slightly adduct both hips; at the same time, lift the femur and apply pressure to the trochanter • Check arms, hands and palmar crease • Palpate clavicles in newborn and arm ROM: smooth, even, regular • C-shape to spine of infant; lumbar lordosis in toddler • Inspect spine: smooth without dimples, tufts, cyst or mass	

Neurological	• A large part of the examination is observational: smoothness of movement and spontaneous activity
	• Bright, active and alert appearance unless asleep
	• Strong cry and suck in newborn
	• CN assessment for newborn:
	  – CN II, III, IV, VI: optic blink reflex to bright light
	  – CN V: rooting and sucking reflex
	  – CN VII: facial movements
	  – CN VIII: Moro (startle reflex) or acoustic blink reflex
	  – CN IX, X: swallowing, gag reflex, co-ordinated suck
	  – CN XII: pinch nose and mouth will open with tongue rise in midline
	• Note/monitor newborn reflexes (rooting, Moro, sucking, plantar and palmar grasp, Babinski, tonic neck, placing, stepping Galant)
	• Note developmental milestones: fix/follow, head lag/head control, sitting, loss of primitive reflexes, fine motor development
		• Jerkiness, tremors, flaccidity
		• Altered level of consciousness
		• Weak cry and/or poor suck
		• Hyper/hyporeflexive newborn
		• Absence or poor response
		• Persistence of primitive reflexes
		• Lack of milestone achievement

Genitourinary

- **Male:** keep warm with nappy on before exam (cremasteric reflex is strong)
- Inspect penis (size, circumcized/non-circumcized)
- Meatus at midline and at tip slightly voiding in straight stream (by history)
- Foreskin tight until 3 months of age (DO NOT RETRACT)
- Testicles descended bilaterally (block inguinal canal)
- Have toddler sit cross-legged to block canals (migratory testes common due to strength of cremasteric reflex)
- Fluid in scrotum in children <2 years of age is common (transilluminate for hydrocoele)
- Palpate for inguinal hernia
- **Female:** external genitalia may be engorged at birth (and for a few weeks following birth) with slight sanguineous drainage from maternal oestrogen effect
- Inspect external genitalia for position, intact structures and presence of vagina
- Smooth, shiny mucosa without excoriation/irritation

- **Male:** red inflamed or oozing penile tip
- Ambiguous genitalia
- Poor stream, pinpoint meatus and/or hypospadias or epispadias
- Phimosis/paraphimosis
- Cryptorchidism
- Hydrocoele > age 2 or if accompanied by pain, non-illumination or increase in size
- Inguinal hernia
- **Female:** ambiguous genitalia
- Anatomical/structural abnormality
- Excoriation, irritation, foul odour or discharge or signs/symptoms of abuse

Rectum/anus

- Patency
- Anal reflex
- Absence of fissure, redness, lesions
- Nappy dermatitis common

- Imperforate anus
- Lack of sphincter tone
- Fissure, redness, lesions, signs/symptoms of sexual abuse
- Severe nappy dermatitis, candidiasis, or staphylococcal superinfection

Table 12.2 Physical examination of the child

System	Normal variants	Abnormal variants
General appearance • Parent/carer/child interaction • Behaviour • Mobility • Gross/fine motor skills • Speech • Hygiene • Nutritional status • Weight • Height	• Well-nourished, well-developed, bright-eyed and active child in no apparent distress; positive parent/carer/child interaction • Weight gain: 2 kg/year from 1 to 10 years of age – PLOT • Height gain: 6–8 cm/year (height at 2 years of age ~ half adult height) – PLOT • Growth can be characterized by steady gains along predictable trajectory	• Uninterested attitude of parent/carer, lack of mutual response between child and parent/carer • Dysmorphic features, facies and/or movements • Foul or unusual odour from child • Rapidly growing or non-growing child • Weight loss of failure to gain weight • Wide discrepancy between height and weight
Vital signs (observations) • Temperature • Apical pulse • Respiratory rate • B/P	• Vital signs within expected range • Axillary or tympanic temperature measurement • Count apical pulse for 60 seconds – sinus arrhythmic normal (rate accelerates on inspiration) • Use palpation or flush techniques if unco-operative	• Vital signs outside expected range

| Skin, nails, hair, head, neck, lymph nodes, eyes, ears, nose, mouth and throat | • Warm skin with pink undertones
• Skin slightly dry without rashes, hyperpigmentation or lesions
• Café-au-lait spots common
• Assess turgor on abdomen
• Pink nailbeds with good capillary refill
• Shiny, firm, elastic hair
• No lice
• Head has rounded shape and is held erect
• No discomfort on palpation of sinuses
• Supple neck that moves easily
• Cervical lymph nodes often normally palpable in children: soft, red, slightly boggy non-tender (diffuse cervical nodes common)
• Inguinal nodes often palpable
• Epitrochlear and axillary nodes usually not palpable
• Bright clear eyes, white sclera, no discharge
• Tiny dark flecks in sclera of black and Asian children is common
• Grey blue or 'muddy' colour of sclera in black children
• Pupils equal, round, reactive to light and accommodation (PERRLA)
• Eyeball reaches adult size by 8 years of age (vision 6/9 by 4 years and 6/6 by 7) | • Poor colour or cyanosis
• Excessive sweating in children may accompany hypoglycaemia, heart disease or hyperthyroidism
• 6 or >6 café-au-lait spots requires evaluation (neurofibromatosis)
• Bruising/unusual marks
• Poor turgor/lack of subcutaneous fat
• Discoloured nailbeds or clubbing
• Exceptionally dry or brittle hair (nutritional deficiencies)
• Lice
• Asymmetry with swelling or bruising
• Head consistently held to one side (investigate vision/strabismus)
• Tenderness over sinuses
• Resistance or pained crying with ROM of neck and/or head tilt
• Firm/hard, warm, red, tender, enlarged nodes
• Supraclavicular node (investigate)
• Purulent discharge from eyes
• Lack of papillary response
• Vision outside age-appropriate norms |

Table 12.2   *(continued)*

System	Normal variants	Abnormal variants
Skin, nails, hair, head, neck, lymph nodes, eyes, ears, nose, mouth and throat *(continued)*	<ul><li>Symmetry of corneal light reflex</li><li>Negative cover test</li><li>Optic disc creamy yellow/orange with sharp margins</li><li>Sharp vessels</li><li>Palpebral conjunctivae pink and glossy</li><li>Tip of pinna at height of outer corner of eye and 10° from vertical (posteriorly)</li><li>Canal with some soft cerumen</li><li>Pearly TM with sharp landmarks, cone of light, and gentle movement</li><li>TM will redden with crying (fades on inspiration)</li><li>Patent nares (check for breath on stethoscope with one naris blocked)</li><li>Firm pink membranes</li><li>Moist, pink, firm and smooth oral mucosa</li><li>Teeth in good repair/condition; appropriate number and alignment</li><li>Tonsils usually large and may have crypts</li><li>Uvula at the midline</li></ul>	<ul><li>Asymmetry of corneal light reflex</li><li>No movement of uncovered eye and steadiness of covered eye</li><li>Pallor to disc, opacities, irregular shape or blurred margins of disc</li><li>Congested/dilated vessels</li><li>Cobblestone appearance in allergic children</li><li>Pallor of outer eye canthus in anaemia</li><li>Low-set ears with deviation in alignment</li><li>Foul or sweet odour from canal</li><li>Excoriated or inflamed canal</li><li>Abnormal light reflex, contour, lack of landmarks or movement, red/purple colour</li><li>Nasal flaring</li><li>Boggy, pale or grey mucosa = allergy</li><li>Red, inflamed mucosa = infection</li><li>Bleeding, lesions, swelling of gums</li><li>Dry mucous membranes</li><li>Dental caries</li></ul>

		• Poor hygiene • Red, swollen inflamed tonsils with white membrane or plaques • +3 to +4 tonsils • Deviation of uvula (? upper motor neurone lesion) or absence of movement (investigate) • Variations in shape, symmetry or movement • Supernumerary nipple(s)
Breasts/chest	• Symmetrical thoracic cage that is wider than it is thick • after 7 years of age, breathing is largely thoracic in females but remains abdominal in males • 2nd rib attaches at sternal angle (angle of Louis) • Symmetrical nipples placed (slightly lateral of midclavicular line (between 4th or 5th ribs) with flat nipple and slightly darker pigmentation to areola	
Pulmonary (respiratory)	• Count rate for 30 seconds • Palpation yields no masses or lumps • Percussion only helpful in older children (dullness is heard over liver and heart) • Crying can enhance auscultation of breath sounds (listen closely on expiration) • Auscultate all fields systematically and symmetrically from apices to bases • Bronchovesicular sounds throughout lung fields	• Rate within normal limits for age • Nasal flaring or sternal/intercostal retractions • Adventitious sounds: discontinuous sounds (crackles) or continuous sounds (wheezes = high-pitched hissing or shrill quality and ronchi = low pitched and have a snoring quality)

Table 12.2 *(continued)*

System	Normal variants	Abnormal variants
Pulmonary (respiratory) *(continued)*	• Transmission of upper airway sounds common • Breath sounds may sound louder/harsher due to thinness of chest wall • Upper airway sounds easily transmitted (listen at nose, sounds will be louder) • Paediatric stethoscope makes auscultation easier (less 'noise' since diaphragm is smaller)	• Diminished or absent breath sounds, tubular sounds over lung fields/prolonged expiratory phase (indicating consolidation)

Cardiovascular	• Inspect nailbeds (hands and feet) = pink with good capillary refill
	• Note any extracardiac signs (pallor, cyanosis, distress)
	• Inspect and palpate the precordium
	• Palpate the apical impulse (PMI) = roll onto left side
	  – 4th ICS lateral to MCL at age 4
	  – 4th ICS at MCL age 4–6 years
	  – 5th ISC medial to MCL > age 7
	• Auscultate one sound at a time (S_1 or S_2) for quality, rate, intensity and rhythm
	• Auscultate in 'Z' pattern over thorax
	• Auscultate supine and sitting (left lateral, standing, squatting, standing after squatting = useful positions in evaluation of murmurs)
	• Innocent murmurs common (soft, short, systolic, vibratory, heard best at left sternal border without radiation)
		• Poor refill or absence of pink undertones
		• Thoracic bulging or thrills
		• Signs and symptoms of CHF (respiratory distress, wet lungs, enlarged liver, tachycardia and poor growth)
		• A_2 moves laterally with cardiac enlargement
		• Abnormal sounds and/or S_4
		• Very loud, holosystolic (pansystolic) or diastolic murmurs
		• Murmurs without innocent qualities

Abdomen

- Functional murmurs (physiological murmurs) common with fever
- Sinus arrhythmic normal (accelerates with inspiration)
- Heart sounds louder due to thin chest wall
- Contour of preschool abdomen may be slightly protuberant when standing but flat when supine
- School-age with slim abdominal shape as potbelly lost
- Slight peristaltic waves may be visible in thin children
- + bowel sound (all 4 quadrants)
- Tympani over stomach with dullness at liver edge
- Liver span changes with age/growth
- Soft abdomen (use child's hand to start if ticklish)
- Caecum easily palpable in RLQ and sigmoid colon (soft sausage in left inguinal area that moves)
- May feel spleen tip 1–2 cm below left costal margin (roll onto left side)
- Palpate for femoral pulses (strong and equal bilaterally)
- Palpate for femoral hernia (3 fingers spread medially from pulse)

- Scaphoid shape or distended shape
- Marked peristaltic waves (obstruction)
- Absent or diminished bowel sounds
- Engorged or enlarged liver
- Crying or obvious pain with palpation
- Masses or lumps or bulges (umbilical hernia closed by 4 years of age)
- Enlarged spleen (feels like a water balloon)
- Full, bounding or absent femoral pulses
- Femoral hernia

Musculoskeletal

- Observe movement, general symmetry and muscle strength/tone
- Note gait (base narrow, arms by sides, shoes with wear on outside of heels and inside of toes)

- Hyper/hypotonia and scissoring
- Abnormal gait or limp
- Asymmetry of shoulders or unevenness of scapulae

Table 12.2 *(continued)*

System	Normal variants	Abnormal variants
Musculoskeletal *(continued)*	• Note 'plumb line' down back: back of head, along spine to middle of sacrum • Shoulders level and scapulae even • Preschool child: slight genu valgum (<2.5 cm between medial malleoli when knees together) • Preschool child: may look flat-footed (pes planus) until 36 months due to fat pads at arch • Normal Trendelenburg sign (progressive subluxation of the hip): even iliac crests when weight is shifted from one leg to the other • Full ROM of remaining joints • Check for tibial torsion: with legs hanging over exam table place fingers on malleoli (all 4 malleoli should be parallel or less than 20° out of straight with medial malleolus anterior to lateral malleolus)	• 2.5 cm between medial malleoli • Marked pronation of the foot past 36 months • Subluxation of the hip: uneven iliac crests when weight shifted from one leg to the other (when child stands on 'affected leg' the pelvis drops) • Pain, tenderness, swelling or restricted movement in any joint • Tibial torsion after 3 years of age
Neurological	• A large part of the examination is observational: smoothness of movement, spontaneous activity and behaviour • Bright, interactive • Gross and fine motor skills appropriate for age (able to balance on one foot and hop by 4 years of age and accurate finger-to-nose test with eyes open and closed by 5)	• Jerkiness, tremors, flaccidity, bizarre behaviour • Altered level of consciousness • Delays in fine or gross motor skills • Hyperactivity or decreased/absent reflexes • Absent or poor response

	• Deep tendon reflexes (DTRs) difficult to assess in children under the age of 5
	 • CN assessment in older children as adult:
	   – CN II: fundoscopic
	   – CN III, IV, VI: PERRLA and EOMs
	   – CN V: clenching teeth
	   – CN VII: smile
	   – CN VIII: hearing screen
	   – CN IX, X: rise of uvula with 'ahhhhh'
	   – CN XII: clear speech 'light, tight, dynamite'
		• Persistence of primitive reflexes
		 • Lack of milestone achievement

Genitourinary	• **Male:** inspect penis (size, circumsized/non-circumsized) • Meatus at midline and at tip slightly voiding in straight stream (by history) • Foreskin retractable by 4–5 years of age • Testicles descended bilaterally (block inguinal canal) • Palpate for inguinal hernia • **Female:** inspect external genitalia for position, intact structures and presence of vagina and patent hymen • Smooth shiny mucosa without excoriation/irritation	• **Male:** red inflamed or oozing penile tip • Poor stream, pinpoint meatus and/or hypospadias or epispadias • Phimosis/paraphimosis • Cryptorchidism • Inguinal hernia • **Female:** abnormal anatomical structures • Excoriation, irritation, foul odour or discharge or signs/symptoms of abuse
Rectum/anus	• Absence of fissure, redness, lesions	• Fissure, redness, lesions, signs/symptoms of sexual abuse

Table 12.3   Physical examination of the young person

System	Normal variants	Abnormal variants
General appearance • Hygiene • Dress • Behaviour, mobility • Gross/fine motor skills • Speech • Nutritional status • Weight • Height	• Well-nourished young person in no apparent distress • Parent/carer may or may not be present (as young person prefers) • Weight gain (females) from age 10 to 14 years ~17.5 kg – PLOT • Weight gain (males) from age 12 to 16 years ~23.7 kg – PLOT • Height gain (females) from 11 to 15 years height ~16 cm; 95% of adult height achieved by menarche – PLOT • Height gain (males) from 12 to 16 years ~22 cm; 95% of adult height achieved by 16 years – PLOT • Growth can be characterized by rapid gains with endocrine and hormonal changes, increased bone growth and muscle mass • Females typically double their body weight between 8 and 15 years of age • Males double their body weight between 10 and 17 years of age • Steady gains along predictable trajectory • Vital signs within expected range	• Distressed appearance • Homelessness • Intoxication or under the influence of drugs • Dysmorphic features, facies, and/or movements • Foul or unusual odour from young person • Weight loss or failure to gain weight • Wide discrepancy between height and weight • Vital signs outside expected range
Vital signs (observations) • Temperature • Apical pulse • Respiratory rate • B/P		

Skin, nails, hair, head, neck, lymph nodes, eyes, ears, nose, mouth and throat	• Skin, nails, hair, head, neck, lymph nodes, eyes, ears, nose and throat as adult • Note: acne: location, severity, extent, type (comedones, pustules, cysts), healing or active and any other lesions (peak at 14–16 for girls and 16–19 in boys) • Mouth – underside of teeth without pitting	• Severe acne: cysts, nodules, severe pustules • Pitting, erosion of enamel related to bulimia (exposure of teeth to stomach acids)
Breasts/chest	• **Male:** gynaecomastia is common finding in young males, often presents as tender nodule and may persist for several years • **Female:** Young females may present with cystic changes or fibroadenomas • Tanner staging of female breasts (sexual maturity rating) • Asymmetry in female breast development common	• Variation in shape, symmetry or movement • Cysts or nodule lesion that persists at midpoint of menstrual cycle may require investigation • Breast development <8 years of age requires evaluation • No female breast development by 13 years of age requires evaluation
Pulmonary (respiratory)	• As adult	• As adult
Cardiovascular	• As adult • 20–40% of young people with precordial murmur (evaluate as for children)	• As adult • Murmur without qualities of innocent or functional murmurs
Abdomen	• As adult	• As adult

Table 12.3 *(continued)*

System	Normal variants	Abnormal variants

Musculoskeletal	• As adult
	• Scoliosis screen (standing upright and bent forward):
	  – symmetrical appearance to posterior ribs
	  – equal elevation of shoulders, scapulae and iliac crests
	  – no areas of prominence on one side of back
		• Asymmetry of ribs, shoulders, scapulae or areas of the back

Neurological
Genitourinary
	• As adult
	• **Male:** sexual maturity rating:
	  – enlargement of testes
	  – pubic hair growth (Tanner staging of pubic hair growth)
	  – darkening of scrotal colour
	  – roughening of scrotal skin
	  – increase in penile length and width
	  – axillary hair growth
	• **Female:** sexual maturity rating:
	  – presence of pubic hair (Tanner staging of pubic hair growth)
	  – axillary hair
	  – darkening/dulling of genitalia mucosa
	  – pelvic exam indicated in history of sexual activity
		• As adult
		• **Male:** no development of secondary sex characteristics by 14 years
		• **Female:** no development of secondary sex characteristics by 13 years

Rectum/anus	• As adult (internal examination rarely indicated)	• As adult

Information for tables extracted from Aylott, 2006a,b, 2007a,b; Barkauskas *et al.*, 2002; Barnes, 2003; Bickley & Szilagyi, 2007; Epstein *et al.*, 2008; Swartz, 2006.

References

Aylott, M. (2006a) Developing rigour in observation of the sick child: Part 1. *Paediatric Nursing*, **18**(8): 38–44.

Aylott, M. (2006b) Observing the sick child: Part 2. *Paediatric Nursing*, **18**(9): 38–44.

Aylott, M. (2007a) Observing the sick child: Part 2b Respiratory palpation. *Paediatric Nursing*, **19**(1): 38–45.

Aylott, M. (2007b) Observing the sick child: Part 2c Respiratory auscultation. *Paediatric Nursing*, **19**(3): 38–45.

Barkauskas, V., Baumann, L. & Darling-Fisher, C. (2002) *Health and Physical Assessment*, 3rd edn. Mosby, London.

Barnes, K. (1998) *Lecture Notes on a Developmental Approach to the Assessment of the Paediatric Patient.* City University, London.

Barnes, K. (ed) (2003) *Paediatrics: a Clinical Guide for Nurse Practitioners.* Butterworth Heinemann, London.

Barnes, K. & Smart, F. (2003) A developmental approach to the history and physical examination in paediatrics. In: Barnes, K. (ed) *Paediatrics: A Clinical Guide for Nurse Practitioners.* Butterworth Heinemann, London.

Bickley, L. & Szilagyi, P. (2007) *Bates' Guide to Physical Examination and History Taking*, 5th edn. Lippincott, Philadelphia.

Department of Health (2004) *The National Service Framework for Children, Young People and Maternity Services Core Standards: Standard 1 Promoting Health and Well-being, Identifying Needs and Intervening Early.* Department of Health, London.

Engle, J. (2002) *Paediatric Assessment*, 4th edn. Mosby, London.

Epstein, O., Perkin, G., de Bono, D. & Cookson, J. (2008) *Clinical Examination*, 4th edn. Mosby, London.

Gill, D. & O'Brien, N. (2007) *Paediatric Clinical Examination Made Easy*, 5th edn. Churchill Livingstone, Edinburgh.

Swartz, M. (2006) *Physical Diagnosis, History and Examination*, 5th edn. Saunders, London.

Todd, S. & Barnes, K. (2003) Anatomical and physiological differences in paediatrics. In: Barnes, K. (ed) *Paediatrics: A Clinical Guide for Nurse Practitioners.* Butterworth Heinemann, London.

CHAPTER 13

Assessment of Disability Including Care of the Older Adult

General examination

Introduction

It is important, particularly in the older adult, to **assess whether the patient has a disability**. The older adult requires a lot of attention. Not only is depression a prevalent factor but, according to Swartz (2006) and Thompson (2002), older adults are faced with changes in their self-image and the way they are perceived by others. The nurse must never assume that older adults' complaints are 'natural for their age' (Swartz, 2006: 42). The nurse should question whether the complaint:

- interferes with normal life and aspirations
- makes the patient dependent on others
  - requires temporary assistance for specific problems
  - occasional or regular assistance long-term
  - supervised accommodation
  - assisted living accommodation
  - nursing home with 24-hour care.

It is necessary to assess the following in a patient:

- **ability to do day-to-day functions**
- **mental ability, including confusion or dementia (consideration should be given to Alzheimer's disease)**
- **emotional state and drive.**

The descriptive terms used for disability have specific definitions in a World Health Organization classification (WHO, 1980).

- **Impairment** – any loss or abnormality of anatomical, physiological or psychological function, i.e. **systems or parts of body that do not work**.
- **Disability** – any restrictions or lack of ability (due to an impairment) to perform an activity within the range considered normal, e.g. **activities that cannot be done**.
- **Handicap** – a limitation of normal occupation because of impairment or disability, e.g. **social consequences**.

Thus:
- **a hemiparesis is an impairment**
- **an inability to wash or dress is a disability**
- **an inability to do an occupation is a handicap.**

It is important to note that disability and handicap are not always given due attention and are the practical and social aspects of the disease process. It is a mistake if the nurse is preoccupied by impairments, since the patient often perceives disability as the major problem.

The impairments, disability and handicap should have been covered in a normal history and examination, but it can be helpful to bring together important facts to provide an overall assessment.

A summary description of a patient may include the following.
- **aetiology**
  - familial hypercholesterolaemia
- **pathology**
  - atheroma
  - right middle cerebral artery thrombosis
- **impairment**
  - left hemiparesis
  - paralysed left arm, fixed in flexion
  - upper motor neurone signs in left arm and face
  - hearing loss/deafness
- **disability**
  - difficulty during feeding
  - cannot drive his car
- **handicap**
  - can no longer work as a travelling salesman
  - embarrassed to socialize
- **social circumstances**
  - partner can cope with day-to-day living, but lack of income from his occupation and withdrawal from society present major problems (Barkauskas *et al.*, 2002; Bickley & Szilagyi, 2007; Epstein *et al.*, 2008; Talley & O'Connor, 2006).

Assessment of impairment

The routine history and examination will often reveal impairments. Additional standard clinical measures are often used to assist quantification, e.g.:
- treadmill exercise test
- peak flow meter
- Medical Research Council scale of muscle power (Hatton & Blackwood, 2003)

- making five-pointed star from matches (to detect dyspraxia in hepatic encephalopathy).

Questionnaires can similarly provide a semi-quantitative index of important aspects of impairment and give a brief shorthand description of a patient. The role of the questionnaire is partly as a checklist to make sure the key questions are asked.

Cognitive function

In the older adult, impaired cognitive function can be assessed by a standard 10-point **mental test score** introduced by Hodkinson (1972). The test assumes normal communication skills. One mark each is given for correct answers to 10 standard questions (**see Appendix 3 for questionnaire**).

- age of patient
- time (to nearest hour)
- address given, for recall at end of test, e.g. 42 West Street or 92 Columbia Road
- recognize two people
- year (if January, the previous year is accepted)
- name of place, e.g. hospital or area of town if at home
- date of birth of patient
- start of World War I
- name of monarch in UK, president in USA
- count backwards from 20 to 1 (no errors allowed unless self-corrected)
- (check recall of address).

This scale is a basic test of gross defects of memory and orientation and is designed to detect cognitive impairment. It has the advantages of brevity, relative lack of culture-specific knowledge and widespread use. In the older adult, 8–10 correct answers is normal, 7 is probably normal, 6 or less is abnormal.

Specific problems, such as confusion or wandering at night, are not included in the mental test score, and indicate that the score is a useful checklist but not a substitute for a clinical assessment. Most dementias are associated with Alzheimer's disease in 50–85% of cases or vascular multi-infarct dementia in 10–20% of cases (Bickley & Szilagyi, 2007). Dementia frequently has a slow, insidious onset and families and clinicians may not detect it, especially in the early stages of cognitive impairment. You should look for problems with memory early on and then for changes in cognitive function and/or activities of daily living (ADLs) later on. Take note when a family member mentions or complains about new or unusual behaviour, and investigate any possible contributing factors such as medications, depression, metabolic abnormalities or other medical and psychiatric conditions (Bickley & Szilagyi, 2007; Swartz, 2006).

Affect and drive

Motivation is an important determinant of successful rehabilitation. Depression, accompanied by lack of motivation, is a major cause of disability. In older adults depression is often underdiagnosed and undertreated. Asking the question: 'Do you often feel sad or depressed?' is 'approximately 80% sensitive and specific' therefore positive responses should indicate the need for further investigation (Bickley & Szilagyi, 2007: 408–409).

Enquire about symptoms of depression and relevant examination, e.g. 'How is your mood? Have you lost interest in things?'

Making appropriate lifestyle changes, recruiting help from friends or relatives, can be key to increasing motivation. Pharmaceutical treatment of depression can also be helpful.

Assessment of hearing

According to Bickley & Szilagyi (2007), more than one-third of adults over the age of 65 have detectable hearing deficits. The Royal National Institute for Deaf People (RNID) indicates that around the age of 50 the proportion of deaf people begins to increase sharply and that by the age of 60, 55% are deaf or hard of hearing. Being deaf or hard of hearing means different things to different people. Many older adults will not notice that their hearing has deteriorated until considerable hearing loss has occurred. Commonly, older adults develop an ability to lip read to a degree as their hearing deteriorates. It has been estimated that there are 9 million deaf and hard-of-hearing people in the UK. This number is rising as the number of people over the age of 60 increases. Most of these 9 million people have developed a hearing loss as they have grown older. Presbyacusis is the term used for age-related hearing loss. It is the most common type of deafness in older adults.

There are two primary types of deafness. These are:

- conductive deafness, where sound has difficulty passing through the outer or middle ear
- sensorineural deafness, where the cause of deafness is in the cochlea or hearing nerve.

According to the RNID (2009), some people may have the same type and degree of hearing loss in each ear whilst for others it may be different in each ear. It is recommended that a hearing test is conducted to identify the type of deafness a person has. Older adults who need hearing aids should be told they can get them free of charge on the NHS.

Assessment of disability

Assessing restrictions to daily activities is often the key to successful management.
- **Make a list of disabilities separate from other problems, e.g. diagnoses, symptoms, impairments, social problems.**
    This list can assist with setting priorities, including which investigations or therapies are most likely to be of benefit to the patient.

Activities of daily living (ADL)

These are key functions which in the older adult affect the degree of independence. Several scales of disability have been used. One of these, the **Barthel Index of ADL**, records the following disabilities that can affect self-care and mobility (see Appendix 4 for questionnaire):
- continence – urinary and faecal
- ability to use toilet
- grooming
- feeding
- dressing
- bathing
- transfer, e.g. chair to bed
- walking
- using stairs.

The assessment denotes the current state and not the underlying cause or the potential improvement. It does not include cognitive functions or emotional state. It emphasizes independence, so a catheterized patient who can competently manage the device achieves the full score for urinary continence. The total score provides an overall estimate or summary of dependence, but between-patient comparisons are difficult as they may have different combinations of disability. Interpretation of score depends on disability and facilities available.

Instrumental activities of daily living (IADL)

These are slightly more complex activities relating to an individual's ability to live independently. They often require special assessment in the home environment.
- preparing a meal
- doing light housework
- using transport
- managing money
- shopping

- doing laundry
- taking medications
- using a telephone

Communication

In the older adult, difficulty in communication is a frequent problem, and impairment of the following may need special attention.
- deafness (do the ears need syringing? is a hearing aid required?)
- speech (is dysarthria due to lack of teeth?)
- an alarm to call for help when required
- aids for reading, e.g. spectacles, magnifying glass
- resiting or adaptation of doorbell, telephone, radio or television

Analysing disabilities and handicaps and setting objectives

After writing a list of disabilities, it is necessary to develop a possible treatment plan with specific objectives. The plan needs to be realistic. A multidisciplinary team approach, including social workers, physiotherapists, occupational therapists, nurses and doctors, is usually essential in the rehabilitation of older adult patients.
The overall aims in treating the older adult include the following.
- to make diagnoses, if feasible, particularly for treatable illnesses
- to comfort and alleviate problems and stresses, even if one cannot cure
- to add life to years, even if one cannot add years to life
Specific aspects which may need attention include the following.
- alleviate social problems if feasible
- improve heating, clothing, toilet facilities, cooking facilities
- arrange support services, e.g. help with shopping, provision of meals, attendance at day centre
- arrange regular visits from district/public health nurse or other helper
- make sure family, neighbours and friends understand the situation
- treat depression
- help with sorting out finances
- provide aids, e.g.
- large-handled implements
- walking frame or stick
- slip-on shoes
- handles by bath or toilet
- help to keep as mobile as feasible
- facilitate visits to hearing aid centre, optician, chiropodist, dentist
- ensure medications are kept to a minimum, and the instructions and packaging are suitable

A major problem arises if the disability leads to the patient being unwelcome. This depends on the reactions of others and requires tactful discussion with all concerned.

Identifying causes for disabilities

Specific disabilities may have specific causes which can be alleviated. In the older adult, common problems include the following.

Confusion
This is an impairment. Common causes are:
- infection
- drugs
- other illnesses, e.g. heart failure
- sensory deprivation, e.g. deafness, inability to see, darkness.

Assume all confusion is an acute response to an unidentified cause.

Incontinence
- toilet far away, e.g. upstairs
- physical restriction of gait
- urine infection
- faecal impaction
- uterine prolapse
- diabetes

'Off legs'
- neurological impairment
- unsuspected fracture of leg
- depressed
- general illness, e.g. infection, heart failure, renal failure, hypothermia, hypothyroid, diabetes, hypokalaemia

Falls
- carpet that is not secure
- dark stairs
- poor vision, e.g. cataracts
- postural hypotension
- cardiac arrhythmias
- epilepsy
- neurological deficit, e.g. Parkinson's disease, hemiparesis
- cough or micturition syncope
- intoxication

References

Barkauskas, V., Baumann, L. & Darling-Fisher, C. (2002) *Health and Physical Assessment*, 3rd edn. Mosby, London.

Bickley, L. & Szilagyi, P. (2007) *Bates' Guide to Physical Examination*, 5th edn. Lippincott, Philadelphia.

Epstein, O., Perkin, G., de Bono, D. & Cookson, J. (2008) *Clinical Examination*, 4th edn. Mosby, London.

Hatton, C. & Blackwood, R. (2003) *Lecture Notes on Clinical Skills*, 4th edn. Blackwell Science, Oxford.

Hodkinson, H. (1972) Evaluation of a mental test score for assessment of mental impairment in the elderly. *Age and Ageing*, **1**: 233–238. Available at: http://en.wikipedia.org/wiki/Abbreviated_mental_test_score.

Royal National Institute for Deaf People (2009) Available at: www.rnid.org.uk/information_resources/factsheets/hearing_aids/factsheets_leaflets/buying_a_hearing_aid.htm.

Swartz, M. (2006) *Physical Diagnosis, History and Examination*, 5th edn. Saunders, London.

Talley, N. & O'Connor, S. (2006) *Clinical Examination: A Systematic Guide to Physical Diagnosis*, 5th edn. Churchill Livingstone, London.

Thompson, S. (2002) Older people. In: Thompson, N. (ed) *Loss and Grief*. Palgrave, Basingstoke.

World Health Organization (1980) *International Classification of Impairments, Disabilities, and Handicaps*. World Health Organization, Geneva.

CHAPTER 14

Basic Examination, Notes and Diagnostic Principles

Basic examination

Introduction

In practice, you cannot attempt to elicit every single physical sign for each system. Your examination will be guided by the patient's chief complaint and presenting history. Basic signs should be sought on every examination, and if there is any hint of abnormality, additional physical signs can be elicited to confirm your suspicion. Listed below are the basic examinations of the systems which will enable you to complete a routine examination adequately but not excessively.

- **General examination**
    - general appearance
    - is the patient well or ill?
    - look at temperature chart or take patient's temperature
    - any obvious abnormality?
    - mental health state, mood, behaviour
- **General and cardiovascular system**
    - observation – dyspnoea, distress
    - blood pressure
    - hands
    - temperature
    - nails, e.g. clubbing, leuconychia, koilonychias, palmar erythema
    - pulse – rate, rhythm, character
    - axillae – lymph nodes
    - neck – lymph nodes
    - face and eyes – anaemia, jaundice
    - tongue and fauces – central cyanosis
    - jugular venous pulse (JVP)/distension (JVD) – height and v-wave
    - apex beat/point of maximal impulse (PMI) – position and character
    - parasternal – heave or thrills
    - stethoscope

- heart sounds (S_1 and S_2), added sounds (clicks or snaps), splits (? physiological split), murmurs
- listen in all five areas with stethoscope using the bell and diaphragm
- lay patient on left side and with the bell of stethoscope listen for mitral stenosis (MS)
- sit patient up, lean forward, breathe out, with bell of stethoscope listen for aortic incompetence (AI)

- **Respiratory system**
  - observation (scars, lesions, ecchymoses)
  - trachea – position
  - **front of chest**
    - movement (respiratory excursion; flail)
    - palpate (lumps, crepitus, fremitus)
    - percuss – compare sides
    - auscultate – compare sides
  - **back of chest**
    - movement (respiratory excursion)
    - palpate (lumps, crepitus, fremitus)
    - percuss – particularly level of bases (diaphragmatic excursion); compare sides
    - auscultate – compare sides
    - examine sputum
- **Examine spine** (? lordosis, kyphosis, scoliosis, gibbus)
- **Abdomen**
  - lay patient flat (knees bent to relax abdomen)
  - look at abdomen – ask if pain or tenderness
  - auscultate in all four quadrants (include aortic, iliac and femoral arteries/? bruits)
  - palpate abdomen gently
    - generally all over; ? masses
    - liver – then percuss
    - spleen – then percuss
    - kidneys
    - (shifting dullness – ascites if indicated)
  - feel femoral pulses and inguinal lymph nodes
  - herniae
  - males – genitals
  - per rectum (PR; only if given permission) – usually at end of examination
  - per vaginam (PV; only if given permission) – usually at end of examination
- **Legs**
  - observation
  - arterial pulses (joints if indicated)
  - neurology

– reflexes	– knees – ankles – plantar responses	tone power co-ordination	⎫ ⎬ only if ⎭ indicated
– sensation	– pinprick – vibration	position cotton-wool temperature	

- **Arms**
  - posture: outstretched hands, eyes closed, rapid finger movements
  - finger–nose co-ordination

– reflexes	– triceps – biceps – supinator	tone power	⎫ ⎬ only if ⎭ indicated
– sensation	– pinprick	vibration position cotton-wool temperature	

- **Cranial nerves**
  - I (if indicated)
  - II: eyes
    - reading print/acuity
    - fields
    - pupils – torch and accommodation
    - ophthalmoscope – sclera, cornea, anterior chamber and posterior fundi
  - III, IV, VI: eye movements (EOM)
    - 'Do you see double?'
    - note nystagmus
  - V, VII
    - open mouth
    - grit teeth – feel masseters
    - sensation – cotton-wool
    - (corneal reflex – if indicated)
    - (taste – if indicated)
  - VIII: hearing
    - watch at each ear
    - (Rinne, Weber tests if indicated)
  - IX, X: fauces movement
  - XI: shrug shoulders
  - XII: put out tongue
- **Walk** – look at gait
- **Herniae and varicose veins**

Example of notes

You may find using the SOAPIER format or POMR useful in documenting your findings (Clark, 1999; Epstein *et al.*, 2008; Swartz, 2006).

Patient's name: **Age:**   **Occupation:**
Date of admission:
Complains of (chief complaint):
 – list, in patient's words
History of present illness:
 – detailed description of each symptom (even if appears irrelevant)
 – last well
 – chronological order, with both actual date of onset and time previous to admission
 – (may include history from informant – in which case, state this is so)
 – then detail other questions which seem relevant to possible differential diagnoses
 – then **functional enquiry**, 'check' system for other symptoms
 – (minimal statement in notes – weight, appetite, digestion, bowels, micturition, menstruation, if appropriate)
Past history:
 – chronological order
Family history:
 – include genogram
Personal and social history:
 – must include details of home circumstances, dependants, patient's occupation
 – effect of illness on life and its relevance to foreseeable discharge of patient
 – smoking, alcohol, drug misuse, medications
Medications:
 – list all medications the patient is presently taking
Physical examination:
 – general appearance
 – then record findings according to systems
Minimal statement:

Healthy, well-nourished woman (or man)
Apyrexial (afebrile), not anaemic, icteric or cyanosed
No enlargement of lymph nodes
No clubbing
Breasts/chest and thyroid normal
Cerebrovascular system (CVS):   Blood pressure, pulse rate and rhythm
                                   JVP not raised
                                   Apex position
                                   Heart sounds 1 and 2, no murmurs

Respiratory system:	Chest and movements normal
	Fremitus normal
	Percussion note normal
	Breath sounds bilateral/vesicular
	No other (adventitious) sounds
Abdominal system:	Tongue and fauces normal
	Abdomen normal, no tenderness
	Liver, spleen, kidneys, bladder impalpable
	No masses felt
	Hernial orifices normal
	Rectal examination normal
	Vaginal examination not performed
	Testes normal
Central nervous system (CNS):	Alert and intelligent
	Pupils equal, regular, react equally to light and accommodation (PERRLA)
	Fundi normal
	Normal eye movements
	Other cranial nerves normal
	Limbs normal

Knee jerks	+	+
Ankle jerks	+	+
Plantar reflexes	↓	↓

Touch and vibration normal

Spine and joints normal

Gait normal

Pulses (including dorsalis pedis, posterior tibial and popliteal) palpable

Summary

Write a few sentences only:
- salient positive features of history and examination
- relevant negative information
- home circumstances
- patient's mental state
  - understanding of illness
  - specific concerns

Problem list and diagnoses

After your history and examination, **make a list of**:
- **the diagnoses you have been able to make**
- **problems or abnormal findings which need explaining.**

For example:
- symptoms or signs
- anxiety
- poor social background
- laboratory results
- drug sensitivities.

It is best to separate the current problems of actual or potential clinical significance requiring treatment or follow-up from the inactive problems. An example is:

Active problems	Date
1 Unexplained episodes of fainting	1 week
2 Angina	since 1990
3 Hypertension – blood pressure 190/100 mmHg	1990
4 Chronic renal failure – plasma creatinine 200 μmol/l	August 1996
5 Widower, unemployed, lives on own	
6 Anxious about possibility of being injured in a fall	
7 Smokes 40 cigarettes per day	

Inactive problems	Date
1 Thyrotoxicosis treated by partial thyroidectomy	1976
2 ACE inhibitor-induced cough	1991

When you initially begin examining patients you will have difficulty knowing which problems to put down separately, and which can be covered under one diagnosis and a single entry. It is therefore advisable to rewrite the problem list if a problem resolves or can be explained by a diagnosis. When you are more experienced, it will be appropriate to fill out the problems on a complete problem list at the front of the notes. (Do not include the nursing diagnosis in the medical notes. Use medical diagnoses in the medical notes. Document the nursing diagnosis on the nursing care plan.)

Active problems	Date	Inactive problems	Date
Include symptoms, signs, unexplained abnormal investigations, social and psychiatric problems		Include major past illness, operation or hypersensitivities; do not include problems requiring active care	

From the problem list, you should be able to determine:
- **differential diagnoses**, including that which you think is most likely. Remember:

- **common diseases occur commonly**
- **an unusual manifestation of a common disease** is more likely than an uncommon disease
- **do not necessarily be put off by some aspect which does not fit**
- **possible diagnostic investigations** you feel are appropriate
- **management and therapy** you think are appropriate
- **prognostic implications.**

Diagnoses

The diagnostic terms which are used often relate to different levels of understanding.

Disordered function	Immobile painful joint ↑	Breathlessness ↑	Angina ↑
Structural lesion	Oste-oarthritis ↑	Anaemia ↑	Narrow coronary artery ↑
Pathology	Iron-deposition fibrosis (haemochromatosis) ↑	Iron deficiency ↑	Aortitis ↑
Aetiology	Inherited disorder of iron metabolism – homozygous for C282Y with A-H	Bleeding duodenal ulcer	*Treponema pallidum* (syphilis)

Different problems require diagnoses at different levels, which may change as further information becomes available. Thus, a patient initially may be diagnosed as *pyrexia of unknown origin*. After a plain X-ray of the abdomen, he may be found to have a *renal mass* which on a computed tomography (CT) scan becomes *perinephric abscess*, which from blood cultures is found to be *Staphylococcus aureus* infection. For a complete diagnosis all aspects should be known, but often this is not possible.

Note that many terms are used as a diagnosis but, in fact, cover considerable ignorance; for example, *diabetes mellitus* (originally 'sweet-tasting urine' but now also diagnosed by high plasma glucose) is no more than a descriptive term of disordered function. *Sarcoid* relates to a pattern of symptoms and a pathology of non-caseating granulomata, of which the aetiology is unknown.

Progress notes

The electronic patient record is becoming the norm in many healthcare environments. It is now accessible in GP surgeries as well as outpatient clinics and in hospitals. A single patient record that can be accessed from any setting is rapidly becoming the norm in the NHS.

In the GP surgery or clinic, full progress notes should be kept to give a complete picture of:

- how the diagnosis was established
- how the patient was treated
- the evolution of the illness
- any complications that occurred.

These notes are as important as the account of the original examination. In acute cases, record daily changes in signs and symptoms. In chronic cases, the relevant systems should be re-examined at least once a week and the findings recorded.

It is useful to separate different aspects of the illness:

- symptoms
- signs
- laboratory investigations
- general assessment, e.g. apparent response to therapy
- further plans, which would include educating the patient and his family about the illness.

Objective findings such as alterations in weight, improvement in colour, pulse, character of respirations or fluid intake and output are more valuable than purely **subjective statements** such as 'feeling better' or 'slept well'.

When appropriate, daily blood pressure readings or analyses of the urine should be recorded.

An account of all procedures such as aspirations of chest should be included. Specifically record:

- the findings and comments of the physician, surgeon or nurse consultant managing the case
- results of a case conference
- an opinion from another department.

Serial investigations

The results of these should be collected together in a **table** on a special sheet. When any large series of investigations is made, e.g. serial blood counts, erythrocyte sedimentation rates or multiple biochemical analyses, the results can also be expressed by a **graph**.

Operation notes

If you are working in a team where patients are undergoing surgical treatment, you may be required to write an operation note following surgery. An operation note must be written immediately after the operation. Do not trust your memory for any length of time as several similar problems may be operated on at one session. Even if you are distracted by an emergency, the notes must be written up the same day as the operation. These notes should contain definite statements on the following facts:

- name of surgeon performing the operation and his or her assistant
- name of anaesthetist and anaesthetic used
- type and dimension of incision used
- pathological condition found, and mention of anatomical variations
- operative procedures carried out
- method of repair of wound and suture materials used
- whether drainage used, material used, and whether sutured to wound
- type of dressing used.

Postoperative notes

Within the first 2 days after an operation note:

- the general condition of the patient
- any complication or troublesome symptom, e.g. pain, haemorrhage, vomiting, distension, etc.
- any treatment.

Discharge note from hospital

A full statement of the patient's condition on discharge should be written:

- final diagnosis
- active problems
- medication and other therapies
- plan
- specific follow-up points, e.g. persistent depressive disorder, blood pressure monitoring
- what the patient has been told
- where the patient has gone, and what help is available
- when the patient is next being seen
- an estimate of the prognosis.

References

Clark, C. (1999) Taking a history. In: Walsh, M., Crumbie, A. & Reveley, S. (eds) *Nurse Practitioners, Clinical Skills and Professional Issues.* Butterworth Heinemann, Oxford.

Epstein, O., Perkin, G., de Bono, D. & Cookson, J. (2008) *Clinical Examination,* 4th edn. Mosby, London.

Swartz, M. (2006) *Physical Diagnosis, History and Examination,* 5th edn. Saunders, London.

CHAPTER 15
Presenting Cases and Communication

Presentations to doctors, nurses, allied health professionals and patients

Introduction

Nursing and medicine are disciplines in which you have to be able to communicate effectively. The more practice you get, the better you will become and the more confident you will appear in front of doctors, nurses, allied health professionals and patients. Confidence displayed by you is an important aspect of therapy and the value to the patient of a nurse who can speak lucidly is enormous.

Practise talking to yourself in a mirror, avoiding any breaks or interpolating the word 'er'. Open a textbook, find a subject and give a little talk on it to yourself. Even if you do not know anything about the subject, you will be able to make up a few coherent sentences once you are practised.

A presentation is not the time to demonstrate you have been thorough and have asked all questions, but to show that you can intelligently assemble the essential facts. In all presentations, give the salient positive findings and the relevant negative findings. For example:

- in a patient with progressive dyspnoea, state if patient has ever smoked
- in a patient with icterus, state whether patient has been abroad, has had any recent injections or drugs, or contact with other jaundiced patients.

Three types of presentations are likely to be encountered: presentation of a case to a meeting, presentation of a new case on a ward round and a brief follow-up presentation.

Presentation of a case to a meeting

This must be properly prepared, including visual aids as necessary. The principal details, shown on a PowerPoint® presentation or overhead projector, are helpful as a reminder to you, and the audience may more easily remember the details of a case if they 'see' as well as 'hear' them. An advantage of

PowerPoint® is the ability to print out the full presentation as a series of slides with spaces for the audience to write notes.

- Practise your presentation from beginning to end several times. Leave nothing to chance.
- Do not speak to the screen; speak to the audience.
- Do not crack jokes, unless you are confident that they are apposite.
- Do not make sweeping statements.
- Remember what you are advised to do in a court of law – dress up, stand up, speak up, shut up.
- Read up about the disease or problem beforehand so that you can answer any queries.
- Read a recent leading article, review or research publication on the subject and refer to this during your presentation.

In many clinical settings it is expected that you present an **apposite, original article**. Be prepared to evaluate and criticize the manuscript. If your seniors or colleagues cannot provide you with references, look up the subject in CINHAL, Medline, British Nursing Index, Assia, Cochrane, *Index Medicus* or recently published textbooks (published references should be within the past 5 years). Always ask the librarian for advice. Laboriously repeating standard information from a textbook is often a turn-off. A recent series or research paper is more educational for you and more interesting for the audience.

A PowerPoint® slide or overhead should summarize any presentation.

| Mr A. B. | Age: *x* years | Brief description, e.g. occupation |

Complains of
(state in patient's words – for *x* period)
History of present complaint
- essential details
- other relevant information, e.g. risk factors
- relevant negative information relating to possible diagnoses
- extent to which symptoms or disease limit normal activity
- other symptoms – mention briefly

Past history
- briefly mention inactive problems
- historical information about active problems, or inactive problems relevant to present illness
- record allergies, including type of reaction to drugs

Family history
- brief information about parents, otherwise detail only if relevant (present a genogram for the audience to review).

Social history
- brief unless relevant
- give family social background

- occupation and previous occupations
- any other special problems
- tobacco or ethanol abuse, past or present

Treatment
- note all drugs with doses

Chief complaint
- note in the patient's words what the patient indicates the problem is

On examination

General description
- introductory descriptive sentence, e.g. well, obese man (indicate BMI)
- clinical signs relevant to disease
- relevant negative findings

    Remember these findings should be descriptive data rather than your interpretation.

Problem list

Differential diagnoses

Put in order of likelihood.

Investigations
- relevant positive findings
- relevant negative findings
- tables or graphs for repetitive data
- scan an electrocardiogram or temperature chart for the PowerPoint® presentation or photocopy an electrocardiogram or temperature chart for overhead presentation

Progress report

Plan

Subjects which are often discussed after your presentation include:
- other differential diagnoses
- other features of presumed diagnosis that might have been present or require investigation
- pathophysiological mechanisms
- mechanisms of action of drugs and possible side effects

Presentation of a new case on a ward round

- Good written notes are of great assistance. Do not read your notes word for word – use them as a reference.
- Highlight, underline or asterisk key features you wish to refer to, or write up a separate note-card for reference.
- Talk formally and avoid speaking too quickly or too slowly. Speak to the whole assembled group rather than a tête-à-tête with the consultant.
- Stand upright and look presentable – it helps to make you appear confident.
- If you are interrupted by a discussion, note where you are and be ready to resume, repeating the last sentence before proceeding.

History

The format will be similar to that on PowerPoint® or an overhead, with emphasis on positive findings and relevant negative information. A full description of the initial main symptom is usually required.

Examination

Once your history is complete, the consultant may ask for the relevant clinical signs only. Still add in relevant negative signs you think are important.

Summary

Be prepared to give a problem list and differential diagnoses.

If you are presenting the patient at the bedside, ensure the patient is comfortable. If the patient wishes to make an additional point or clarification, it is best to welcome this. If it is relevant it can be helpful. If irrelevant, politely say to the patient you will come back to him in a moment, after you have presented the findings. Do not appear to disagree with the patient in his presence.

Brief follow-up presentation

Give a brief, orienting introduction to provide a framework on which other information can be placed. For example:

A *xx*-year-old man who was admitted *xx* days ago.

Long-standing problems include *xxxxx* (list briefly).

Presented with *xx* symptoms for *x* period.

On examination, had *xx* signs.

Initial diagnosis of *xx* was confirmed/supported by/not supported by *xx* investigations.

He was treated by *xx*.

Since then *xx* progress:

- symptoms
- examination

    Start with general description and temperature chart and, if relevant, investigations.

If there are multiple active problems, describe each separately, e.g.

- first in regard to the *xxxx*
- second in regard to the *xxxx*

The outstanding problems are *xxxx*.

The plan is *xxxx*.

Aides-mémoire

These are basic lists that provide brief reminders when presenting patients and diseases. Organizing your thoughts along structured lines is helpful.

History
- principal symptom(s)
- history of present illness
- note chronology
- present situation
- functional enquiry
- past history
- family history
- personal and social history

Pain or other symptoms
- site
- radiation
- character
- severity
- onset/duration
- frequency/periodicity or constant
- precipitating factors
- relieving factors
- associated symptoms
- getting worse or better

Lumps
Inspection
- site
- size
- shape
- surface
- surroundings

Palpation
- soft/solid consistency
- surroundings – fixed/mobile
- tender
- pulsatility
- transmission of illumination

Local lymph nodes
About the disease
- incidence
- geographical area
- gender/age
- aetiology
- pathology

- macroscopic
- microscopic
- pathophysiology
- symptoms
- signs
- therapy
- prognosis

Causes of disease
- **genetic**
- **infective**
  - virus
  - bacterial
  - fungal
  - parasitic
- **neoplastic**
  - cancer
    - primary
    - secondary
  - lymphoma
- **vascular**
  - atheroma
  - hypertension
  - other, e.g. arteritis
- **infiltrative**
  - fibrosis
  - amyloid
  - granuloma
- **autoimmune**
- **endocrine**
- **degenerative**
- **environmental**
  - trauma
  - iatrogenic – drug side effects
  - poisoning
- **malnutrition**
  - general
  - specific, e.g. vitamin deficiency
  - perinatal with effects on subsequent development

Diagnostic labels

- aetiology, e.g. tuberculosis, genetic
  ↓

- pathology, e.g. sarcoid, amyloid
  $\downarrow$
- disordered function, e.g. hypertension, diabetes
  $\downarrow$
- symptoms or signs, e.g. jaundice, erythema nodosum

People – including patients

A significant number of disasters, a great deal of irritation and a lot of unpleasantness could be avoided in the GP surgery, outpatient clinics and hospitals by proper communication. You must remember that you are part of a multidisciplinary team, all of whom significantly help the patient. You must be able to communicate properly with the medical staff, nursing staff, physiotherapists, occupational therapists, administrators, ancillary staff and, above all, the patients.

Remember these points.

- **Time** – when you talk to anyone, try not to appear in a rush or they will lose concentration and not listen. A little time taken to talk to somebody properly will help enormously. One minute spent sitting down can seem like 5 minutes to the patient; 5 minutes standing up can seem like 1 minute.
- **Silence** – in normal social interaction, we tend to avoid silences. In a conversation, as soon as one person stops talking (or even before), the other person jumps in to say his or her bit. When interviewing patients, it is often useful, if you wish to encourage the patient to talk further, to remain silent a moment longer than would be natural. An encouraging nod of the head or an echoing of the patient's last word or two (reflection) may also encourage him to talk further.
- **Listen** – active listening to someone is not easy but is essential for good communication. Many people stop talking but not all appear to be listening. Sitting down with the patient is advantageous, both in helping you to concentrate and in transmitting to the patient that you are willing to listen.
- **Smile and use facilitative body language** – grumpiness or irritation is the best way to stop a patient talking. A smile and display of interest will often encourage a patient to tell you problems he would not normally disclose. This behaviour helps everybody to relax.
- **Reassurance** – if you appear confident and relaxed, this helps others to feel the same. Being calm without excessive body movements can help. Note how a good nurse consultant has a reassuring word for patients and allows others in the team to feel they are (or are capable of) working effectively.
- **Advocacy** – as a nurse, you are the patient's advocate. Advocacy is essential in order to preserve the nurse/patient relationship.

CHAPTER 16

Imaging Techniques and Clinical Investigations

General procedures

Introduction

This chapter begins with a general description of the major techniques used in imaging and clinical investigations. It addresses the basic principles of diagnostic imaging techniques and is followed by additional specialized investigations in cardiology (supported by Chapter 3), respiratory medicine (supported by Chapter 4), gastroenterology (supported by Chapter 5), renal medicine and neurology (supported by Chapter 9).

Diagnostic imaging

Diagnostic imaging consists of a range of procedures and use of sophisticated equipment to produce high-quality images to view various body organs and systems that aid identification, evaluation and monitoring of disease processes, soft tissue and skeletal abnormalities and trauma. The range of techniques includes the following.

- Ultrasound – uses high-frequency sound. This technique is increasingly used in obstetrics, including fetal monitoring throughout pregnancy, gynaecology, abdominal, paediatrics, cardiac, vascular and musculoskeletal medicine.
- X-rays – used to look through tissue to examine bones, cavities and foreign objects.
- Fluoroscopy – used to image the GI tract, providing a real-time image with X-rays.
- Angiography – to investigate blood vessels and organ perfusion after injecting a contrast agent which aids visualization of the cardiovascular system.
- CT (computed tomography) – provides cross-sectional views (slices) of the body.
- MRI (magnetic resonance imaging) – builds a two- or three-dimensional map of different tissue types within the body.

- Nuclear medicine – uses radio-active pharmaceuticals which can be administered to examine how the body and organs function.

Ultrasound

High-frequency (2.5–10 MHz) ultrasound waves are produced by the piezo-electric effect within ultrasound transducers. These transducers, which both produce and receive sound waves, are moved over the skin surface and images of the underlying organ structures are produced from the reflected sound waves. Structures with very few interfaces, such as fluid-filled structures, allow through transmission of the sound waves and therefore appear more **black** on the screen. Structures with a large number of interfaces cause significant reflection and refraction of the sound waves and therefore appear **whiter**. Air causes almost complete attenuation of the sound wave and therefore structures deep to this cannot be visualized.

Ultrasound scanning is a real-time examination and is dependent on the experience of the operator for its accuracy. The diagnosis is made from the real-time examination, although a permanent record of findings can be recorded on X-ray-like film.

The technique has the advantage of being safe, using non-ionizing radiation, being repeatable, painless and requiring little, if any, pre-preparation of the patient. It is also possible to carry out the examination at the patient's bedside and to evaluate a series of organs in a relatively short period of time.

Ultrasound is used in many different situations, including the following.

Abdomen
- **liver** – tumours, abscesses, diffuse liver disease, dilated bile ducts, hepatic vasculature
- **gallbladder** – gallstones, gallbladder wall pathology (Fig. 16.1)
- **pancreas** – tumours, pancreatitis
- **kidneys** – size, hydronephrosis, tumours, stones, scarring
- **spleen** – size, focal abnormalities
- **ovaries** – size, cysts, tumours
- **uterus** – pregnancy, tumours, endometrium
- **aorta** – aneurysm
- **bowel** – inflammation, tumours, abscesses

Brain
- possible in the infant before the anterior fontanelle closes

Heart
See Echocardiography in this chapter.

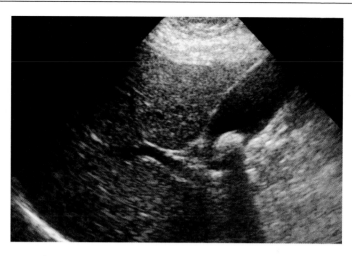

Fig. 16.1   Ultrasound scan showing a stone within the gallbladder, casting an acoustic shadow.

Blood vessels
  – aneurysms, stenoses, clots in veins

Neck
  – thyroid – characterization of masses

Scrotum
  – tumours, inflammation

Musculoskeletal
  – joint effusions, soft tissue masses

Radiography

Conventional X-rays visualize only four basic radiographic densities: air, metal, fat and water. Air densities are black; metal densities (the most common of which are calcium and barium) are white with well-defined edges; fat and water densities are dark and mid grey.

There can be difficulty in visualizing a three-dimensional structure from a two-dimensional film. One helpful rule in deciding where a lesion is situated is to note which, if any, adjacent normal landmarks are obliterated. For example, a water density lesion which obliterates the right border of the heart must lie in the right middle lobe and not the lower lobe. A different view, e.g. lateral chest radiograph, is needed to be certain of the position of densities.

Apart from skeletal imaging of limbs and spine, the most common radiographic examinations are the chest radiograph and abdominal radiograph.

Chest radiograph

Use a systematic approach to evaluate the image
- Posteroanterior (PA) chest radiograph is the standard view (anteroposterior (AP) is only done when the patient is in a bed) (Fig. 16.2). The correct name for the usual chest study is 'a PA chest radiograph'. This means that the anteriorly situated heart is as close to the film as possible and its image will be minimally enlarged. Generally this view is taken with the patient standing facing toward the X-ray film.

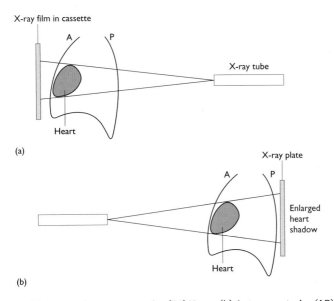

Fig. 16.2 (a) A normal posteroanterior (PA) X-ray. (b) Anteroposterior (AP) chest X-ray for chest radiographs of patients in bed.

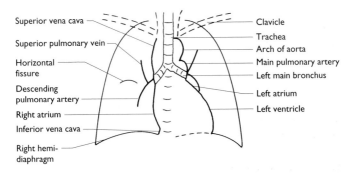

Fig. 16.3 Review particularly lungs, apices, costophrenic angles, hilar, behind heart.

- When reviewing the image (Fig. 16.3) follow a logical progression from centre of film to periphery.
  - interfaces are only seen in silhouette when adjacent tissues have different attenuation properties of X-rays; thus the heart border becomes invisible when there is collapse or consolidation in the adjacent lung
- **Technical factors**
  - positioning – apices and costophrenic angles should be on the film
  - inspiration – at least six posterior ribs seen above right diaphragm
  - penetration – midcardiac intervertebral disc spaces visible
  - rotation – medial end clavicles equidistant from spinous processes
  - note any catheters, tubes, pacing wires, pneumothorax
- **Heart**
  - size
    - normal <50% cardiothoracic ratio (maximum diameter of heart to maximum internal diameter of thoracic ribs as per cent)
    - males <15.5 cm, females <15 cm diameter
  - shape – any chamber enlarged?
    - PA radiograph: LV and RA
    - lateral radiograph: RV and LA
  - calcification – in valves (better seen on lateral chest X-ray) or arteries
- **Pericardium**
  - globular suggests *pericardial effusion* (general examination of the patient will show distended neck veins and muffled heart sounds)
  - calcification suggests *tuberculosis*
- **Aorta**
  - large in aneurysms, small in *atrial septal defect*
  - calcification in intima, >6 mm inside outer wall suggests *dissection*
- **Mediastinum**
  - ?widening – look at lateral chest X-ray to locate
- **Hila**
  - right at horizontal fissure, left 0–2.5 cm higher
    - displacement suggests loss of lung volume, e.g. *collapse, fibrosis*
  - enlargement
    - if lobulated – a mass or lymph nodes
    - ?vascular dilation
  - density – ?mass projected over hilum
- **Pulmonary vessels**
  - large in intracardiac or peripheral shunts – prominent in outer third (plethora)
  - large in *pulmonary hypertension* with small vessels in outer third (pruning) – *shunts, hypoxia, emboli, chronic lung disease*
  - segmental avascularity – *pulmonary emboli*
  - small in *congenital heart disease, right ventricular/pulmonary artery atresia*
- **Lung parenchyma**
  - lungs should be equally transradiant (black)

- alveolar shadows – ill-defined or confluent and dense
    - air bronchogram – water, pus, blood, tumour around patent bronchi, often seen end on, as a circle, near hila
- nodular shadows, e.g. *granuloma, tuberculosis*
- reticular shadows – *fibrotic lung disease*
        Note uniformity, symmetry, unilateral or bilateral, upper or lower zones.
- masses
    - define position (request lateral chest radiograph), edge, shape, size
    - *tumour, abscess, embolus, infection*
- **Pleura**
    - fluid
        - homogeneous, opaque shadow, usually with lateral meniscus
        - if air–fluid interface, *empyema* or after thoracocentesis
    - pneumothorax
        - peripheral space devoid of markings with edge of lung visible
        - look for mediastinal (shift) displacement – *tension pneumothorax*
    - masses
        - lobulated shadows – loculated fluid or tumour
- **Skeleton**
    - sclerosis, focal – ?*metastases*, e.g. *breast, prostate, stomach, kidney, thyroid, lymphoma*
        – *myelofibrosis, Paget's disease*
    - lytic – ?metastases, e.g. *lung, colorectal, myeloma*
    - osteopenia (only visible when advanced) – osteoporosis and osteomalacia cannot be distinguished on radiographs, except Looser's zones (pseudofracture) in osteomalacia
    - look for fractures
- **Other areas**
    - hiatus hernia, behind heart
    - left lower lobe collapse (pneumothorax), behind heart
    - lungs behind dome of diaphragm
    - gas below diaphragm on erect chest radiograph – *perforated viscus, recent surgery*
    - apices – ?lung visible above clavicle

Abdominal radiograph

This is less satisfactory than chest radiography because there are fewer contrasting densities as most of the tissues being imaged are soft tissues. Air in the gut is helpful, as are the psoas lines. Try to find as many organ outlines as possible.

- supine (AP) radiograph is the standard view.
- erect radiograph:
    - for air–fluid levels (AFLs)

- <5 short AFLs normal
- many – *obstruction*
- also in *paralytic ileus, coeliac disease, jejunal diverticula*
- **Visceral organs** (Fig. 16.4)
  - liver
    - usually <18 cm long – inferior surface outlined by fat
    - ?gas in biliary tree centrally
  - spleen – enlargement displaces stomach gas bubble to midline
  - kidneys – normally 3–3.5 vertebrae long

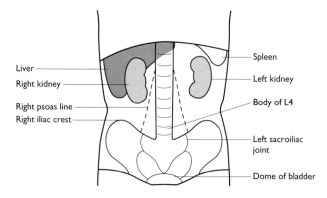

Fig. 16.4   Visceral organs.

- **Bowel gas pattern**
  - stomach
    - normally small air bubble (gastric bubble)
    - dilated in *pyloric stenosis* and *proximal small bowel obstruction*
  - small bowel
    - central position
    - small loops, valvulae across lumen, no faeces
    - dilated when >3.5 cm proximally, >2.5 cm distally – suggests *obstruction*
  - large bowel
    - vertical in flanks and across top of abdomen
    - wider loops, haustral folds do not cross lumen ± faeces
    - dilated when >5.5 cm – suggests obstruction
    - >9 cm – suggests perforation risk
  - hernial orifices – ?bowel air pattern below femoral neck indicates herniae
- **Abnormal gas**
  - pneumoperitoneum
  - both sides of bowel defined as thin lines
  - loss of liver density from gas anteriorly

  - bowel wall – thin streaks of gas suggest infarction or gas-producing bacteria
- **Abnormal calcification**
  - 30% gallstones are radiopaque – can be anywhere in abdomen
  - pancreas calcification – follows oblique line of pancreas and suggests *chronic pancreatitis*
  - renal stones – usually radiopaque
  - nephrocalcinosis – *medullary sponge kidney* or *metabolic calcinosis*
  - in pheboliths or faecoliths in diverticulae
- **Other soft tissues**
  - psoas lines
    - outlined by retroperitoneal fat
    - absent in 20% of normal patients
    - unilateral absence suggests *retroperitoneal mass* or *haematoma*
  - ascites
    - uniformly grey appearance
    - bowel gas 'floats' centrally (abdominal examination shows tympani on percussion centrally with lateral dullness)

Arteriography and venography

A series of X-ray images is taken after a radiopaque contrast has been injected into a blood vessel (Fig. 16.5):
  - coronary arteriography, e.g. *coronary artery disease*
  - cerebral angiography, e.g. *aneurysm* after *subarachnoid haemorrhage*
  - carotid angiography, e.g. *stenoses*
  - pulmonary angiography, e.g. *pulmonary embolus* or *fistula*

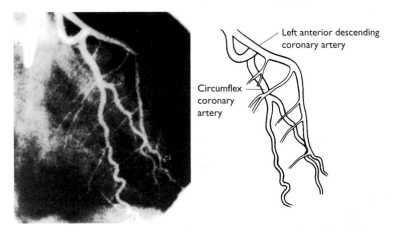

Fig. 16.5   Left coronary artery angiogram viewed from right.

- renal angiography, e.g. *renal artery stenosis, arteriovenous fistula*
- aortography and iliofemoral angiography, e.g. *aortic aneurysm, iliofemoral artery atheroma*
- leg venogram, e.g. *deep venous thrombosis*

Concurrent venous blood sampling may help localize an endocrine tumour, e.g. parathormone from an occult parathyroid tumour, catecholamines from a phaeochromocytoma, or to confirm the significance of renal artery stenosis using renal vein renin analyses.

Computed tomography

A CT scan uses X-rays to take a series of pictures of the body at slightly different angles, as the apparatus rotates through 360°, and uses a computer to put them together to produce very detailed pictures of the inside of the body (Fig. 16.6). Attenuation of X-rays depends on tissue – water is arbitrary 0, black is −1000 and white is +1000 Hounsfield units. Different 'windows' are chosen to display different characteristics, e.g. soft tissue window, lung window, bone window.

CT can be used:

- for organs and masses in abdomen and thorax
- to diagnose tumours, infarcts and bleeds in cerebral hemispheres
- for posterior fossa lesions – less easy to visualize because of bony base of skull
- to visualize disc prolapse and neoplasm in spinal cord, but adjacent bones interfere; intrathecal contrast medium is often required for cord tumours

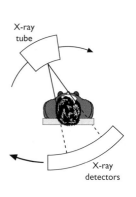
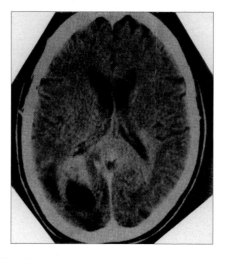

Fig. 16.6 CT scan across cerebral hemispheres.

Variants of CT:
- intravenous contrast
  - iodine based
  - opacifies blood vessels
  - shows leaky vessels or increased number of vessels
- oral contrast
  - opacifies gut contents
- spiral CT
  - X-ray tube constantly rotated with patient moving through scan gentry
  - computer segments image data into slices
  - advantages – faster, more detail, can use intravenous contrast medium
  - becoming the investigation of choice for pulmonary embolism
  - multi-slice CT which takes a number of CT 'slices' at the same time to speed up the scanning process

Nuclear medicine studies

These studies use radio-active isotopes (mostly technetium 99 m) coupled to appropriate pharmaceuticals or monoclonal antibodies designed to seek out different organ systems or pathology to obtain pictures of the body with a gamma camera. The studies yield functional rather than anatomical information. They are sensitive but not specific. Lesions present as either photon-abundant areas (as in bone or brain) or photon-deficient areas (as in liver, lung, heart, etc.). The following are the most common investigations routinely available.

Skeletal system

Any cause of increased bone turnover or altered blood flow to bone, e.g. tumour, infection, trauma, infarction. Used mostly for detection of metastases.

Pulmonary system

The diagnosis of pulmonary emboli using perfusion scintigraphy, when emboli cause defects which do not correspond to water densities in the same position on simultaneous chest radiographs. Usually only indicated when chronic obstructive airways disease is present.

Cardiovascular system

For the measurement of ventricular function, e.g. ejection fractions, and for examining myocardial integrity. Ischaemia or scarring causes 'cold' areas

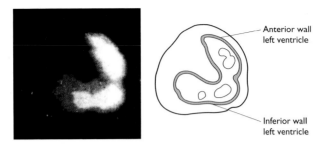

Fig. 16.7   Thallium 201 study of the heart.

on myocardial scintigrams. Studies are usually carried out at rest and after exercise (Fig. 16.7).

Urogenital system

Renography (an activity–time curve of the passage of radio-active tracer through the kidney) for detecting abnormalities of renal blood flow, parenchymal function and excretion. Renal scintigraphy will detect scarring and is used to measure divided renal function. Chromium-51 EDTA (ethylene diamine tetra-acetic acid) clearance measurements yield accurate assessment of glomerular filtration rate. Methods are also available for detecting testicular torsion.

Cerebral scintigraphy

For the detection of abnormalities associated with certain neuropsychiatric disorders, notably the dementias, schizophrenia and epilepsy.

Thyroid

For estimation of the size, shape and position of the gland, detecting the presence of 'hot' thyrotoxic nodules or 'cold' nodules caused by adenoma, carcinoma, cysts, haemorrhage or any combination thereof. Iodine uptake can also be estimated simultaneously.

Adrenals

The detection of autonomously functioning Conn's tumours (cortex) and phaechromocytoma (medulla).

Reticuloendothelial system

Mapping of the bone marrow and lymphatic flow. Occasionally used to visualize the liver and spleen if ultrasound not available.

In addition, radiolabelled white cells can be used to search for infection or inflammation, notably in bone, suspected inflammatory bowel disease and after abdominal surgery.

Tracers are also available for detecting certain tumours, notably lymphoma, colonic carcinoma, ovarian carcinoma and malignant melanoma. Labelled red cells can detect sites of gastrointestinal bleeding. Oesophageal and gastric emptying studies are also available.

Magnetic resonance imaging

Also known as nuclear magnetic resonance (NMR). Magnetic resonance imaging (MRI) uses a strong magnetic field and radio waves to produce detailed pictures of the inside of the body.

Provides cross-sectional images (MRI) or spectroscopic information on chemicals in tissues (magnetic resonance spectroscopy, MRS).

A small trolley carries the patient into a super-conducting magnet that provides a strong external magnetic field (Fig. 16.8). The axes of individual hydrogen ions usually lie at random but can be lined up at a particular angle by a strong magnetic field (position a). When subjected to a second radio-frequency magnetic field, the angle is changed (to position b). When the radiowaves cease, position a is restored by the continuing magnetic field and a radiowave is emitted and detected.

MRI scans can show muscles, joints, bone marrow, blood vessels, nerves and other structures within the body. The images the scans produce are usually

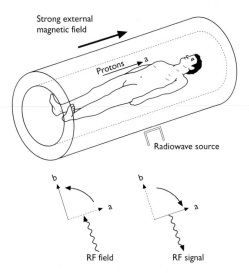

Fig. 16.8 Magnetic resonance imaging.

two-dimensional but, in some cases, several different scans can be taken to build up a three-dimensional image that can be displayed on a computer screen.

Hydrogen is the most plentiful element in the body. MRI can detect differences between the concentration of hydrogen ions in different tissues, notably fat (-CH2-) and water (HOH).

Excellent for examination of the head and spinal cord:

- the brain for demonstrating tumours, multiple areas of demyelination of white matter in multiple sclerosis (Fig. 16.9), in spinal cord lesions, including disc prolapse
- bone and softtissue tumours

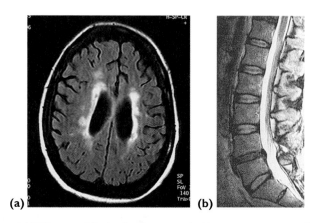

(a)   **(b)**

Fig. 16.9   (a) MRI scan of the brain. The central white areas are areas of demyelination in multiple sclerosis. (b) MRI (sagittal section) of the lumbar spine showing white central spinal fluid surrounding the spinal cord.

MRI will show detailed cross-sectional anatomical detail similar to CT scanning but can also provide coronal and sagittal planes in addition to the standard axial plane available from CT scanning.

Images can be obtained that accentuate different characteristics:

- **spin echo T$_1$-weighted**
  - fat – white (bright)
  - fluid – dark
  - cortical bone – black
- **spin echo T$_2$-weighted**
  - fat – grey
  - fluid – white (bright)

- **gradient echo**
  - flowing blood – white
  - used for MRI angiography
- **intravenous contrast**
  - gadolinium based
  - leaky vessels from inflammation
  - increased number of vessels from neoplasm
- **oral contrast**
  - to label bowel

N.B. Patients with pacemakers should not be subjected to MRI. Patients with metal implants may not be able to undergo MRI and must be discussed with a radiologist. MRI has an expanding role in many fields of medicine and the indications for its use are likely to increase.

PET scanning

Positron emission tomography (PET) is imaging using 18-F-dioxyglucose (FDG). FDG uptake correlates with glucose metabolism. Malignant tumours actively metabolize glucose, making it possible to image tumours using this technique. PET scanning is undergoing further evaluation and is useful in oncology.

A PET scan produces three-dimensional, colour images of the body using radiation. It can be used to diagnose a health condition or find out more about how a condition is developing. It can also be used to measure how well treatment for a condition is working.

A PET scan works by detecting radiation inside the body, and makes images that show how the radiation is being broken down. Radiation is given to the body safely as a medicine called a radiotracer, which goes to the part of the body that needs to be examined. The level of radiation is very small, so it does not damage the body.

Endoscopy

An endoscopy is a procedure in which the internal organs are directly visualized, usually with a fibreoptic endoscope. An endoscope is a thin, long, flexible tube that contains a light source and a video camera, so that images of the inside of the body can be relayed to an external monitor (screen).

Gastroscopy

A flexible scope is inserted via the patient's mouth after intravenous diazepam for direct vision of oesophagus, stomach and duodenum. Refer to Endoscopic retrograde cholangiopancreatography (ERCP) in this chapter.

Proctoscopy

With the patient lying in a left lateral position, with knees and hips flexed, a short tube is introduced through the patient's anus with a removable obturator lubricated with a gel. This is used to investigate **rectal bleeding** – haemorrhoids or anal carcinoma.

Sigmoidoscopy

With the patient in left lateral position, either a rigid tube with a removable obturator or a flexible fibreoptic endoscope is introduced. The bowel is kept patent with air from a hand pump. This is used to investigate:

- **bleeding, diarrhoea or constipation** – ulcerative colitis, other inflammatory bowel disease or carcinoma
- **inflamed area or lumps**, which can be biopsied.

Colonoscopy

After the bowel is emptied with an oral purgative and a washout if necessary, the whole of the colon and possibly the terminal ileum can be examined. This is used to investigate **bleeding, diarrhoea or constipation** – *inflammatory bowel disease, polyps* or *carcinoma*.

Bronchoscopy

After intravenous diazepam, the major bronchi are observed. This is used to investigate **haemoptysis or suspected bronchial obstruction** – *bronchial carcinoma* and for clearing *obstructed bronchi*, e.g. peanuts, plug of mucus.

Laparoscopy

After general anaesthetic, organs can be observed through a small abdominal incision, aspirated for cells or organisms, or biopsied. Laparoscopic surgery includes sterilization, ova collection for *in vitro* fertilization and laparoscopic cholecystectomy.

Cystoscopy

After local anaesthetic, a cystoscope is inserted into the urethral meatus. This is used for the following:

- **urinary bleeding or poor flow** – *bladder tumours*
- under direct vision, catheters can be inserted into ureters for retrograde pyelograms.

Colposcopy

Examination of the cervix, usually to take a cervical smear. This is used to investigate **premalignant changes** or **cancer**.

Needle biopsy

Core biopsy

A small core of tissue (30×1 mm) is obtained through needle puncture of organs for histological diagnosis. This is used to investigate:

- liver – *cirrhosis, alcoholic liver disease, chronic active hepatitis*
- kidney – glomerulonephritis, interstitial nephritis
- lung – *fibrosis, tumours, tuberculosis*

Fine-needle aspiration

A technique to obtain cells for diagnosis of tumours or for microbiological diagnosis. The needle position is guided by ultrasound, computed tomographic (CT) or magnetic resonance imaging (MRI) scan. For investigation of many unexplained lumps, e.g. pancreas or breast lumps, to diagnose carcinoma.

Cardiological investigations

Electrocardiogram

See Chapter 17.

Chest radiograph

See earlier in this chapter.

Exercise electrocardiography (stress testing)

- Exercise may reveal cardiac dysfunction not apparent at rest.
- Most commonly used in suspected coronary artery disease.

Connected to a 12-lead electrocardiograph (ECG) machine, with resuscitation equipment available, the patient exercises at an increasing workload on a treadmill (or bicycle). **Bruce protocol**: 3-minute stages of increasing belt speed and treadmill gradient. Take ECG every minute, blood pressure every 3 minutes. This assesses:

- exercise capacity
- haemodynamic response
- symptoms
- ECG changes.

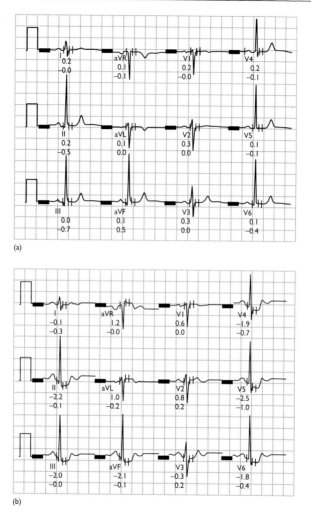

(a)

(b)

Fig. 16.10   Example of a strongly positive exercise test – signal-averaged recordings before exercise (a) and at peak effort (b). There is a marked horizontal ST depression in the inferolateral leads, II, III, aVF and V$_{4-6}$.

Exercise for as long as possible, stopping when there are:
- marked symptoms
- severe ECG changes
- ventricular arrhythmias
- fall in blood pressure.

Myocardial ischaemia causes ST segment depression. A high false-positive rate occurs in absence of angina (c. 20%). False-positive incidence depends on age and sex, with young females having the highest rate, even in the presence of typical symptoms of angina.

Clinically important abnormalities are:
- horizontal or downward sloping ST depression (Fig. 16.10)
- deep ST depression
- ST changes with typical anginal symptoms.

A definitely negative test at a high workload denotes an excellent prognosis.
- **Angiography is indicated** if only a low workload is achieved before important abnormalities occur.
- **Medical treatment of angina** may be appropriate if three or four stages are completed.

Echocardiography

This visualizes structures and function of the heart. Uses ultrasound (2.5–7.5 MHz) to reflect from interfaces in the heart, e.g. ventricle and atrial walls, heart, valves, major vessels. The higher frequency gives better discrimination but lower tissue penetration. The time delay between transmission and reception indicates depth.

Two-dimensional echocardiography

Two-dimensional echocardiography (2D) (Fig. 16.11) uses a scanning beam swept backwards and forwards across a 45° or 60° arc to construct a picture of the anatomy of the heart.

Two-dimensional (2D) echocardiography is excellent for demonstrating:
- valvular anatomy
- ventricular function, e.g. poor contraction, low ejection fraction, akinetic segment, paradoxical motion in aneurysm
- structural abnormalities:
  - pericardial effusion
  - ventricular hypertrophy
  - congenital heart disease.

Quantifying valvular function is better achieved by Doppler echocardiography.

M-mode echocardiography

M-mode echocardiography (Fig. 16.12) uses a single pencil beam, and movements of the heart in that beam are visualized on moving sensitized paper. It predates 2D echocardiography but is useful for measuring ventricular diameters in systole/diastole.

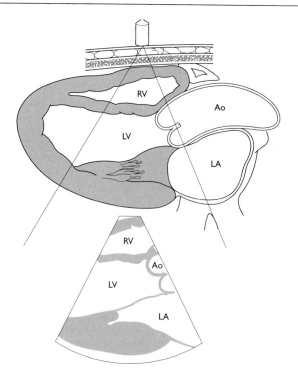

Fig. 16.11 Two-dimensional echocardiograph. Ao, aorta; LA, left atrium; LV, left ventricle; RV, right ventricle.

Doppler ultrasound cardiography

- Velocity of blood movement in the heart and circulation assessed by Doppler shift.
- Blood accelerates through an obstruction, e.g. a stenosed valve. The peak velocity is proportional to the haemodynamic gradient.
- Reverse flow pattern in valvular reflux.

Multigated Doppler or colour flow Doppler
- Rapid method of detecting abnormal blood flow due to a leaking valve or an intracardiac shunt, e.g. ventricular septal defect.
- Doppler ultrasound provides functional assessment to complement the anatomical assessment of 2D echocardiography.
- Echo machine calculates the direction and velocity of flow, pixel by pixel, within a segment of the image and codes it in colour.
- It superimposes flow on the 2D image.

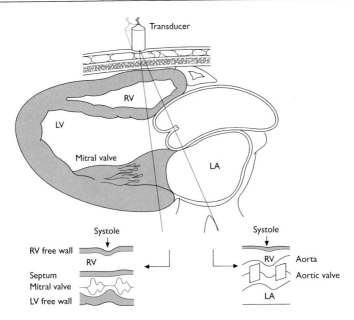

Fig. 16.12 M-mode echocardiographs, with two examples showing mitral and aortic valves opening and closing. LA, left atrium; LV, left ventricle; RV, right ventricle.

Radionuclide imaging in cardiology

Radionuclides can be used in the assessment of cardiac disease in three main ways.

Myocardial perfusion scintigraphy

- **Demonstrates abnormal blood flow in coronary artery disease** in conjunction with exercise testing. Thallium 201 is extracted from the blood in proportion to flow.
- Ischaemic myocardium appears as a cold spot on the scan taken immediately after injection of thallium.
- If the area is not infarcted, the cold spot 'fills in' as thallium redistributes in the following 4 hours.
- Thallium scanning is a more reliable diagnostic investigation than exercise testing and the number and extent of defects correlate with prognosis.

Radionuclide ventriculography (multiple gated acquisition (MUGA) scanning)

– Assesses ventricle function.

The patient's blood (usually red blood cells) is labelled with technetium 99 m (half-life 6 hours). A gamma camera and a computer generate a moving image of the heart by 'gating' the computer to the patient's ECG.

Systolic function of the left ventricle is quantified by the ejection fraction (normally 0.50–0.70):

$$\text{Ejection fraction} = \frac{\text{stroke volume}}{\text{end-diastolic volume}}$$

i.e. the proportion of the total diastolic volume that is ejected in systole.

Images can be collected during exercise as well as at rest, to assess the effect of stress on left ventricular function.

Pyrophosphate scanning

– Demonstrates recent myocardial infarction, e.g. 1–10 days after event.

Technetium 99 m pyrophosphate is taken up by areas of myocardial infarction producing a hot spot, maximal at 3 days. Indicated when:

- the ECG is too abnormal to demonstrate infarction (e.g. left bundle branch block)
- the patient has presented after the plasma enzyme changes, e.g. at 3 days.

Cardiac catheterization

An invasive assessment of cardiac function and disease in which fine tubes are passed, with mild sedation under operating theatre conditions:

- retrograde through arteries to left side of heart and coronary arteries
- anterograde through veins to right side of heart and pulmonary arteries
  - to make diagnosis, e.g. is valve critically stenosed?
  - is chest pain due to coronary artery disease?
  - to plan cardiac surgery, particularly coronary artery bypass grafting

It entails a major radiation dose. Major complications (one in 2000 cases) include:

- access artery dissection (2%)
- myocardial infarction (0.1%)
- air or cholesterol emboli can cause stroke or myocardial infarction
- death (0.01%).

Risks must be outweighed by the benefit the patient receives.

The most common approach is **cannulation of the right femoral vessels by the Seldinger technique**. A percutaneous fine-gauge needle punctures the vessel, through which a soft guidewire is passed. The needle is

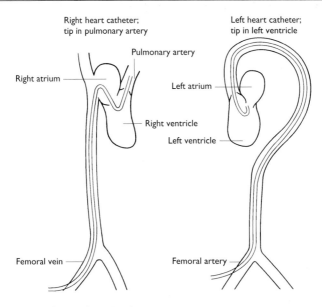

Right heart catheter;
tip in pulmonary artery

Left heart catheter;
tip in left ventricle

Pulmonary artery

Right atrium

Left atrium

Right ventricle

Left ventricle

Femoral vein

Femoral artery

Fig. 16.13 Cardiac catheterization.

withdrawn and an introducer sheath and catheter are inserted over the guidewire which is then withdrawn. Haemostasis is achieved by compression. The technique is not suitable if the patient is on anticoagulant drugs, has severe peripheral vascular disease or an abdominal aortic aneurysm (Fig. 16.13).

Alternative approach: **brachial vessels at elbow through a skin incision**. Closure of arterotomy by sutures allows use in anticoagulated patients.

Pressure measurements

Cardiac haemodynamics and gradients across individual valves, e.g. by pulling the catheter back across the **aortic valve**, whilst systolic pressures is recorded (Fig. 16.14).

Mitral stenosis is quantified by the diastolic pressure difference between the left ventricle (**left heart catheter**) and left atrium measured indirectly via the **right heart catheter** in the 'wedge' position – passed through the pulmonary artery to occlude a pulmonary arteriole so the pressure at the tip reflects the left atrial pressure transmitted through the pulmonary capillaries (Fig. 16.15).

The **cardiac output** is calculated either by the **Fick principle** (cardiac output is inversely proportional to difference between systemic arterial and mixed venous blood oxygen saturation) or by the **thermodilution** technique.

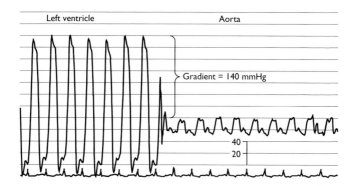

Fig. 16.14 Aortic stenosis. The systolic pressure falls as the catheter tip leaves the left ventricle, crossing the stenosed aortic valve. Diastolic pressure is prevented from falling by the aortic valve.

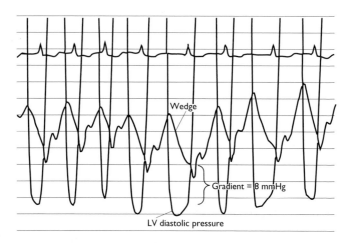

Fig. 16.15 Mitral stenosis. Left ventricular (LV) pressure trace expanded to show low diastolic pressures. A pressure difference between the wedge trace and LV diastolic trace reflects obstruction to flow into the left ventricle due to mitral stenosis. The rhythm is atrial fibrillation.

Radiopaque contrast

Radiopaque contrast (iodine based) is:
- injected into chambers to assess their systolic function and to detect valve regurgitation, e.g. left ventricular injection for mitral regurgitation
- injected into coronary ostia to detect coronary artery disease, with X-ray images of different projections.

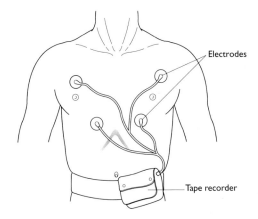

Fig. 16.16   The arrangement for the 24-hour ECG tape recorder.

Twenty-four hour ECG tape recording

ECG worn for 24 hours (or 48 hours) (Fig. 16.16) obtains on tape a continuous ECG recording during normal activities. For diagnosis of:
 – palpitations
 – dizzy spells
 – light-headedness or black-outs of possible cardiac origin.
May show episodes of:
 – atrial asystole
 – atrial or ventricular tachycardias
 – complete heart block
 – ST segment changes during angina or silent ischaemia.

Twenty-four hour blood pressure recording

Blood pressure is measured intermittently with an upper arm cuff and microphone, with recording on a tape. Allows evaluation of blood pressure during everyday activities without the 'white coat' effect of anxiety at the doctor's surgery increasing measured blood pressure.

Hypertension is defined as day-time average >140/>90 mmHg. Absence of lower blood pressure during the night ('dip') suggests secondary hypertension.

Respiratory investigations
pH and arterial blood gases

See Chapter 19 for values in type I and type II respiratory failure. Normal ranges (Fig. 16.17):

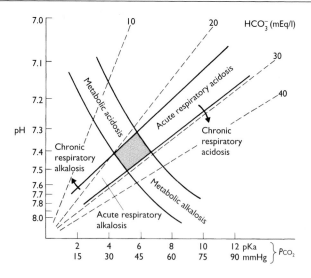

Fig. 16.17   Descriptive clinical terms. Shaded area is normal range.

- pH 7.35–7.45
- P_{CO_2} 4.6–6.0 kPa
- P_{O_2} 12–14 kPa
- HCO_3- 22–26 mmol/l
- base excess is the amount of acid required to titrate pH to 7.4.

In ventilatory failure:
- P_{O_2} low
- P_{CO_2} high.

In respiratory failure from lung disease often:
- P_{O_2} low
- normal P_{CO_2} due to high carbon dioxide (CO_2) solubility and efficient transfer in lungs.

  For example, in asthma, raised CO_2 signifies tiredness and decreased ventilation from reduced muscular effort.

Respiratory acidosis

CO_2 retention from:
- respiratory disease with right-to-left shunt
- ventilatory failure
  - neuromuscular disease
  - physical causes, e.g. flail chest, kyphoscoliosis.

  Raised CO_2 leads to increased bicarbonate:

$$CO_2 + H_2O = H_2CO_3 = H^+ + HCO_3-$$

In chronic respiratory failure, renal compensation by excretion of H^+ and retention of HCO_3^- leads to further increased HCO_3^- (i.e. maintenance of normal pH with compensatory metabolic alkalosis).

Respiratory alkalosis
CO_2 blown off by hyperventilation due to:
- hysteria
- brainstem stimulation (rare).

In respiratory alkalosis:
- Po_2 normal
- Pco_2 low.

If chronic, compensated by metabolic acidosis with renal retention of H^+ and excretion of HCO_3^-.

Metabolic acidosis
Excess H^+ in blood:
- ketosis – 3-OH butyric acid accumulation in diabetes or starvation
- uraemia – lack of renal H^+ excretion
- renal tubular acidosis – lack of H^+ or NH_4^+ excretion
- acid ingestion – aspirin
- lactic acid accumulation – shock, hypoxia, exercise, biguanide
- formic acid accumulation – methanol intake
- loss of base – diarrhoea.

Usually compensatory respiratory alkalosis, e.g. Kussmaul respiration of diabetic coma (hyperventilation with deep breathing):
- Po_2 normal
- Pco_2 low
- to assist diagnosis, measure the anion gap:

$$[Na^+] + [K^+] - [Cl^-] - [HCO_3^-] = 7{-}16 \text{ mmol/l}$$

If the anion gap >16 mmol/l, unestimated anions are present, e.g. 3-OH butyrate, lactate, formate.

Metabolic alkalosis
Loss of H^+ due to:
- prolonged vomiting
- potassium depletion – secondary to renal tubular potassium–hydrogen exchange
- ingestion of base – old-fashioned sodium bicarbonate therapy of peptic ulcers.

Usually compensatory respiratory acidosis with hypoventilation:
- Po_2 low
- Pco_2 high.

Peak flow (Fig. 16.18)

- Blow into machine as hard and fast as you can.
- Records in litres per minute. Useful for diagnosing and observing asthma. Normal range is 300–500 l/min.
- Improvement with β-agonist, e.g. isoprenaline, indicates reversible airway disease, i.e. asthma.

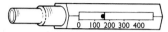

Fig. 16.18 Peak flow machine.

Spirometry (Fig. 16.19)

- Blow into machine, a **vitalograph**, as hard as you can – measures pattern of air flow during forced expiration.
- To distinguish between restrictive lung disease, e.g. *emphysema, fibrosis,* and *obstructive lung disease*, e.g. *asthma, chronic obstructive airways disease.*

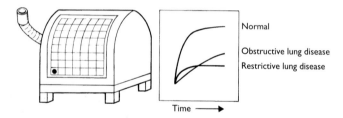

Fig. 16.19 A vitalograph.

Skin testing for allergens

Drops of a weak allergen solution are placed on the skin and a superficial prick of the skin, with a short lancet through the liquid, inoculates the epidermis. Special lancets coated with freeze-dried allergen can be used. A local wheal indicates an allergic response.

Carbon monoxide transfer factor

The rate of uptake of carbon monoxide from inspired gas determines the lung diffusion capacity. It is reduced in alveolar diseases, e.g. *pulmonary fibrosis.*

Chest radiograph

See earlier in this chapter.

Ventilation/perfusion scan

Ventilation (*V*) scan
Inhalation of an isotope allows a picture of the parenchyma of the lungs to be taken by a gamma camera.

Perfusion (*P*) scan
Injection of isotope into the bloodstream demonstrates the blood flow in the lungs.

Mismatch of the scans is used to diagnose pulmonary embolism, i.e. air reaches all parts of the lung, while the blood does not (Fig. 16.20). Matching defects occur with other lung pathologies, e.g. *emphysema*.

N.B. A perfusion scan showing an area of ischaemia with a normal chest X-ray is generally sufficient to diagnose a pulmonary embolus. A *V/Q* scan is needed if there is other lung pathology suspected or seen on X-ray (e.g. chronic bronchitis/emphysema), but in practice the results are difficult to interpret.

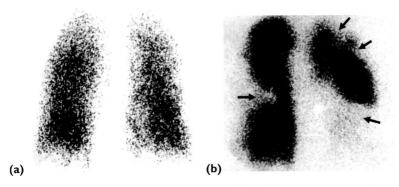

(a) **(b)**

Fig. 16.20 *V/Q* scan of pulmonary embolism: (a) ventilation scan – normal; (b) perfusion scan (arrows mark perfusion defects).

Bronchoscopy

Flexible bronchoscopy – under mild sedation, e.g. intravenous diazepam with local anaesthetic spray to pharynx and larynx. Vision by fibreoptics.
- Obstructions can be visualized.
- Biopsies can be taken for neoplasms.
- Aspiration samples, sometimes after lavage with saline, can be taken for organisms and malignant cells.

Gastrointestinal investigations

Abdominal radiograph

See earlier in this chapter.

Abdominal ultrasound

See earlier in this chapter.

Upper gastrointestinal endoscopy

A flexible fibreoptic tube is introduced into the oesophagus, stomach and duodenum after mild sedation, e.g. intravenous diazepam, with local anaesthetic to the pharynx.

Direct vision of the gastrointestinal tract to investigate:

- **dysphagia** – oesophageal tumour or stricture
- **haematemesis or melaena** – oesophageal varices, gastric and duodenal ulcers, superficial gastric erosions, gastric carcinoma
- **epigastric pain** – peptic ulcer, oesophagitis, gastritis, duodenitis
- **unexplained weight loss** – gastric carcinoma.

Endoscopic retrograde cholangiopancreatography (Fig. 16.21)
Through a fibreoptic endoscope, with a picture on a video, under direct vision, a tube is inserted through the ampulla of Vater at the opening of the common bile duct, and introduction of a radiopaque contrast medium allows X-ray visualization of:

- **biliary tree**, for stones, tumours, strictures, irregularities
- **pancreatic ducts**, for chronic pancreatitis, dilated ducts or distortion from a tumour.

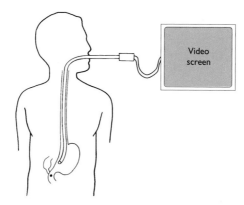

Fig. 16.21 Endoscopic retrograde cholangiopancreatography.

The endoscope can be used for surgery, including **sphincterotomy** of the ampulla for removal of gallstones in the bile duct or the introduction of a rigid tube, **a stent**, through a constricting tumour to allow biliary drainage.

Barium swallow, meal, enema

Barium is drunk (swallow for oesophagus, meal for stomach/duodenum) or introduced rectally (enema) or via a catheter into the duodenum (small bowel enema). X-rays are taken with barium coating the mucosa. Air may be introduced to distend organs and to give double-contrast films.

- It outlines physical abnormalities:
    - strictures, e.g. *fibrosis, carcinomata*
    - filling defects, e.g. *polyps, carcinomata*
    - craters, e.g. *ulcers, diverticula*
    - mucosal irregularities
    - mucosal folds radiating from *peptic ulcer*
    - clefts in *Crohn's disease of ileum and colon*
    - featureless mucosa of *early ulcerative colitis*
    - islands of mucosa in *severe ulcerative colitis.*

An irregularity on a single film needs to be seen on other views before an abnormality is confirmed, as peristalsis or gut contents can mimic defects.

Hydrogen breath tests

- **Lactulose breath test for bacterial overgrowth**. Oral lactulose is given, and excess gut flora in the small bowel or blind loop cause prompt metabolism to provide exhaled hydrogen.
- **Lactose breath test for lactase deficiency.**
- Oral lactose with subnormal exhaled hydrogen.

Renal investigations

Urine testing

Testing the urine is part of the routine physical examination. It is most simply done using one of the combination dipsticks.

- Dip the stick in the urine and compare the colours with the key at the times specified. Of particular interest are:
    - pH
    - protein content (**N.B.** does not detect Bence Jones protein)
    - ketones
    - glucose
    - bilirubin
    - urobilinogen
    - blood/haemoglobin.

Urine microscopy

Urine should be sent to the laboratory (sterile) for 'M, C and S':
- M (microscopy) – for the presence of red cells, white cells, casts and pathogens
- C (culture) – using appropriate media to detect bacteria and other pathogens
- S (sensitivity) – to determine the sensitivity of bacteria to antibiotics.

Creatinine clearance

Precise measurements of the **glomerular filtration rate** are made isotopic-ally, e.g. chromium EDTA clearance. The creatinine clearance is easier to organize, although less accurate.
- Collect a blood sample for plasma creatinine.
- Collect a 24-h urine sample for creatinine.

Formula:

$$\frac{U \times V}{P \times T}$$

$$\frac{\text{Urine creatinine (mmol)}}{\text{Plasma creatinine (mmol)}} \times \frac{\text{Urine volume (ml)} \times 10^3}{\text{Duration collection (min)}} = \text{Clearance (ml/min)}$$

Normal value: 80–120 ml/min.

Abdominal radiograph

See earlier in this chapter.

Abdominal ultrasound

See earlier in this chapter.

Intravenous urogram

An initial plain film to show renal or ureteric stones. Contrast medium is injected intravenously, concentrated in the kidney and excreted.
- nephrogram phase – kidneys are outlined
  - observe position, size, shape, filling defects, e.g. tumour
- excretion phase – renal pelvis
  - renal papillae may be lost from chronic pyelonephritis, papillary necrosis

- calyces blunted from hydronephrosis
- pelviureteric obstruction – large pelvis, normal ureters
- ureters – observe position – displaced by other pathology?
  - size – dilated from obstruction or recent infection
  - irregularities – may be contractions and need to be checked in sequential films.
- bladder-observe outline and any indentations or shadows.

Neurological investigations

Electroencephalogram

Approximately 22 electrodes are applied to the scalp in standard positions and cerebral electrical activity is amplified and recorded. There are marked normal variations and differences between awake and sleep.

Main uses
- epilepsy
  - primary, generalized epilepsy – generalized spike and slow-wave discharges
  - partial epilepsy – focal spikes
- disorders of consciousness or coma
  - encephalopathy
  - encephalitis
  - dementia.

The main value of this technique is in showing episodes of abnormal waves compatible with epilepsy. Large normal variation makes interpretation difficult.

Lumbar puncture

A needle is introduced between the lumbar vertebrae (Fig. 16.22), through the dura into the subarachnoid space, and cerebrospinal fluid is obtained for examination. Normal cerebrospinal fluid is completely clear.

The major diagnostic value of this technique is in:
- subarachnoid haemorrhage – uniformly red, whereas blood from a 'traumatic' tap is in the first specimen
- xanthochromia – yellow stain from haemoglobin breakdown
- meningitis – pyogenic, turbid fluid, white cells, organisms on culture, low glucose and raised protein
- raised pressure may indicate a tumour.

CT scanning

See earlier in this chapter.

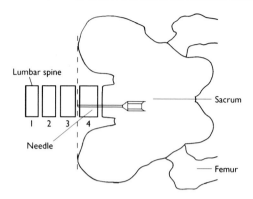

Fig. 16.22   The lumbar puncture needle is positioned between L3 and L4 to one side of the supraspinous ligament.

Magnetic resonance imaging

See earlier in this chapter.

Myelogram

Contrast medium is injected into cerebrospinal fluid in the subarachnoid space to demonstrate thoracic or cervical disc prolapses or cord tumours. Largely replaced by MRI.

Lumbar radiculogram

Contrast medium is injected to demonstrate lumbar disc prolapses. Largely replaced by MRI.

CHAPTER 17

The 12-Lead Electrocardiogram

General principles

Introduction

The electrocardiogram (ECG) tracings arise from the electrical changes, depolarization and repolarization that accompany muscle contraction. With knowledge of the relative position of the leads to the electrodes, the ECG tracings provide direct information of the cardiac muscle and its activity.

Six **standard leads** – I, II, III, aVR, aVL, aVF – are recorded from the limb electrodes (aV = augmented voltage) and examine the heart from different directions (Fig. 17.1). The standard leads examine the heart in the **vertical** plane (Fig. 17.2).

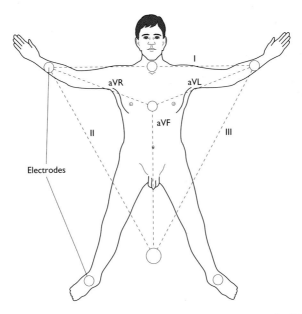

Fig. 17.1   The positioning of the limb electrodes and the six standard leads.

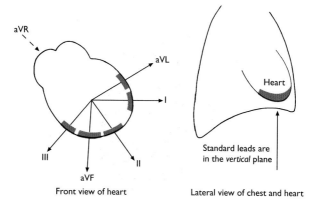

Fig. 17.2 Examining the vertical plane.

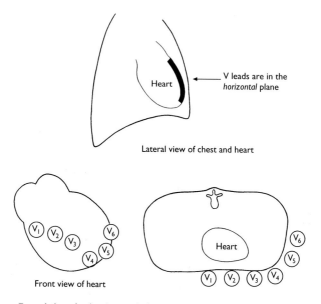

Fig. 17.3 Examining the horizontal plane.

Six **chest leads**, V leads, attached by sticky electrodes to the chest wall, are all in the **horizontal** plane (Fig. 17.3).

Obstruction of arteries gives appropriate specific patterns of ischaemia:

- left anterior descending coronary artery – *anterior ischaemia* or *infarct* (V_{1-6})
- circumflex coronary artery – *lateral ischaemia* or *infarct* (I, aVL)
- right coronary artery – *inferior ischaemia* or *infarct* (II, III, aVF) (Fig. 17.4).

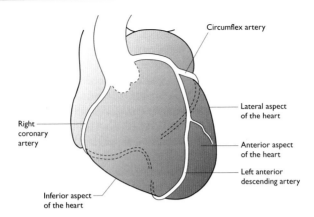

Fig. 17.4 Coronary arteries.

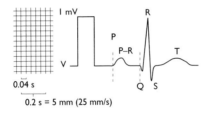

Fig. 17.5 Standardising the ECG tracing. P, atrial depolarization; QRS, ventricular depolarization; T, repolarization.

Every ECG tracing must first be standardized by making sure the 1 mV mark deviates the pointer 10 small squares on the paper (Fig. 17.5).

Normal ECG (Fig. 17.6)

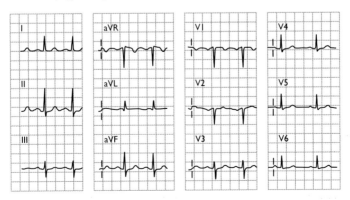

Fig. 17.6 A normal electrocardiogram.

Normal ECG variants

- T waves can be inverted in leads III, aVF, V_{1-3}.
- T waves and P waves are always inverted in aVR (if not, leads are misplaced).
- In a young athletic person:
  - ST segments may be raised, especially in leads V_{1-5}
  - right bundle branch block (RBBB) may occur
  - electrical criteria of left ventricular hypertrophy may be present
  - bradycardia <40 beats/min
  - physiological Q waves.
- Ectopics of any type, including ventricular, are rarely of significance.
- Raised ST segments are common in Afro-Caribbean subjects.
- P mitrale is overdiagnosed:
  - P wave in V_1 is often biphasic.

Electrophysiology of cardiac contractions

All cardiac muscle has a tendency to depolarization, leading to excitation and contraction.

Initial electrical discharge from the sinoatrial (SA) node (under the influence of sympathetic and parasympathetic control) spreads to the atrioventricular (AV) node and via the bundle of His to the ventricles (Fig. 17.7).

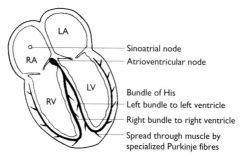

Fig. 17.7   Conduction system (electrical pathway).

The deflection of the ECG tracing indicates the average direction of all muscle activity at each moment.

Depolarization spreads:
- towards lead – ECG tracing moves up the paper
- away from lead – tracing moves down paper.

P wave (Fig. 17.8)

- depolarization spreads from SA node to AV node through the atrial muscle fibres (1 in Fig. 17.8)
- best seen in leads II and V₁
- usually small, as atria are small

Normal P wave <2.5 mm high, <2.5 mm wide.

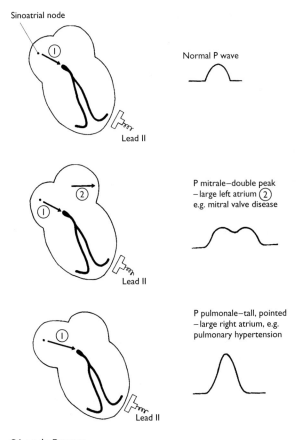

Sinoatrial node

Lead II

Normal P wave

P mitrale—double peak
– large left atrium (2)
e.g. mitral valve disease

Lead II

P pulmonale—tall, pointed
– large right atrium, e.g.
pulmonary hypertension

Lead II

Fig. 17.8 SA node P wave.

QRS complex (Fig. 17.9)

The QRS deflections have a standard nomenclature:

    Q – any initial deflection downwards.

    R – any deflection upwards, whether or not a preceding Q.

    S – any deflection downwards after an R wave, whether or not a preceding Q.

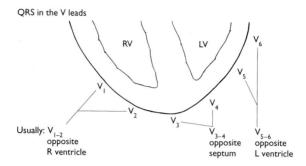

QRS in the V leads

Usually: V$_{1-2}$ opposite R ventricle

V$_{3-4}$ opposite septum

V$_{5-6}$ opposite L ventricle

Fig. 17.9 QRS in the V leads.

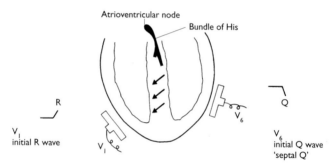

V$_1$ initial R wave

V$_6$ initial Q wave 'septal Q'

Fig. 17.10 Depolarization of the septum.

The septum depolarizes first from left to right (Fig. 17.10). The ventricles then depolarize from inside outwards. The large left ventricle then normally dominates (Fig. 17.11).

The transition point where R and S are equal is the position of the septum (Fig. 17.12).

V$_6$ S wave after R wave as depolarization spreads around ventricle away from V$_6$.

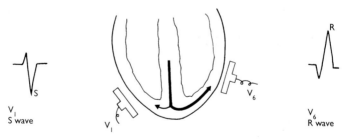

V$_1$ S wave

V$_6$ R wave

Fig. 17.11 Depolarization of the ventricles.

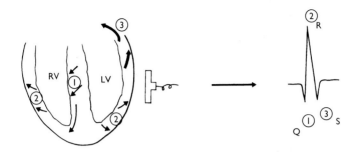

Fig. 17.12   The transition point.

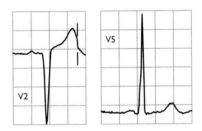

Fig. 17.13   Left ventricular hypertrophy.

Left ventricle hypertrophy (LVH)

V_5 or V_6 – R wave >25 mm.
V_1 or V_2 – S wave deep.
Tallest R wave + deepest S wave >35 mm (Fig. 17.13).

- Voltage changes on their own are not enough – thin people with a thin ribcage can have big complexes.
- Obese people have small complexes.
- Also look for R wave in V_1
    - rotation to right of transition point left axis deviation.
- T wave inversion in V_5, V_6 in the presence of LVH is termed left ventricular 'strain pattern' and indicates marked hypertrophy (Fig. 17.14).

Right ventricle hypertrophy (RVH)

The left ventricle is no longer dominant.
V_1 – R wave > S wave.
V_6 – deep S wave (Fig. 17.15).
Also look for:

- right axis deviation
- peaked P of right atrial hypertrophy
- T wave inversion in V_2 and V_3 – right ventricular 'strain pattern'.

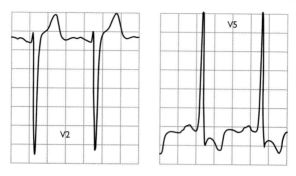

Fig. 17.14   Left ventricular hypertrophy strain pattern.

Fig. 17.15   Right ventricular hypertrophy.

Myocardial infarction (MI) – full thickness of ventricle

Infarction is the term for dead muscle. See Table 17.1 for the time sequence of ECG changes in myocardial infarction.

Table 17.1   Classic time sequence of onset of ECG changes in myocardial infarction

Approximate time of onset after chest pain		ECG changes
Immediately	1. May be normal	ECG may be normal. Occasionally ST segment changes occur immediately pain develops, or even before
0–2 h	2. 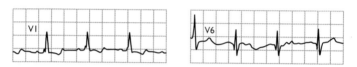	ST segments rise – occluded artery → injury pattern

Table 17.1 (*continued*)

Approximate time of onset after chest pain		ECG changes
3–8 h	3.	Injured tissue remains Some dies (Q waves = myocardium death) Some improves to become ischaemic only (T wave inversion) Full infarct pattern: – Q waves – raised ST segments – inverted T waves
8–24 h	4.	Injured tissue either dies → Q wave or improves and abnormal ST segments disappear Inverted T waves remain
After 1–2 days	5.	Ischaemia disappears T waves upright again Q waves usually remain, as dead tissue will not come alive again Q waves may subsequently disappear if scarred tissue contracts

Pathological Q wave:
   – width = or > 0.04 s (one small square)
   – depth > one-third height of R wave
   – smaller Q waves are physiological from septum depolarization
   – as ventricles depolarize from inside, an electrode in the ventricle cavity would record contraction as Q wave
   – through 'dead' window, this is seen as if from inside the heart, i.e. the depolarization of the far ventricle wall away from the electrode gives a negative deflection (Fig. 17.16).

Acute myocardial ischaemia – raised ST segments
Damaged but potentially salvageable myocardium:
   – ST segment – normally within 0.5 mm of isoelectric line
   – ST elevation in V_1 and V_2 may be normal – high 'take-off' of j point
   – ST elevation elsewhere is normal.

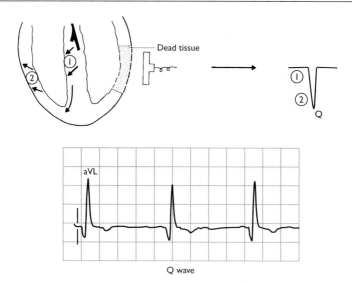

Fig. 17.16   Pathological Q wave.

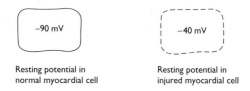

Fig. 17.17   Normal baseline.

Normal baseline:
Resting myocardial cell potential approximately −90 mV. In an injured cell, failing cell membrane only allows potential of perhaps −40 mV (Fig. 17.17).

   If two electrodes record from different areas of the resting heart, one normal and one injured, a galvanometer would register −50 mV (i.e. the difference between −90 mV and −40 mV). This depresses the baseline below normal over the injured area, although this cannot be recognized until after the QRS complex (Fig. 17.18).

Raised ST segment:
   − acute ischaemic injury of ventricle
   − pericarditis
   − normal athletes
   − normal Afro-Caribbeans.

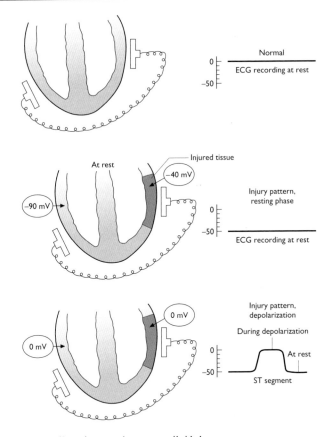

Fig. 17.18 Baseline changes in myocardial injury.

Anterior infarction (Figs 17.19, 17.20)
- changes in leads V_{1-6}
- occlusion of left anterior descending coronary artery

Inferior infarction (Fig. 17.21)
- changes in leads II, III, aVF
- occlusion of right coronary artery

Lateral infarction
- changes in leads I, aVL
- occlusion of circumflex artery

Septal infarction
- changes in leads V_{2-3}
- occlusion of septal branches of left anterior descending coronary artery

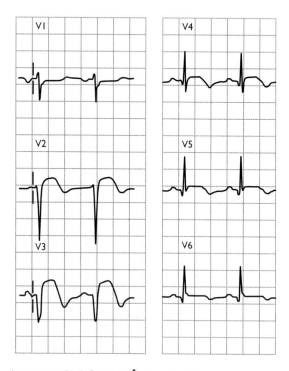

Fig. 17.19 Acute anterior infarct: ST ↑ V_{2-6} at 3–8 hours.

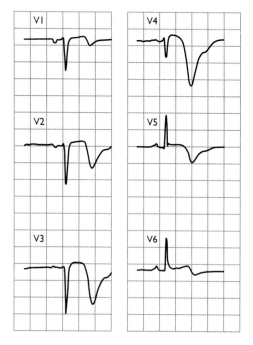

Fig. 17.20 Ten hours after anterior myocardial infarct.

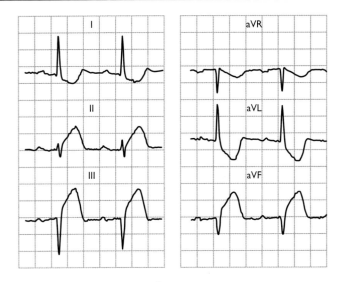

Fig. 17.21 Acute inferior infarct: ST ↑ in II, III, aVF with reciprocal depression in other leads.

Posterior infarction
- changes in lead V_1 (e.g. R wave, ST depression)
- occlusion of branches of right coronary artery

Chronic myocardial ischaemia
Reduced oxygen supply to muscle:
- ST depression
- T wave inversion
- occasionally tall pointed T wave

These changes can also occur during an exercise tolerance test when ischaemia develops (Fig. 17.22).

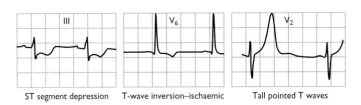

ST segment depression   T-wave inversion–ischaemic   Tall pointed T waves

Fig. 17.22 Chronic myocardial ischaemia.

QRS axis

- The direction of depolarization of the heart is sometimes helpful in diagnosis.
- Note that the axis deviation on its own is rarely significant but alerts you to look for right or left ventricular hypertrophy.
- Look at the standard leads for the most equiphasic QRS complex (R and S equal). The axis is approximately at right angles to this in the direction of the most positive standard lead (largest R wave) (Fig. 17.23).

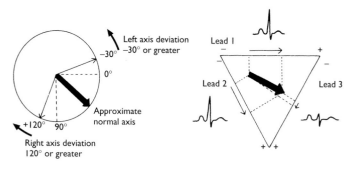

Fig. 17.23   QRS axis.

Pattern recognition
Left axis deviation

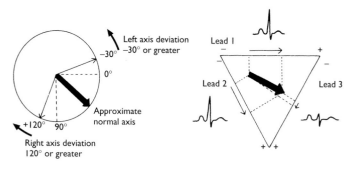

Fig. 17.24   Left axis deviation.

Right axis deviation

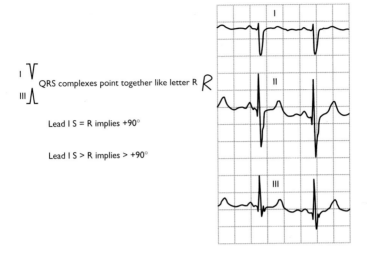

Fig. 17.25   Right axis deviation.

QRS complex

- Normal if width <0.12 s (three small squares).
- If >0.12 s – bundle branch block.
- An apparently wide QRS complex, <0.12 s wide – partial bundle branch block or interventricular conduction defect.
- Left bundle branch block (LBBB) is usually associated with some form of heart disease.
- RBBB is often a normal variation, especially in athletes. Immediately after a myocardial infarction, the development of RBBB may be serious.

Left bundle branch block
- M pattern in V_6.
- Throughout ECG, slurred ST segment and T wave inversion opposite to major deflection of QRS.
- Lead V_6
    - depolarization of septal muscle from right bundle gives positive deflection
    - right heart depolarization gives negative deflection
    - left heart depolarization gives positive deflection (Fig. 17.26)
- Standard leads
    - left axis deviation as impulse spreads from right bundle up to left ventricle
    - also occurs if only anterior fascicle of left bundle blocked
    - left anterior hemiblock

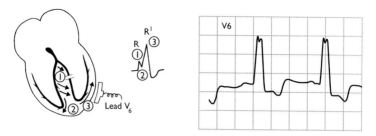

Fig. 17.26 Left bundle branch block.

Right bundle branch block
- M pattern in V_1.
- Lead V_1
  - depolarization of septal muscle from left bundle gives positive deflection
  - left heart depolarization gives negative deflection
  - right heart depolarization gives positive deflection (Fig. 17.27)
- Standard leads
  - axis usually normal, as depends on large muscle mass of left ventricle
  - if RBBB is associated with left axis, there is block of anterior fascicle of left bundle – bifascicular block
    All heart is being excited via remaining posterior fascicle of left bundle.

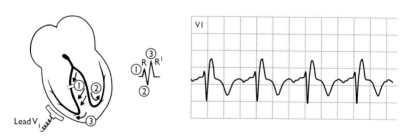

Fig. 17.27 Right bundle branch block.

Arrhythmias

- sinus arrhythmia
- ectopics
- tachycardias
- bradycardias

Sinus arrhythmia

Normal variation with respiratory rate – increase rate on inspiration (Fig. 17.28).

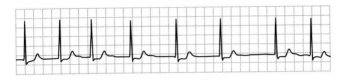

Fig. 17.28   Sinus arrhythmia.

Ectopics

Atrial ectopics

Ectopic focus anywhere in atria. Depolarization spreads across atrium to AV node like any normal beat:
- P wave is abnormal shape
- normal QRS complex

The atrial ectopic focus must fire early or would be entrained by normal excitation:
- appears early on rhythm strip
- followed by compensatory pause – waiting for normal SA node cycle (Fig. 17.29)

Junctional or nodal ectopics

Ectopic at AV node; no P wave (Fig. 17.30).

Ventricular ectopics

Ectopic anywhere in ventricles. Depolarization occurs first in that ventricle then spreads to other ventricle:
- no P wave
- wide complex
- bundle branch block pattern
  - left focus – RBBB pattern
  - right focus – LBBB pattern

Atrial and junctional ectopics are invariably innocent when picked up on a random ECG. The majority of ventricular ectopics are also innocent except after a myocardial infarction. Ventricular ectopics picked up on routine monitoring of healthy patients are approximately proportional to age, i.e. 30% of 30 year olds, 50% of 50 year olds and almost 100% of 70 year olds. Innocent ventricular ectopics usually disappear on exercise (Fig. 17.31).

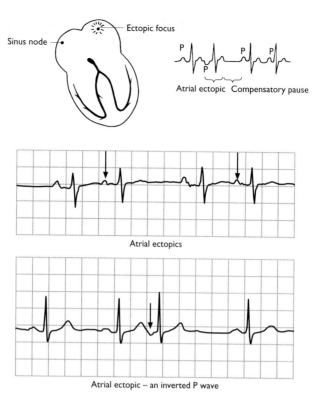

Fig. 17.29   Atrial ectopics.

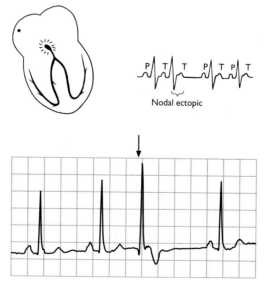

Fig. 17.30   Junctional or nodal ectopics.

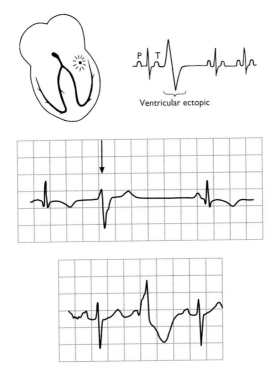

Fig. 17.31   Ventricular ectopics.

Tachycardias

Classification of tachycardias

- Tachycardias are divided into:
    - **narrow-complex regular** – QRS complex up to 0.08 s – two little squares on ECG
        - sinus tachycardia (Fig. 17.32)
        - supraventricular tachycardia, atrial tachycardia, atrial flutter
    - **narrow-complex irregular**
        - atrial tachycardia with varying block, atrial fibrillation

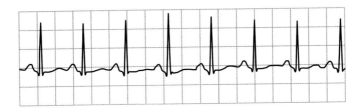

Fig. 17.32   Sinus tachycardia.

- **broad-complex** – QRS complex about 0.12 s – three small squares
  - ventricular arrhythmias and occasionally supraventricular with aberrant (delayed) conduction
- Deciding whether a tachycardia is **atrial** or **ventricular** is not easy. Here are some pointers.
  - Narrow-complex tachycardias are usually atrial and broad-complex usually ventricular, **but not always**.
  - When acute ischaemic heart disease is present, tachycardias are usually ventricular. In the absence of ischaemic heart disease tachycardias are usually atrial, **but not always**.
  - If there is independent atrial activity (random appearance of p values), the tachycardia is ventricular.
  - Look at the patient's preceding ECGs or rhythm strip. If the tachycardia looks like a previous ectopic beat in shape, it will be that type of tachycardia.
  - Vagal stimulation (rubbing carotid, etc.) will only be effective in atrial rhythms.
  - The regularity or irregularity is not helpful in distinguishing ventricular from atrial arrhythmias.

Atrial fibrillation

The electrical impulse and contraction travel randomly around the atria:
- 'bag-of-worms' quivering atria
- irregular little waves on ECG – best seen V$_1$ (Fig. 17.33).

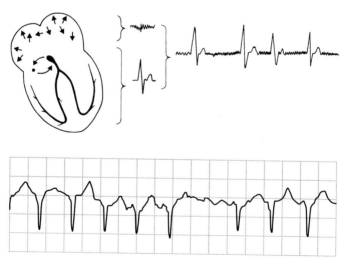

Fig. 17.33 Atrial fibrillation.

When it first develops, often 150+, fibrillation waves are difficult to see:
- AV node fires irregularly
- normal QRS complexes
    If irregular rate, no P waves, normal QRS – likely to be atrial fibrillation.

Digoxin is still the drug of choice – it decreases transmission of impulses down the bundle of His.

Atrial flutter

Atria contract very rapidly, 200–250 beats/min, giving a sawtooth pattern, but the ventricles only respond to every second or third or fourth contraction (2:1, 3:1, 4:1 block) (Fig. 17.34).

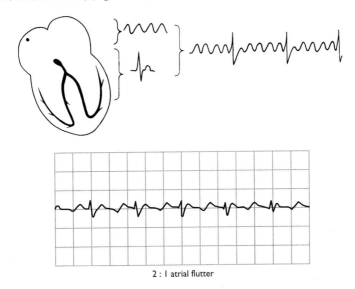

2 : 1 atrial flutter

Fig. 17.34   Atrial flutter.

Treated with digoxin, normally changes to atrial fibrillation.

Supraventricular tachycardia (SVT)
- Arises near AV node, 170 beats/min or more, regular.
- Complexes are identical, normal width or wide if also bundle branch block.
- Common in young patients (20–30 years).
- Rarely represents heart disease.
- Sudden onset and finish.
- Last few minutes to several hours.
- Patient may be tired, light-headed, uncomfortable.
- In older patients SVTs more likely to represent heart disease (Fig. 17.35).

Vagal stimulation (rubbing carotid sinus) can terminate attack.

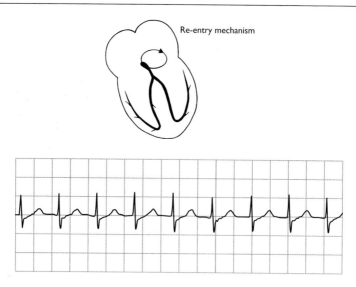

Fig. 17.35 Supraventricular tachycardia.

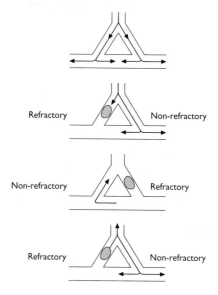

Fig. 17.36 The mechanism of re-entry tachycardias.

Re-entry is the most common mechanism for tachycardias (Fig. 17.36). Assumes two conduction pathways lead to ventricles. Normally conduction passes equally quickly down both pathways.

Problems arise when one pathway recovers more slowly than the other. When this happens the next conduction passes down only one pathway.

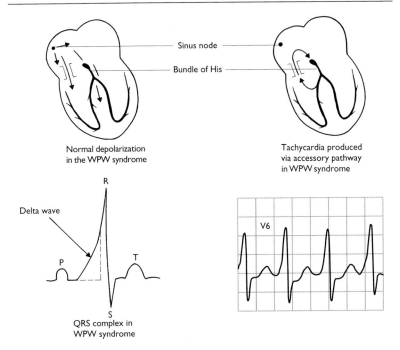

Fig. 17.37   Wolff–Parkinson–White syndrome.

Conduction subsequently passes retrogradely up the other pathway, which is no longer refractory. This pathway then becomes refractory while the first pathway conducts again and the impulse races round the pathways to give a tachycardia.

Wolff–Parkinson–White syndrome

This is the classic re-entry arrhythmia. There are two separate pathways from the atria to the ventricles. In the resting ECG the early entry, by the aberrant conduction pathway bypassing the bundle of His, is seen as a delta wave (Fig. 17.37).

Ventricular tachycardia

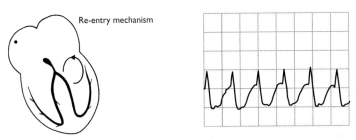

Fig. 17.38   Ventricular tachycardia.

- Potentially dangerous rhythm which can develop into ventricular fibrillation.
- Rapid but not as fast as SVT (usually <170 beats/min).
- Often slightly irregular.
- Patient often looks collapsed.
- Always wide QRS complex
    - LBBB pattern – right focus
    - RBBB pattern – left focus.

Treatment is with lidocaine 100 mg intravenously at once with transfer of the patient to hospital.

Bradycardias

Pulse rate <60 beats/min.

Sinus

Normal P wave and QRS complexes.

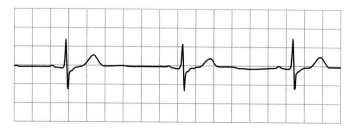

Fig. 17.39   Sinus bradycardia.

- **Causes:**
    - athletic heart
    - β-blockers
    - hypothyroidism
    - raised intracranial pressure
    - pain with vagal response
        - dental pain
        - glaucoma
        - biliary colic (Fig. 17.40).

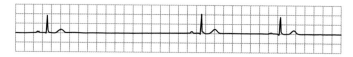

Fig. 17.40   Sinus arrest with vagal stimulation.

First-degree heart block
- PR interval (beginning of P wave to beginning of QRS complex) >0.22 s (5.5 little squares).
- Depolarization delayed in the region of AV node (Fig. 17.41).

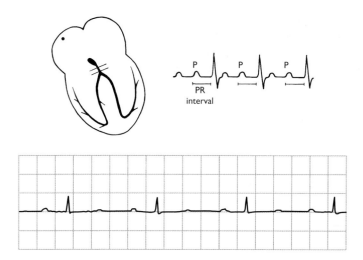

Fig. 17.41 First-degree heart block.

Wenckebach heart block
In a cycle of three or four beats, the PR interval gradually lengthens until a P wave appears on its own with no QRS complex. The cycle then repeats itself (Fig. 17.42).

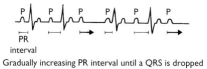
Gradually increasing PR interval until a QRS is dropped

Fig. 17.42 Wenckebach heart block.

2:1 Block
The QRS complexes only respond to every other P wave, i.e. every other P wave has no QRS complex (Fig. 17.43).

Complete heart block
- No relation between P waves and QRS complex.
- Inherent ventricular rate about 40 beats/min.
- QRS complex abnormal as it arises in a ventricular focus (Fig. 17.44).

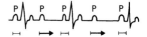

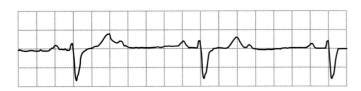

Fig. 17.43   2:1 block.

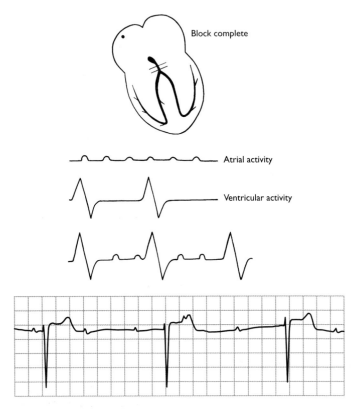

Fig. 17.44   Complete heart block.

Pacemakers

- When conduction defects cause asystolic pauses or very slow heart
  rates, pacemakers can stimulate either the atrium or ventricle and
  restore rhythm.
- Pacemakers can be basic or very sophisticated.

Ventricle-only pacemakers

These are the most common type of pacemaker (80%+) (Fig. 17.45).

If the ventricle fails to produce an electrical signal (QRS complex), the
pacemaker senses this and fires at approximately 60–70 beats/min. It is
inhibited when the ventricle's QRS complex returns at an adequate rate.

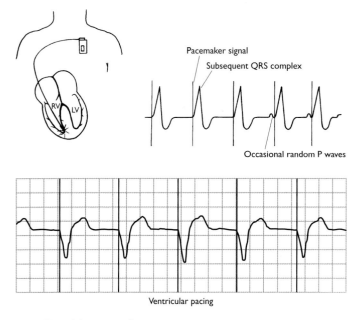

Fig. 17.45 Ventricle pacemakers.

Atrial-only pacemakers

In the sick sinus syndrome, the P wave fails to materialize but conduction in
the AV node and bundle of His is normal. Pacing the atrium restores normal
function.

Sequential pacemakers

These pacemakers cause the sequential contraction of the atrium and ventricle in a more normal physiological way. This may provide a better cardiac output (Fig. 17.46).

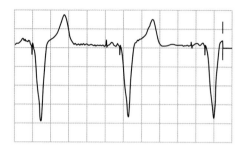

Fig. 17.46   Sequential pacing.

Looking at the ECG

Examine logically, reading complexes from left to right.
- **Rhythm:**
    - sinus rhythm ± ectopics; ignore sinus arrhythmia
    - regular
    - slow complete heart block
    - sinus bradycardia
    - fast sinus tachycardia
    - supraventricular tachycardia
    - ventricular tachycardia
    - regular atrial flutter
    - irregular
        - atrial fibrillation
        - atrial tachycardia with varying block
- **Rate:** add up the number of large squares between two successive beats. Divide into 300. For example:

$$\frac{300}{\text{5 large squares}} = 60 \text{ beats/min}$$

1.5 squares	= 200 beats/min	3.5	= 85 beats/min
2	= 150 beats/min	4	= 75 beats/min
2.5	= 120 beats/min	5	= 60 beats/min
3	= 100 beats/min	6	= 50 beats/min

If the simple formula does not work for irregular rhythm then add up the number of complexes in 6 seconds (sometimes marked on the paper) and multiply by 10.

- **Complex shape** – brief guide:
  - P wave: abnormal shape
    - atrial ectopics, P mitrale, P pulmonale
    - 0.10–0.22 s (2.5–5.5 squares)
  - PR interval: prolonged
    - >0.22 s: first-degree heart block
    - <0.1 s: Wolff–Parkinson–White syndrome
  - QRS complex
    - large Q wave – full-thickness infarct?
    - wide QRS >0.12 s: branch block
    - R wave if large: ventricular hypertrophy?
  - ST segment: elevated or depressed – ischaemia or other causes?
  - T wave: if inverted – ischaemia or other causes?

In summary, particularly look for:

- abnormal rhythm
- abnormal rate
- abnormal QRS – especially ischaemia, infarct, hypertrophy

CHAPTER 18

Interpretation of Investigations

Sensitivity, specificity and efficiency

Introduction

These terms have specific meanings which indicate the clinical usefulness of investigations. Sensitivity and specificity assess the frequency of results in relation to the correct answers.

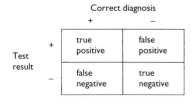

Correct diagnosis

		+	−
Test result	+	true positive	false positive
	−	false negative	true negative

- **Sensitivity** – how often the correct positive answer is obtained in those who have the disease:

$$= \frac{\text{True-Positive}}{\text{True-positive} + \text{false-negative}}, \text{ i.e.}$$

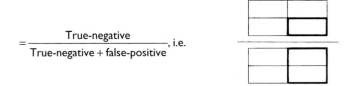

It also expresses the likelihood that a negative test result correctly indicates disease is not present: 95% sensitivity means five false-negatives in 100 patients with the disease.

- **Specificity** – how often the correct negative answer is obtained in those who do not have the disease:

$$= \frac{\text{True-negative}}{\text{True-negative} + \text{false-positive}}, \text{ i.e.}$$

It also expresses the likelihood that a positive test result will correctly indicate disease: 90% specificity means 10 false-positives in 100 subjects tested who do not have the disease.

Thus, a large heart on X-ray is a fairly sensitive test for severe mitral regurgitation (most patients with mitral regurgitation have a large heart) but it is not a specific test (because many heart diseases produce a large heart).

- **Efficiency** – how often the investigation gives the correct answer:

$$= \frac{\text{True-positive} + \text{true-negative}}{\text{All tests}}, \text{i.e.}$$

- **Predictive value of a positive test**

$$= \frac{\text{True-positive}}{\text{True-positive} + \text{false-positive}}, \text{i.e.}$$

Interpretation

The reliance put on the result of an investigation depends on the *a priori* chance of the result being abnormal. Thus a high plasma calcium in a woman with breast cancer would be taken to indicate either bone metastases or the non-metatastic hypercalcaemia (due to tumour production of a parathormone-like peptide), whereas a similar value in an apparently normal nursing student would be regarded as being a false-positive until rechecked. Where the prior probability of an event is known, Bayes' theorem can be used to calculate the current probability. The prevalence of an abnormality in the population therefore assists interpretation of an individual patient's results.

Prevalence and incidence

Please note the difference between prevalence and incidence.
- **Prevalence** – the number of cases of a disease in a designated population, e.g. 10% of males aged 40–60 years.
- **Incidence** – the number of new cases during a specific period, e.g. 10 per 100 000 population per annum.

CHAPTER 19

Laboratory Results – Reference Values

General tests

Introduction

Reference intervals (ranges) are the most common expression of normal ranges. In some situations, **specific diagnostic reference intervals** are appropriate, e.g. twice normal values of plasma creatine kinase for diagnosing Duchenne muscular dystrophy.

Action limits can be set for various situations, which aid decision taking, e.g. a cholesterol value of <5.2 mmol/l can be considered low risk. The treatment of higher cholesterol values will depend on other risk factors such as weight and family history.

Patient-specific reference intervals are sometimes required for therapeutic purposes, e.g. specific glucose control criteria for different types of diabetic patients.

It is important to recognize that methods and instrumentation vary from laboratory to laboratory and that all laboratories publish their own ranges. Ranges vary according to the sex, age and ethnicity of the reference population. The following results are a general guide for adult values (Newham Healthcare NHS Trust, 2003). You are strongly advised to consult the laboratory reference values that have produced the data you are reviewing.

Blood chemistry and haematology 'tests' offered by most laboratories represent an economical way to gain significant information about a patient's physical condition at the time of testing. These results, following review and interpretation with other patient findings, play an important part in moving from a differential diagnosis to formal diagnosis.

Haematology

Test	Male	Female	Male/female
Haemoglobin	12.5–17.5 g/dl	11.5–15.5 g/dl	(Age and sex related)
Packed cell volume (PCV) (haematocrit)	40–54%	37–47%	
Red cell count	$4.5–6.5 \times 10^{12}/l$	$3.9–5.6 \times 10^{12}/l$	
Mean cell volume (MCV)			78–96 fl
Mean cell haemoglobin			27–32 pg
Mean cell haemoglobin concentration			32–36 g/dl
Reticulocyte count			0.2–2.5%
White cell count			$4.0–11.0 \times 10^{9}/l$
D-dimer (FDP = fibrinogen degradation products)			0–0.5
Platelets			$150–400 \times 10^{9}/l$
Prothrombin time			10–14 s (dependent on reagents and instrumentation)
Activated partial thromboplastin time			30–40 s (dependent on reagents and instrumentation)
International normalized ratio (INR) therapeutic range for treatment of deep vein thrombosis			2.0–3.0
Erythrocyte sedimentation rate (ESR) Westergren at 1 h	0–10 mm	0–15 mm	(Higher values of ESR may occur in normal elderly patients)

Cerebrospinal fluid

Cells	0–5 white cells/0 red cells ($<5/mm^3$)
Glucose	2.0–4.0 mmol/l
Pressure	70–180 mmH$_2$O
Protein	0.10–0.40 g/l

Clinical chemistry (in SI units)
Serum or plasma

ACE (angiotensin-converting enzyme)	Up to 52 IU/l
ACTH (adrenocorticotrophic hormone)	<50 µg/l
Albumin	35–55 g/l (adult)
Aldosterone, recumbent (doubles after 30 min in upright posture)	100–4500 pmol/l
Alkaline phosphatase (adult)	80–306 IU/l (dependent on sex)
	64–306 (female age dependent)
α1-antitrypsin	1.1–2.0 mg/dl (age dependent)
Amylase	0–90 IU/l
Anion gap	7–16 mmol/l
Aspartate aminotransferase (AST)	10–34 IU/l male
	10–30 IU/l female
Bicarbonate	21–28 mmol/l
Bilirubin (total)	0–19 µmol/l
	0–227 (7-day-old infant)
Bilirubin in babies (toxic value)	Action point >227 µmol/l
Bilirubin (conjugated)	10% of total
C-peptide (fasting – interpret with glucose value)	0.2–0.8 nmol/l
C-reactive protein	<10 mg/l adults
	<5.0 mg/l paediatrics
Caeruloplasmin	0.2–0.4 g/l
Calcitonin	<0.46 µg/l
Calcium (adjusted to albumin 40 glc)	2.02–2.60 mmol/l
Carbon monoxide – non-smoker	Up to 3%
Carbon monoxide – smoker	Up to 8%
Carcinoembryonic antigen (CEA)	0–4 µg/l
Catecholamines	Noradrenaline and adrenaline normally tested on urine
Chloride	95–105 mmol/l
Cholesterol	<5.0 mmol/l is considered low risk
Copper	12–20 µmol/l
Cortisol (09.00 hours)	138–499 nmol/l
Cortisol (midnight)	55–3600 nmol/l
Creatine kinase	White male 29–200 IU/l
(UK population reference)	White female 32–160 IU/l
	Afro-Caribbean male 82–600 IU/l
	Afro-Caribbean female 67–400 IU/l
Creatinine (age related)	62–106 µmol/l (adult)
DHEAS (dehydroepiandrosterone sulphate)	0.7–11.5 µmol/l (20–40 years)
	0.8–6.9 µmol/l (41–61 years)
	0.4–4.7 µmol/l (>60 years)
	(age related)

Ferritin	25–300 U/mg/ml men
	10–130 U/mg/ml women
	25–300 U/mg/ml menopausal
α-Fetoprotein (AFP)	0–7 kU/l
Folate (serum)	3–12 µg/l
Folate (red cell)	160–640 µg/l
Follicle-stimulating hormone (female luteal)	1.5–9 U/l
Follicle-stimulating hormone (postmenopausal women)	23–116 U/l
Follicle-stimulating hormone (men)	1.4–18.10 U/l
Gastrin (fasting)	<40 pmol/l
Gastroinhibitory peptide (fasting) (PP)	<300 pmol/l
Glucagon (fasting)	<50 pmol/l
Glucose (plasma, fasting)	<6.0 mmol/l
Glucose (plasma, random)	Up to 7.8 mmol/l
γ-Glutamyl transpeptidase	10–49 IU/l men
	7–32 IU/l women
Haemoglobin A_{1c}	Up to 7.0 good
	Control 8.0–8.9 poor, >8.9 very poor
HDL (high-density lipoprotein) cholesterol	1.0 mmol/l men
	<1.0 mmol/l women
Human chorionic gonadotrophin (hCG)	0–10 IU/l (tumour marker)
17α-Hydroxyprogesterone	<20 nmol/l
Immunoglobulin A	0.8–2.8 g/l (age related)
Immunoglobulin E	<8 g/l
Immunoglobulin G	5.4–16.1 g/l (adult)
Immunoglobulin M	0.5–1.9 g/l (adult)
Insulin (fasting – interpret with glucose value)	3–17 mU/l
Lactate (fasting)	0.6–2.4 mmol/l
Lactate dehydrogenase	220–450 IU/l
Lead (blood)	0.0–0.6 µmol/l
Luteinizing hormone (female luteal)	0.5–17 U/l
Luteinizing hormone (postmenopausal women)	16–54 U/l
Luteinizing hormone (men)	1.5–9.3 U/l
Magnesium	0.70–1.00 mmol/l (adult)
β-Oestradiol (female luteal)	121–550 pmol/l
β-Oestradiol (men)	0–198 pmol/l
Osmolality	280–298 mosmol/kg
Parathyroid hormone (PTH)	1.1–6.8 pmol/l
Phosphate	0.83–1.49 mmol/l (adult)
Potassium	3.5–5.0 mmol/l (adult)
Progesterone (day 21 of normal menstruating female)	8–89 IU/l

Prolactin	60–620 IU/l
Prostate-specific antigen (PSA)	Up to 3.0 mg/ml at 49 years
(age dependent)	Up to 4.1 mg/ml at 59 years
	Up to 6.9 mg/ml at 69 years
	Up to 7.0 mg/ml over 69 years
Protein (total)	66–82 g/l (adult)
Renin (recumbent/overnight)	1.1–2.7 pmol/ml/h
Renin (upright)	0.5–3.1 pmol/ml/h
Sex hormone-binding globulin	14.9–103 mmol/l men
	30–90 mmol/l women
Sodium	135–147 mmol/l
Testosterone	8.4–29 nmol/l men
	0.5–2.6 nmol/l women
Thyroxine, free (FT_4)	10.3–19.4 pmol/l
Transaminase (GPT, ALT)	Up to 35 IU/l
Triglyceride (fasting)	<2.0 mmol/l
Tri-iodothyronine, free (FT_3)	3.5–6.5 pmol/l
TSH (thyroid-stimulating hormone)	0.2–5.5 mU/l
Urate	0.19–0.45 mmol/l men
	0.13–0.40 mmol/l women
Urea	3.3–6.7 mmol/l (adult)
VIP (vasoactive intestinal polypeptide)	<30 pmol/l
Vitamin B_{12}	211–911 ng/l
Vitamin D	15–100 mmol/l
Vitamin E	12–28 µmol/l
Zinc	11–18 µmol/l

24-hour urine

Aldosterone	10–50 nmol/24 h
δ-Amino laevulinic acid	<3.8 µmol/mmol creatinine
Calcium	2.5–7.5 mmol/24 h
Chloride	170–250 mmol/24 h
Copper	0.0–1.0 µmol/24 h
Coproporphyrin	<115 nmol/24 h
Cortisol	79–591 nmol/24 h
Creatinine clearance	90–150 ml/min
Creatinine, 24 h	9–17 mmol/24 h
5-HIAA (5-OH indoleacetic acid)	<6.4 µmol/24 h
Microalbumin	<2.5 µmol/mmol creatinine, men
	<3.5 µmol/mmol creatinine, women
Microalbumin, 24 h	<20 mg/l normal
	30–300 mg/l microalbuminuria
	>300 mg/l proteinuria

Oxalate	0.10–0.46 mmol/24 h
Phosphate	15–50 mmol/24 h
Porphyrin	<35 µmol/mmol creatinine
PBG (porphobilinogen)	<1.5 µmol/mmol creatinine
Potassium	40–120 mmol/24 h
Protein	<0.1 g/24 h
Sodium	100–250 mmol/24 h
24 h UA	3.5–4.2 mmol/24 h
Urea	250–600 mmol/24 h

Drugs in serum

The following are usual therapeutic ranges. The value related to the time of ingestion is crucial for some drugs, e.g. plasma paracetamol 200 mg/l gives a risk of liver damage but the decision interval of the plasma level for therapy decreases with time after an overdose.

Amiodarone before dose	0.5–2.0 mg/l
Carbamazepine before dose	4–12 mg/l (therapeutic)
Carbon monoxide, non-smoker	Up to 3%
Carbon monoxide, smoker	Up to 8%
Clonazepam before dose	Target range <35 µg/l
Digoxin at least 6 h after last dose	0.5–2.0 µg/l
Ethosuximide before dose	40–80 mg/l (therapeutic)
Lithium	0.4–1.0 mmol/l
Phenobarbitone before dose	10–40 mg/l (therapeutic)
Phenytoin before dose	10–20 mg/l (therapeutic)
Salicylate	<350 mg/l (therapeutic)
Theophylline before dose	10–20 mg/l (therapeutic)
Valproate before dose	50–100 mg/l (therapeutic) or 350–700 µmol/l

Toxic levels

Barbiturate – potentially fatal	Positive or negative
Ethanol (physiological <0.2 nmol/l)	>1500 mg/l = legal limit for driving
Paracetamol – risk of liver damage	<200 mg/l 4-h post ingestion, liver damage unlikely
Salicylate	Up to 350 mg/l (therapeutic)

Miscellaneous

Faecal fat	<18 mmol/day
Extractable nuclear antigen-binding association	
Anti-Ro	SLE, cutaneous lupus
Anti-La	SLE, Sjögren's disease
Anti-Sm	SLE (specific)
Anti-RNP	SLE, mixed connective tissue disease
Anti-Scl-70	Progressive systemic sclerosis
Anti-Jo 1	Polymyositis

Arterial blood gases type I and type II respiratory failure

Arterial blood gas values	Normal	Type I respiratory failure	Type II respiratory failure
pH	7.35–7.45	7.35–7.45	7.35–7.45 (compensated) or <7.35 (respiratory acidosis)
P_aO_2	12–14 kPa	<8 kPa	<8 kPa
P_aCO_2	4.6–6.0 kPa	4.6–6.0 kPa	>6 kPa
S_aO_2	95%	<92%	<92%

(Mickelsons & Esmond, 2001)

Conversion factor from mmHg to kPa (= multiply by 0.13333)

Example: PCO_2 range = 35–45 mmHg

        35 mmHg × 0.13333 = 4.6 kPa
        45 mmHg × 0.13333 = 6.0 kPa
        40 mmHg × 0.13333 = 5.3 kPa

Example: P_aO_2 range = 70–105 mmHg

        70 mmHg × 0.13333 = 9.33 kPa
        105 mmHg × 0.13333 = 13.9 kPa
        98 mmHg × 0.13333 = 13 kPa

References

Mickelsons, C. & Esmond, G. (2001) Respiratory support techniques. In: Esmond, G. (ed) *Respiratory Nursing*. Baillière Tindall, London.
Newham Healthcare NHS Trust (2009) *Laboratory Reference Values Derived From Manufacturer Data*. Newham Healthcare NHS Trust, London.

CHAPTER 20

Common Emergency Treatments

Introduction

Patients may present or their condition may deteriorate, requiring the initiation of emergency treatments in any clinical setting. The following notes provide a guide to therapies. In some emergency situations, treatment may need to be initiated before a formal diagnosis is reached. These therapies are considered appropriate as' first-line' treatments at the time of publication.

Acute coronary syndrome

Acute coronary syndromes is a term encompassing sudden ischaemic disorders of the heart and comprises unstable angina and ST elevation myocardial infarction (STEMI) and non-ST elevation myocardial infarction (NSTEMI). These conditions represent a continuum of a similar disease process and cannot always be differentiated in the first few hours. Differential diagnosis is based on clinical history, electrocardiograph (ECG) changes and the presence of cardiac biochemical markers on investigation.

ST elevation myocardial infarction (STEMI)

Classically, central crushing chest pain with radiation to arms, jaw or neck, which can be associated with pallor, sweating and breathlessness. If the patient has experienced angina previously, it will be reported as being similar but more severe and unrelieved by GTN.

Some patients may present with atypical signs; older people and diabetics are particularly susceptible. Common presentations in this group include confusion, collapse and breathlessness.

- Give oxygen via face mask.
- Attach to cardiac monitor, where defibrillation is readily available.
- Monitor vital signs.
- Give GTN sublingually if not already given.
- Gain intravenous (IV) access, take blood for U&Es, FBC, glucose and cardiac biochemical markers, e.g. troponin, CK-MB.

- Give 300 mg aspirin and 300 mg clopidogrel orally unless contraindicated or given by prehospital personnel.
- Give IV opioid analgesia titrated to pain, e.g. morphine 5–10 mg.
- Give IV antiemetic e.g. metoclopramide 10 mg.
- 12-lead ECG: if ST >2 mm elevation in two or more contiguous chest leads or >1 mm in two contiguous limb leads or new left bundle branch block (LBBB) or posterior infarction initiate the following.
  - **Rapid reperfusion of the myocardium**. The two treatment modalities used to achieve rapid reperfusion of the myocardium, which is marked by normalization of the ST segments on the ECG, are primary percutaneous coronary intervention (PCI) and thrombolysis, of which PCI is the gold standard reperfusion treatment for a STEMI. The clinician should phone the 'Heart Attack Centre' and transfer the patient without delay. This system requires agreed clinical pathways between emergency departments/services and invasive cardiac laboratories.
  - If PCI is unavailable, institute **thrombolysis**. The choice of thrombolytic agent may be determined by local policy (Box 20.1). All patients must be screened to ensure they have no contraindications to thrombolysis, e.g. known bleeding diathesis, active peptic ulceration, active internal bleeding, recent surgery, haemorrhagic stroke, aortic dissection and trauma and/or surgery in the last 2 weeks – consult local policy.
- Give β-blocker, e.g. metoprolol 1–2 mg per minute, repeated after 5 minutes (max 10–15 mg) unless contraindicated, e.g. HR <60, systolic blood pressure (SBP) <100 mmHg, moderate to severe heart failure and chronic obstructive pulmonary disease.
- Commence ACE inhibitor within first 24 hours of presentation.
- Treat arrhythmias – check potassium levels.
- Monitor blood sugar and treat hyperglycaemia.

Non-ST elevation myocardial infarction (NSTEMI) and unstable angina

Diagnosis may be unclear at presentation; close observation of ECG and cardiac biochemical markers is required to detect an evolving NSTEMI.

Positive biochemical markers with the ECG changes stated below are indicative of a NSTEMI.

- ST segment depression of >0.05 mV is indicative of myocardial damage.
- T wave inversion is not specific but may be if >0.3 mV deep.
- There may be new or transient LBBB.
- Rarely, Q waves may evolve.

Unstable angina presents with continued myocardial pain without evidence of raised biochemical markers.

Box 20.1   Thrombolytic agents

Streptokinase – used infrequently

Most effective if given <4 hours since the onset of pain
Associated with allergic reactions and hypotension
Give 1.5 mega units in 100 ml normal saline IV infusion over 1 hour
If patient becomes hypotensive (systolic blood pressure <90 mmHg)
    reduce IV rate and tilt patient's head down

Recombinant tissue plasminogen activator – rtPA

Give if streptokinase given >5 days ago
Give if anterior MI in patient <75 years and <4 hours of symptoms or
    hypotensive (systolic blood pressure <90 mmHg)
Give in accelerated regime = 15 mg IV bolus, followed by 0.75 mg/kg
    (max 50 mg) via IV infusion over 30 min, then 0.5 mg/kg (max 35 mg)
    IV infusion over 60 min
Give LMWH or heparin concomitantly according to local policy

Reteplase

Give as two IV boluses of 10 units, 10 minutes apart

Tenecteplase (modified tPA)

Single IV bolus dose over 10 seconds
Dose adjusted according to weight: <60 kg = 30 mg, 60–69 kg =
35 mg, 70–79 kg = 40 mg, 80–89 kg = 45 mg, >90 kg = 50 mg
Give LMWH/heparin

APSAC (anistreplase)

Give as an IV bolus of 30 mg over 2–5 minutes

- Give oxygen via face mask.
- Attach to cardiac monitor, where defibrillation is readily available.
- Perform serial ECGs.
- Monitor vital signs.
- Gain IV access, take blood for U&Es, FBC, glucose and cardiac biochemical markers.
- Give 300 mg aspirin and 300 mg clopidogrel orally unless contraindicated or given by prehospital personnel.
- Give IV opioid analgesia titrated to pain, e.g. morphine 5–10 mg.
- Give IV antiemetic, e.g. metoclopramide 10 mg.
- Start low molecular weight heparin (LMWH).

- Give glycoprotein IIb/IIIa antagonists in high-risk patients with ongoing ischaemia and elevated troponin, e.g. eptifibatide.
- Consider GTN infusion (50 mg GTN in 50 ml normal saline at 1–10 ml/h) titrated to pain, maintaining SBP >100 mmHg. Reduce dose and lower patient's head if hypotension occurs.
- Commence β-blockers, e.g. metoprolol, if not contraindicated. If evidence of heart failure, a calcium antagonist (amlodipine 5–10 mg) can be used.
- Commence anti-hyperlipidaemia therapy.
- Obtain a CXR to rule out left ventricular failure and a widened mediastinum.

NSTEMI management:
Patients experiencing a NSTEMI may be transferred for a PCI immediately; consult local policies.

Other cardiovascular emergencies
Acute left ventricular failure

Acute breathlessness, tachycardia, raised JVP; inspiratory and expiratory crackles on auscultation. This condition requires urgent treatment.

- Sit patient upright.
- Give high-flow oxygen.
- Attach ECG monitor and check for arrhythmias.
- Monitor vital signs, including SpO_2.
- Gain IV access, take blood for FBC, U&Es, glucose and cardiac biomarkers, e.g. CK-MB or troponin.
- Give opioid, e.g. titrated IV morphine 5–10 mg (not to be given to patients who are very drowsy and fatigued).
- Give antiemetic, e.g. IV metoclopramide 10 mg.
- Give IV nitrate therapy if systolic BP >90 mmHg; monitor blood pressure closely to avoid hypotension.
- Obtain a CXR.
- Obtain arterial blood gas (ABG).
- Commence continuous positive airway pressure (CPAP) if not contraindicated, i.e. patient too drowsy. Consult local protocol.

Arrhythmias

- **Bradycardia:** excessive bradycardia <40 beats/min although patients with a heart rate <60 beats/min may be compromised if they have poor cardiac reserve. Consult www.resus.org.uk.
  Patient may complain of feeling light-headed or blackouts.

- Give high-flow oxygen and obtain IV access.
- In the presence of adverse signs, e.g. SBP <90 mmHg, ventricular arrhythmias or heart failure, consider atropine 0.5 mg IV and repeat to a maximum of 3 mg according to response.
- If symptoms persist, consider transcutaneous pacing and gain expert advice.
- **Tachyarrhythmia:** >120 beats/min in compromised patients, e.g. hypotension, heart failure, chest pain. In all patients give high-flow oxygen and obtain IV access.
- **Narrow-complex tachycardia**: perform vagal manoeuvres, use simultaneous ECG monitoring and printout. If the patient is unstable and the tachycardia persists which is not atrial flutter:
  - give adenosine IV 6 mg bolus
  - if no response, give a further 12 mg bolus
  - if no response, give one further 12 mg bolus.

If adenosine is contraindicated or fails to terminate a regular narrow-complex tachycardia without demonstrating that it is atrial flutter, give a calcium channel blocker, e.g. IV verapamil 2.5–5 mg over 2 min.

If the narrow-complex tachycardia persists and the patient remains stable, give amiodarone 300 mg IV over 20–60 mins, then 900 mg over 24 hours. Amiodarone should be given via a central line as it causes thrombophlebitis peripherally (refer to notes below for administration in an emergency).

If patient is unstable, consider synchronized cardioversion. If cardioversion fails to restore sinus rhythm and the patient remains unstable, give IV amiodarone 300 mg over 10–20 min and re-attempt electrical cardioversion. The loading dose of amiodarone can be followed by an infusion of 900 mg over 24 hours.

- Amiodarone can be administered via a large peripheral vein in an emergency. Consult www.resus.org.uk.
- **Broad-complex tachycardia**:
  - patient unstable: synchronized DC cardioversion for up to three attempts. The patient will require sedation prior to cardioversion
    - then give IV amiodarone 300 mg over 10–20 min and repeat DC shock, followed by amiodarone 900 mg over 24 hours. Consult www.resus.org.uk
  - patient stable: give IV amiodarone 300 mg over 20–60 min, then 900 mg over 24 hours.
- **Ventricular fibrillation or pulseless ventricular tachycardia**: refer to the Resuscitation Council Guidelines: www.resus.org.uk.

Severe hypertension

Defined as: systolic blood pressure >200 mmHg and diastolic pressure >120 mmHg, headaches, confusion, nausea, vomiting and papilloedema.

- Confirm hypertension by rechecking blood pressure.
- Gain IV access.
- Send blood for U&Es, creatinine and glucose.
- Perform an ECG and urinalysis.
- Reduced level of consciousness: exclude stroke or subarachnoid haemorrhage; if suspected, arrange immediate CT of head.
- Refer to medical team for advice on further management.
- Gradual reduction of blood pressure is required to avoid cerebral and cardiac hypoperfusion induced by rapid reduction.
- Alert patients can be treated with oral medication.
    - First-line treatment is β-blockers, unless contraindicated, or a low-dose calcium antagonist.
    - Alternatively, consider IV nitroprusside with arterial monitoring.
- Treat any complications, e.g. pulmonary oedema, encephalopathy.

Pulmonary embolism (PE)

Sudden onset of pleuritic chest pain associated with breathlessness and haemoptysis.
- Provide high-flow oxygen via face mask.
- Monitor vital signs, including SpO_2 and urine output.
- Perform an ECG. 'S1, Q3, T3', right access deviation (RAD) and RBBB are only seen in a massive PE. Attach to cardiac monitor, noting sinus tachycardia.
- Gain IV access.
- If hypotensive, give 0.9% saline IV. If this persists, the patient may require inotropic support and invasive monitoring.
- Gain ICU support early.
- Take blood for FBC, U&Es, ESR and ABG (ideally on air).
- D-dimer should not be performed in high-risk patients but may be of use in local protocols to rule out low-risk patients.
- Low molecular weight heparin (LMWH) should be given to all patients with high or intermediate risk of PE until diagnosis is confirmed.
- Analgesia: oral NSAID may be sufficient, opioid analgesia may be required.
- Imaging: should be instigated within 1 hour for suspected massive PE and within 24 hours for non-massive PE.
    - CTPA should be performed on suspected non-massive PE; patients with a good-quality negative scan do not require further imaging or treatment for PE.
    - Patients with a high/intermediate probability of PE and a negative CTPA should undergo further imaging.
    - Pulmonary angiography is the gold standard investigation when diagnosis cannot be gained from non-invasive measures.

- In patients with co-existing clinical deep vein thrombosis (DVT), leg ultrasound as the initial test is often sufficient to confirm venous thromboembolism.
- A single normal leg ultrasound is not sufficient to exclude a subclinical DVT.
- Massive PE
  - Thrombolysis is the first-line treatment, e.g. alteplase 50 mg bolus IV.
  - Pulmonary embolectomy may be performed when thrombolysis is contraindicated – requires specialist facilities and clinicians.
  - Insertion of an IVC filter may be considered if facilities and expert clinicians are available.
- Non-massive PE
  - Thrombolysis should not be given as first-line treatment.
  - LMWH should be given prior to imaging.
  - Oral anticoagulation should only be commenced when venous thromboembolism (VTE) has been confirmed.
  - The INR should be maintained between 2.0 and 3.0; when achieved, heparin can be discontinued.
- Anticoagulation
  - 4–6 weeks for temporary risk factors
  - 3 months for first idiopathic
  - 6 months for all others

Respiratory emergencies

Acute bronchospasm (asthma)

Breathlessness, wheeze, chest tightness and cough.
The initial assessment should be based on clinical signs, peak expiratory flow and pulse oximetry – consider prehospital assessment and treatment when assessing severity.

Moderate asthma
- Increasing symptoms
- Peak expiratory flow (PEF) >50–75% best or predicted
- No features of acute severe asthma

Acute severe
Any one of:
- PEF 33–50% best or predicted
- Respiratory rate ≥25/min
- Heart rate ≥110/min
- Inability to complete sentences in one breath

Life threatening
In a patient with severe asthma, any one of:
- PEF <33% best or predicted
- SpO_2 <92%
- PaO_2 <8 kPa
- Normal $PaCO_2$ (4.6–6.0 kPa)
- Silent chest
- Cyanosis
- Feeble respiratory effort
- Bradycardia, arrhythmia, hypotension
- Exhaustion, confusion, coma

Near fatal
- Raised $PaCO_2$ and/or requiring mechanical ventilation with raised inflation pressures.

Treatment of asthma
- Admit patients with any feature of a life-threatening or near-fatal attack.
- Admit patients with any feature of a severe attack persisting after initial treatment.
- Patients whose peak flow is greater than 75% best or predicted 1 hour after initial treatment may be discharged from ED, unless there are other reasons why admission may be appropriate.
- Give high-flow oxygen.
- Give nebulized β2-agonist bronchodilators driven by oxygen in hospital, e.g. salbutamol 5 mg.
- In severe asthma where the initial response is poor, consider continuous nebulized β2-agonist bronchodilators.
- Add nebulized ipratropium bromide (0.5 mg 4–6 hourly) to β2-agonist treatment for patients with acute severe or life-threatening asthma or those with a poor initial response to β2-agonist therapy.
- Give steroids to all patients presenting with acute asthma, e.g. prednisolone 30–60 mg orally or hydrocortisone 200 mg IV.
- Take an ABG if SpO_2 <92% or other features of life-threatening asthma.
- **Consider giving a single dose of IV magnesium sulphate for patients with:**
  - acute severe asthma who have not had a good initial response to inhaled bronchodilator therapy
  - life-threatening or near-fatal asthma.
- Routine prescription for antibiotics is not indicated for acute asthma.
- Continue prednisolone 40–50 mg daily for at least 5 days or until recovery.
- IV magnesium sulphate (1.2–2 g IV infusion over 20 minutes) should only be used following consultation with senior medical staff.

- A CXR is indicated only if there is:
  - suspected consolidation
  - life-threatening asthma
  - suspected pneumomediastinum or pneumothorax
  - failure to respond to treatment satisfactorily
  - a requirement for ventilation

For further information, consult www.brit-thoracic.org.uk.

Acute exacerbation of chronic obstructive pulmonary disease (COPD)

Breathlessness, cough, sputum production and coarse crackles or wheeze.

Obtain a history to confirm diagnosis; this should include recent history, specifically noting the time scale of deterioration, worsening symptoms and changes to exercise tolerance. Assess current therapy regime and co-morbidities. Ascertain if there have been any admissions to the intensive care unit (ICU).

- Give oxygen via a Venturi mask – aim to maintain SpO_2 >90% without worsening hypercapnia and respiratory acidosis.
- If there is a history of hypercapnia respiratory failure, administer 24–28% oxygen.
- Monitor vital signs, including SpO_2 and ECG.
- Obtain ABG immediately and adjust oxygen accordingly.
- Treat bronchospasm with β2-agonists, e.g. salbutamol 5 mg via oxygen. If ABG shows CO_2 retention, deliver therapy via air; if patient is hypoxic, give oxygen via nasal cannulae whilst nebulizer is administered.
- Give ipratropium bromide 500 μg 6 hourly via a nebulizer.
- Consider IV theophylline as an adjunct to management of COPD exacerbation if there is an inadequate response to bronchodilators.
- Non-invasive ventilation (NIV) is first-line treatment for acute type 2 respiratory failure in patients with chronic COPD who fail to respond to initial treatment and in whom respiratory acidosis remains.
  - NIV should be considered within the first 60 min of arrival to hospital. There should be a treatment plan, including what to do if NIV fails. Consult local guidelines for inclusion and exclusion criteria.
  - If the patient is unable to tolerate NIV, e.g. life-threatening hypoxaemia, inability to protect airway, confusion and agitation, consider mechanical ventilation – gain expert advice from the anaesthetist.
- Gain IV access.
- Take blood for FBC, U&Es, theophylline levels (if taking theophylline prior to admission) and blood cultures if pyrexial.
- Give steroids – 200 mg hydrocortisone IV or 30–40 mg prednisolone.
- Gain a CXR.
- Culture sputum.

- Consider antibiotics if underlying infection is suspected – consult local antibiotic guidelines.
- Urgent physiotherapy input may be required to expectorate sputum.

Community-acquired pneumonia (CAP)

Cough, pyrexia, chest pain and breathlessness. Auscultation may reveal inspiratory crackles or consolidation (dull to percussion and bronchial breathing), although this is not always present. Consider pneumonia in septic and/or confused patients.

The CURB-65 score directs therapy and supports clinical decision making in relation to admission or discharge. Score 1 point for each of:

Confusion
Urea >7 mmol/l
Respiratory rate >30 breaths/min
SBP <90 mmHg or DBP <60 mmHg
Age >65 years

CURB score 3 or more high risk of death – manage as severe pneumonia.
CURB score 2 increased risk of death – consider for short inpatient stay or hospital-supervised outpatient treatment – clinician discretion
CURB score 0–1 low risk of death – treat as having non-severe pneumonia and may be suitable for home treatment.

- Assess airway and administer high-flow oxygen.
- Monitor vital signs including SpO_2 and ECG.
- Obtain ABG if SpO_2 <96%.
- PEF may reveal co-existing COPD or asthma.
- Gain IV access, take blood for FBC, U&Es, CRP, LFT and blood cultures.
- Check ABG and correct hypoxia.
- Obtain a CXR, observing for diffuse infiltrates, e.g. tuberculosis (TB), carcinoma; cavitations, e.g. fungi, gram-negative bacteria; pleural effusion, e.g. empyema, tuberculosis; focal infiltrates, e.g. pneumococcus, *Legionella* and *Klebsiella*.
- Oral paracetamol or NSAID may suffice, opioid analgesia may be considered if required.

Antibiotic therapy in non-severe CAP, CURB 0-1:

- amoxicillin 500 mg–1 g orally 8 hourly for 5 days. If allergic to penicillin, clarithromycin 100 mg orally 12 hourly.

If CURB score 0–1 and previously treated with antibiotics, or CURB score 2:

- amoxicillin orally 500 mg–1 g 8 hourly plus clarithromycin orally 500 mg 12 hourly for 5 days
- if allergic to penicillin, give clarithromycin 500 mg orally 12 hourly
- CURB score 2, or CURB score 0–1 and previously treated with antibioitics, give moxifloxacin 400 mg orally daily (check contraindications and cautions).

Antibiotic therapy for severe CAP, CURB 3:

- co-amoxiclav 1.2 g IV 8 hourly plus clarithromycin 500 mg IV 12 hourly – change to oral regimen when there is clinical improvement and patient has been apyrexial for 24 hours
- oral regimen: co-amoxiclav orally 625 mg 8 hourly plus clarithromycin 500 mg orally 12 hourly
- if allergic to penicillin give levofloxacin IV 500 mg 12 hourly plus clarithromycin 500 mg IV 12 hourly – change to oral regimen when there is clinical improvement and patient has been apyrexial for 24 hours
- oral regimen: moxifloxacin orally 400 mg once daily – check contraindications/cautions.

> Note that co-amoxiclav is oral penicillin. If the patient is allergic to penicillin then he has to have antibiotics that are not penicillin based intravenously. Thus the patient is given levofloxacin intravenously plus clarithromycin intravenously as well. After 48 hours of intravenous infusions/treatment, the patient is put onto oral antibiotics. The oral antibiotic is moxifloxacin which is not a penicillin derivative.

Patients with co-existing COPD may benefit from continuous positive pressure ventilation (CPAP); seek expert advice.

- Other investigations:
  - Sputum cultures.
  - Pneumococcal antigen urine test should be performed on all severe CAP patients.
  - Legionella antigen urine test should be performed on all severe CAP patients.

Gastrointestinal emergencies

Acute gastrointestinal haemorrhage

Postural dizziness, sudden collapse, haematemesis/coffee ground or red/black sticky, malodorous stools; SBP <100 mmHg, pulse >100 beats/min.

- Check airway and breathing and give high-flow oxygen via face mask.
- Position patient on his side.
- Monitor vital signs closely, check for postural drop in non-shocked patients.
- Obtain IV access (one large-bore cannula in each antecubital fossa).
- Take blood for FBC, U&Es, LFTs, clotting, glucose, and group and cross-match 6–8 units.
- Monitor ABGs closely.
- Give IV fluids to stabilize SBP.

- If SBP <90 mmHg, give 500 ml–1 l of 0.9% sodium chloride or Hartmann's followed by blood as necessary.
- In massive haemorrhage give O rhesus negative blood whilst awaiting cross-matched blood.
- When fluid replacement has begun, a central line should be inserted and central venous pressure (CVP) monitoring commenced (especially in older patients) to avoid circulatory overload.
- Insert urinary catheter and monitor hourly urine output.
- Assess for underlying cause – cirrhosis/portal hypertension, peptic ulcer, non-steroidal anti-inflammatory drugs (NSAID) or other causes.
- Alert surgical/gastrointestinal team and arrange urgent endoscopy if appropriate – keep the patient nil by mouth.
- After endoscopic treatment of ulcers, give proton pump inhibitors (PPI), e.g. omeprazole or pantoprazole IV.
- If oesophageal varices, use Sengstaken tube as interim measure, transfuse blood, fresh frozen plasma and platelets as necessary and administer glypressin 2 mg IV initially followed by 1–2 mg every 4–6 hours until bleeding is controlled, for up to 72 hours.

Acute hepatic failure

Jaundice, foetor, liver flap, confusion.
The aim of assessment and treatment is symptomatic support until acute failure resolves.

- Monitor oxygen saturation, give oxygen if SpO_2 <90%.
- Monitor vital signs, including ECG.
- Gain IV access, take blood for FBC, U&Es, clotting, LFTs, phosphate, group and cross-match and ABG.
- Additional blood tests to aid diagnosis may include: viral serology and drug screen, blood cultures and urine and sputum culture and sensitivity.
- Obtain a CXR.
- If SBP <90 mmHg, give colloid or blood.
- Monitor CVP to avoid fluid overload.
- Monitor blood glucose 2 hourly, give 10% or 50% dextrose to maintain blood sugar >3.5 mmol/l.
- Look for indication of drug overdose, including paracetamol. If suspected, give N-acetylcysteine, within 48 hours following overdose or as soon thereafter as possible.
- Check for signs of infection: septicaemia, chest, urine, ascites.
- Consider giving antibiotics (consult local protocols) and antifungal therapy.
- Check for occult bleeding, including increasing plasma urea: consider fresh frozen plasma to correct clotting.
- Monitor renal function; haemofiltration may need to be considered.
- If patient deteriorates, consult specialist liver unit.

Neurological emergencies

Suspected first seizure

A diagnosis of epilepsy is made using history and witness account. If using a witness account, a detailed history of the event should be written in the patient notes. Gain a personal account when the patient is able to provide one, identifying prodrome/aura.

Ascertain activity prior to onset and detailed medical/family history. Do the signs and symptoms include any of the following: sudden onset, injury/tongue biting, incontinence and slow recovery including confusion?

The treatment detailed below assumes the patient has stopped fitting. If still fitting, see below under status epilepticus.

- Monitor vital signs including Glasgow Coma Scale (GCS).
- Gain IV access, take blood for FBC, U&Es, LFTs, blood glucose, calcium and magnesium.
- Record an ECG.
- Obtain CXR.
- CT head if evidence of abnormal neurology examination or of head injury.
- Decision to admit is at the discretion of clinician; if required, referral to the general medical team is appropriate.
- Criteria for admission include seizure and sustained head injury with loss of consciousness, two generalized tonic clonic seizures within 12 hours, two or more new-onset complex partial seizures within 6 hours and evidence of focal neurology.
- Excluding the above, refer to the 'First seizure clinic' as local policy dictates.

Status epilepticus

- Secure the airway.
- Give high-flow oxygen.
- Nurse the patient on his side.
- Monitor vital signs, including GCS, ECG and SpO_2.
- Gain IV access and take blood for FBC, U&Es, LFTs, blood glucose, calcium and magnesium.
- Correct blood glucose; treat hypoglycaemia with 50 ml of 50% glucose IV.
- Give lorazepam IV 4 mg over 2 min, repeat after 10 min if seizures reoccur.
- If excessive alcohol use is suspected, treat with IV thiamine, i.e. Pabrinex, via IV infusion.
- If overdose/poisoning is suspected, take blood for toxicology.
- Observe for signs of injury, e.g. head injury, and infection, e.g. rash.

- For sustained seizure, treat with phenytoin infusion, 15–2 mg/kg at a rate of 50 mg/min or fosphenytoin infusion at a dose of 15–20 mg phenytoin equivalents (PE)/kg at a rate of 50–100 mg PE/min and/or phenobarbitone bolus at 10–15 mg/kg at a rate of 100 mg/min.
- In refractory status (seizure continuing for 60–90 min after initial therapy), general anaesthesia with either propofol or thiapentone.
- Transfer to ICU.

Consult www.nice.org.uk and www.sign.ac.uk.

Stroke

Sudden onset of focal neurological deficit – patients presenting with a stroke require immediate clinical assessment and treatment. Personnel in prehospital and emergency departments (ED) have assessment tools to aid diagnosis.

- If the patient is unconscious:
  - assess airway, look, suction, manual manoeuvre, insertion of an oropharyngeal airway
  - call anaesthetist and prepare for rapid sequence induction (RSI)
  - record vital signs, including ECG and blood sugar
  - gain IV access, take blood for FBC, ESR, U&Es, CRP, calcium, glucose and cholesterol
  - correct hypoglycaemia with 50 ml of 50% glucose IV
  - CT scan or MRI is indicated immediately or within 1 hour if:
    - there are indications for thrombolysis or early anticoagulation treatment
    - the patient is taking anticoagulant treatment
    - there is a known bleeding tendency
    - there is reduced level of consciousness (GCS <13/15)
    - there are unexplained progressive or fluctuating symptoms
    - there is papilloedema, neck stiffness or fever
    - there is severe headache at onset of stroke symptoms.
- If acute ischaemic stroke is diagnosed, administer thrombolysis, e.g. alteplase, within 3 hours of onset of symptoms.
- Patients presenting with a minor stroke will require carotid imaging (Doppler ultrasound, magnetic resonance angiogram (MRA) or a CT angiogram (CTA).
- If intracerebral haemorrhage refer patient to surgeons.
- Keep the patient nil by mouth. A swallowing assessment must be conducted by an appropriately trained healthcare professional before the patient is given any oral food, fluid or medication.
- Patient should be admitted to a specialist stroke unit.

Consult www.nice.org.uk, www.dh.uk, www.rcplondon.ac.uk.

Unconscious patient

- Clear and maintain airway and give high-flow oxygen.
- Nurse in a prone or recovery position unless airway protected by endotracheal tube.
- Monitor vital signs, GCS and ECG.
- Gain IV access, take blood for FBC, U&Es, consider paracetamol and salicylate levels if overdose suspected; if pyrexial or history of pyrexia, take blood cultures.
- Exclude head injury, neurological deficit, neck stiffness, diabetic hyperglycaemia, overdose or suicide risk.
- Check blood sugar; treat hypoglycaemia if indicated with 50 ml 50% glucose IV.
- If fitting, treat as above.
- If respiratory rate <10 breaths/min, commence assisted ventilation and consider IV naloxone.
- If SBP <90 mmHg, give 500 ml 0.9% sodium chloride IV.
- Check ABG.
- Obtain a CXR.
- Obtain CT scan to diagnose stroke, head injury or subarachnoid haemorrhage.

Meningitis

Symptoms include headache, neck stiffness, vomiting, photophobia, pyrexia and petechial rash. Diagnosis can be difficult in older people or immunosuppressed patients who may present with 'flu-like' symptoms.

Clinicians should wear appropriate personal protective equipment, e.g. an FFP3 mask, when intubating a patient with suspected meningococcal infection.

- Commence treatment immediately if diagnosis is predominantly meningococcal septicaemia – do not wait for investigation results.
- Gain IV access, take blood for FBC, U&Es, glucose, clotting screen, blood cultures and a ethylenediamine tetra-acetic acid (EDTA) bottle for polymerase chain reaction (PCR).
- Administer antibiotics, e.g. ceftriaxone 2 g IV or cefotaxime 2 g IV.
- If known history of anaphylaxis to cephalosporins, chloramphenicol 25 mg/kg 6 hourly (max 1 g qds) is an alternative.
- Check for evidence of raised intracranial pressure, e.g. papilloedema, confusion, hypertension and bradycardia.
- Perform CT of brain if evidence of raised intracranial pressure before performing a lumbar puncture (LP).
- Undertaking an LP:

- Note pressure.
- Cerebrospinal fluid (CSF) for culture-bacterial, PCR for viruses, biochemistry and microscopy.
- Cloudy CSF (white cells) – prompt IV antibiotics after blood cultures (if not already given).
- Bloodstained – assess whether bloody tap, e.g. blood at first then clearing, or subarachnoid haemorrhage (consistent blood with xanthochromia for CSF after centrifuging down red cells).
- Notify communicable disease control.
- Provide prophylaxis for family and close friends.

Other systems

Diabetic ketoacidosis (DKA)

Usually occurs in known insulin-dependent diabetics but may manifest in some type 2 diabetics. DKA may be induced by infection, vomiting or lack of insulin. The patient may complain of polydipsia, polyuria and abdominal pain and may appear drowsy with/without ketotic breath. Occurs over 1–3 days.

- If altered level of consciousness, provide airway support.
- Give high-flow oxygen via a mask and consider the need for anaesthetic support/intubation.
- Monitor vital signs, including blood sugar and urinalysis for glucose and ketones. ECG and cardiac monitoring, observing for hyper/hypokalaemia.
- Gain IV access, take blood for FBC, U&Es, glucose, creatinine and blood cultures.
- Take ABG, monitoring for metabolic acidosis with evidence of respiratory compensation.
- Obtain CXR, observing for infection.
- Fluid replacement, use 0.9% saline +/− potassium until blood glucose <12 mmol/l over 24-h period.
- If hypotensive, give 0.9% saline to restore blood pressure. Then give 1 litre 0.9% saline over first 30 min. Then give 1 l 0.9% saline at 500 ml/h for 1–2 hours; if still hypotensive, the rate may need to be increased. Then give 1 l 0.9% saline 4 hourly until rehydrated.
- Potassium replacement – none if potassium >5.5 mmol/l. Otherwise, add 20–40 mmol/l to each litre of IV saline.
- Switch IV fluid to glucose when blood sugar <12 mmol/l.
- Administer insulin infusion on sliding scale (50 IU Actrapid in 50 ml of 0.9% saline) (Table 20.1); aim to reduce glucose level by 5 mmol/h.

Table 20.1   Sliding scale for insulin infusion

Glucose (mmol/l)	Insulin (IU/h)
>20	6
17–20	5
14–17	4
11–14	3
7–10	2
4–7	1
<4	0.5

- Consider central line to monitor CVP if severely unwell or older patient.
- Insert urinary catheter and monitor urine output hourly.
- If drowsy, insert a nasogastric tube to prevent aspiration.

Hypoglycaemia

Symptoms include confusion, drowsiness/unconsciousness, perspiring and tachycardia, usually in insulin-dependent diabetic. N.B. Many diabetic patients are asymptomatic with hypoglycaemia.
- Assess airway and support as necessary.
- Give high-flow oxygen.
- Check plasma glucose (do not wait for laboratory results – treat immediately).
- If the patient is able to co-operate, give sugar lumps, Dextrosol or high concentrate sugar drink e.g. Lucozade, followed by biscuits.
- If IV access is difficult to obtain, give glucagon 1 mg intramuscularly. Glucagon is not effective if hypoglycaemia is due to liver failure or chronic alcoholism.
- If the intravenous route is readily available, give 50 ml of 50% glucose IV followed by a 50 ml 0.9% saline to flush hypertonic glucose out of vein.
- If the patient fails to recover in 20 min, recheck blood sugar and consider other causes.
- It is safe to discharge the patient if:
  - the patient has fully recovered
  - a cause has been identified and rectified
  - appropriate follow-up has been arranged.

Hyperosmolar non-ketotic hyperglycaemia (HONK)

Hyperosmolar non-ketotic acidosis (HONK) occurs in people with type 2 diabetes, who may be experiencing high blood glucose levels, often over

40 mmol/l. It can develop over a course of days or weeks and symptoms can include polyuria and polydipsia, nausea, reduced skin turgor, disorientation and, in later stages, drowsiness and a gradual loss of consciousness. Mortality rate is up to 30%.

Fluid replacement and insulin are the cornerstones of treatment but the therapy regime is more cautious to avoid fluid overload and rapid reduction in blood sugar.

- If altered level of consciousness, provide airway support.
- Give high-flow oxygen via a mask and consider the need for anaesthetic support/intubation.
- Monitor vital signs, including blood sugar and urinalysis, remembering there may not be ketones present.
- Perform an ECG, observing for STEMI; instigate cardiac monitoring, observing for hyper/hypokalaemia.
- Gain IV access, take blood for FBC, U&Es, glucose, osmolarity, creatinine and blood cultures.
- Measure ABG, monitoring for metabolic acidosis with evidence of respiratory compensation
- Obtain CXR – observing for infection.
- Fluid replacement – should be cautious:
  - 1 l 0.9% saline over the first 60 minutes then
  - 1 l 0.9% saline with potassium every 2 hours for 4 hours then
  - 1 l 0.9% saline with potassium 6 hourly until rehydrated, may take 48 hours.

  N.B. If plasma Na >150 mmol/l give 0.45% saline.
- Give insulin via sliding scale (see Table 20.1), 50 IU Actrapid in 50 ml 0.9% saline. Regime may be different from that of DKA, consult local guidelines.
- When blood glucose <12 mmol/l, change fluid to 5% dextrose, consider stopping IV insulin and commencing oral hypoglycaemic therapy.
- Insert a urinary catheter and monitor urine output hourly.
- Patients are at risk of venous thromboembolism; commence anticoagulation.
- Osmolarity can be calculated before the laboratory result becomes available:

  $2 \times [\text{Na} + \text{K}] + \text{glucose (mmol/l)} + \text{urea (mmol/l)}.$

Severe sepsis

Pyrexia >39°C, heart rate >100 beats per minute, respiratory rate >30 beats per minute, SBP < 90 mmHg. Signs and symptoms include: fever, nausea and vomiting, diarrhoea, reduced level of consciousness and confusion.

***The goal-directed therapy outlined below should be completed
within the first 6 hours of identification of severe sepsis.***
- Assess airway and support as appropriate.
- Give high-flow oxygen.
- Gain IV access, take blood for serum lactate, blood cultures, FBC, U&Es,
  glucose, LFTs, clotting screen, group and save, and amylase.
- Take an ABG.
- Administer broad-spectrum antibiotic, within 3 h of ED admission and
  within 1 h of non-ED admission.
- If hypotensive and/or a serum lactate >4 mmol/l:
  - deliver an initial minimum of 20 ml/kg of crystalloid
  - administer vasoconstricting inotropes for hypotension which is not
    responding to initial fluid resuscitation to maintain mean arterial
    pressure (MAP) >65 mmHg.
- In the event of persistent hypotension despite fluid resuscitation (septic
  shock) and/or lactate > 4 mmol/, aim to achieve:
  - a central venous pressure (CVP) of >8 mmH$_2$O
  - a central venous oxygen saturation (ScvO$_2$) >70% or mixed venous
    oxygen saturation (SvO$_2$) >65%.
- In addition to blood cultures, send urine, stool, sputum, wound swabs,
  throat swabs and line tips.
- Obtain a CXR to check for infection and an USS/CT of the pelvis to
  check for collections, chest and abdomen.
- Get specialist ICU help early.

Consult www.survivingsepsis.org.

Poisoning

- Monitor airway and give high-flow oxygen (do not give in paraquat
  poisoning, increases toxicity).
- Place in recovery position if < level of consciousness.
- Monitor vital signs, including ECG; place on a cardiac monitor.
- Gain IV access, take blood for FBC, U&Es, paracetamol, salicylate.
- Monitor ABG.
- Treat arrhythmia.
- If respiratory rate <10 breaths/min, give naloxone IV.
- If GCS <8/15 which is not reversed by naloxone or flumazanil, patient
  requires intubation and ventilation.
- Correct hypotension; if SBP <90 mmHg, give 500 ml IV 0.9% saline
  over 30 min.
- Gastric lavage may have some benefit in tricyclic antidepressant or
  opioid overdose when gastric emptying is reduced (consult Toxbase).
- Paracetamol overdose:

- administer acetylcysteine according to paracetamol level
- initial dose: give 150 mg/kg in 200 ml dextrose over 15 min then 50 mg/kg in 500 ml over 4 hours then 100 mg/kg in 1 l over 16 h
- side effects including urticarial rash and nausea can occur; give antihistamine, e.g. chlorphenamine 10 mg IV.
- Aspirin overdose:
  - gastric lavage if overdose >4.5 g in the previous hour
  - give 50 g activated charcoal
  - take salicylate levels (if not already done)
  - check U&Es, ABG
  - in severe overdose, observe for CNS features, acidosis
  - get expert help and consider haemodialysis.
  - For all other episodes of poisoning gain expert advice from a poisons unit or Toxbase.

Anaphylactic reaction

- Assess airway for swelling, e.g. lips, tongue, throat; hoarseness and stridor.
- Establish an airway. Get anaesthetic help early, emergency intubation and ventilation may be required.
- Assess breathing for tachypnoea, wheeze, fatigue, cyanosis and SpO_2 <92% and administer high-flow oxygen.
- Consider an inhaled β2-agonist, e.g. salbutamol 5 mg, for bronchospasm.
- Assess circulation for tachycardia. Check for pallor, hypotension, faintness and drowsiness/coma.
- Give IV fluid challenge: 500–1 l 0.9% saline IV.
- Monitor vital signs including SpO_2 and ECG.
- Give adrenaline 1:1000 intramuscularly and repeat after 5 min if no better.
- If profound shock, consider slow IV adrenaline 1:10 000 or 1:100 000 solution – this must only be given by experienced specialists.
- Give chlorphenamine 10 mg slow intravenously.
- Give hydrocortisone 200 mg slow intravenously.
- Second-line therapy includes an H2-antagonist, e.g. ranitidine 50 mg IV tds.
- Give IV fluid, if severe hypotension does not respond to drug therapy; consider rapid infusion of 1–2 l 0.9% saline.
- Admit after initial therapy; patients must be observed for 4–6 hours.

Consult resus.org.uk.

Websites

www.brit-thoracic.org.uk
www.nice.org.uk
www.rcplondon.ac.uk
www.resus.org.uk
www.sign.ac.uk
http://survivingsepsis.org

Appendices

1 Jaeger Reading Chart

Jaeger types assess visual acuity for close tasks. They provide the easiest quick method of assessment. The patient should wear the spectacles normally required for reading. Ask the patient to read the smallest type she can; if read with few mistakes, ask her to read the next size down. Record the size of type that can be read with each eye separately.

Hope, they say, deserts us at no period of our existence. From first to last, and in the face of smarting disillusions we continue to expect good fortune, better health, and better conduct; and that so confidently, that we judge it needless to deserve them. I think it improbable that I shall ever write like Shakespeare, conduct an army like Hannibal, or distinguish

Here we recognise the thoughts of our boyhood; and our boyhood ceased — well, when? — not, I think, at twenty; nor, perhaps, altogether at twenty-five: nor yet at thirty: and possibly to be quite frank, we are still in the thick of that arcadian period. For as the race of man, after centuries of civilisation, still keeps

I have always suspected public taste to be a mongrel product, out of affectation by dogmatism; and felt sure, if you could only find an honest man of no special literary bent, he would tell you he thought much of Shakespeare bombastic and most absurd, and all of him written in very

If you look back on your own education, I am sure it will not be the full, vivid, instructive hours of truancy that you regret: and you would rather cancel some lack-lustre period between sleep and waking in the class. For my own part, I have attended

There is a sort of dead-alive, hackneyed people about, who are scarcely conscious of living except in the exercise of some conventional occupation.

Books are good enough in their own way, but they are a mighty bloodless substitute for life. It seems a pity to sit, like the Lady of Shalott, peering into a mirror,

The other day, a ragged, barefoot boy ran down the street after a marble, with so jolly an air that he set every one he passed

A happy man or woman is a better thing to find than a

"How now, young fellow, what dost thou

"Truly, sir, I

2 Visual Acuity 3 m Chart

The 3 m Snellen chart should be held 3 m from the patient, with good lighting, with each of the patient's eyes covered in turn. Use the patient's usual spectacles for this distance. If the patient cannot read 6/6 (e.g. 6/12 is best vision in one eye), repeat without spectacles and with a 'pinhole' that largely nullifies refractive errors. Note for each eye the best acuity obtained and the method used, e.g. L 6/9 R 6/6 with spectacles.

V H

36

X U A

24

H T Y O

18

V U A X T

12

H A Y O U X

9

Y U X T H A O V

6

X O A T V H U Y

5

3 Hodkinson Ten Point Mental Test Score

A simple test of impaired cognitive function (see Chapter 8).

1	Age	Must be correct
2	Time	Without looking at clock or watch, and correct to nearest hour
3	42 West Street	Give this (or similar) address twice, ask patient to repeat immediately (to check it has registered), and test recall at end of procedure
4	Recognize two people	Point at nurse and other, ask: 'Who is that person? What does she/he do?'
5	Year	Exact, except in January when previous year is accepted
6	Name of place	May ask type of place, or area of town
7	Date of birth	Exact
8	Start of World War I	Exact year
9	Name of present monarch	
10	Count from 20 to 1	Backwards, may prompt with 20/19/18, no other prompts; patient may hesitate and self-correct but no other errors (tests concentration)

Check recall of address
(question 3 above)

Total score out of 10

Communication problems (e.g. *deafness, dysphasia*) or abnormal mood (e.g. *depression*) may affect the mental test score, and should be noted.

(After Qureshi, K. & Hodkinson, H. (1974) Evaluation of a ten-question mental test in the institutional elderly. *Age and Ageing*, **3**: 152.)

4 Barthel Index of Activities of Daily Living

An assessment of disabilities affecting key functions that influence a person's mobility, self-care and independence (see Chapter 13).

Bowels:
  0 = incontinent (or needs to be given enema)
  1 = occasional accident (once per week or less)
  2 = continent (for preceding week)

Bladder:
  0 = incontinent or catheterized and unable to manage alone
  1 = occasional accident (once per day or less)
  2 = continent (for preceding week)

Feeding:
  0 = unable
  1 = needs help cutting, spreading butter, etc.
  2 = independent

Grooming:
  0 = needs help with personal care
  1 = independent face/hair/teeth/shaving (implements provided)

Dressing:
  0 = dependent
  1 = needs help but can do about half unaided
  2 = independent (including buttons, zips, laces, etc.)

Transfer bed to chair and back:
  0 = unable, no sitting balance
  1 = major help (one strong/skilled or two people), can sit up
  2 = minor help from one person (physical or verbal)
  3 = independent

Toilet use:
  0 = dependent
  1 = needs some help, but can do something alone
  2 = independent (on and off, dressing, wiping)

Mobility around house or ward, indoors:
  0 = immobile
  1 = wheelchair independent, including corners
  2 = walks with help of one person (physical, verbal, supervision)
  3 = independent (but may use any aid, e.g. stick)

Stairs:
  0 = unable
  1 = needs help (physical, verbal, carrying aid)
  2 = independent

Bathing:
  0 = dependent
  1 = independent (in and out of bath or shower)

Total score out of 20

Guidelines for the Barthel Index of Activities Of Daily Living (ADL)

1 The index should be used as a record of what a patient actually does, not what a patient *can* do.
2 The main aim is to establish the degree of independence from any help, physical or verbal, however minor and for whatever reason.
3 The need for supervision renders the patient not independent.
4 A patient's performance should be established using the best available evidence. The patient, friends/relatives and nurses are the usual sources, but direct observation and common sense are also important. Direct testing is not necessary.
5 Usually the patient's performance over the preceding 24–48 hours is important, but occasionally longer periods will be relevant.
6 Middle categories imply that the patient supplies over 50% of the effort.
7 The use of aids to be independent is allowed.

(After Collin, C., Wade, D.T., Davies, S. & Horne, V. (1988) The Barthel ADL index: a reliability study. *International Disability Studies*, **10**: 61–63.)

Further Reading

Chapter 1

Barkauskas, V., Baumann, L. & Darling-Fisher, C. (2002) *Health and Physical Assessment*, 3rd edn. London: Mosby

Bickley, L. & Szilagyi P. (2007) *Bates' Guide to Physical Examination*, 5th edn. Philadelphia: Lippincott

Epstein, O., Perkin, G., de Bono, D. & Cookson, J. (2008) *Clinical Examination*, 4th edn. London: Mosby

Hatton, C. & Blackwood, R. (2003) *Lecture Notes on Clinical Skills*, 4th edn. Oxford: Blackwell Science

Seidel, H., Ball, J., Dains, J., & Benedict, G. (2006) *Mosby's Physical Examination Handbook*. St. Louis: Mosby

Swartz, M. (2006) *Physical Diagnosis, History and Examination*, 5th edn. London: W. B. Saunders

Talley, N. & O'Connor, S. (2006) *Clinical Examination: a Systematic Guide to Physical Diagnosis*, 5th edn. London: Churchill Livingstone

Chapter 2

Barkauskas, V., Baumann, L. & Darling-Fisher, C. (2002) *Health and Physical Assessment*, 3rd edn. London: Mosby

Bickley, L. & Szilagyi P. (2007) *Bates' Guide to Physical Examination*, 5th edn. Philadelphia: Lippincott

Epstein, O., Perkin, G., de Bono, D. & Cookson, J. (2008) *Clinical Examination*, 4th edn. London: Mosby

Hatton, C. & Blackwood, R. (2003) *Lecture Notes on Clinical Skills*, 4th edn. Oxford: Blackwell Science

Seidel, H., Ball, J., Dains, J. & Benedict, G. (2006) *Mosby's Physical Examination Handbook*. St. Louis: Mosby

Swartz, M. (2006) *Physical Diagnosis, History and Examination*, 5th edn. London: W. B. Saunders

Talley, N. & O'Connor, S. (2006) *Clinical Examination: a Systematic Guide to Physical Diagnosis*, 5th edn. London: Churchill Livingstone

Chapter 3

Barkauskas, V., Baumann, L. & Darling-Fisher, C. (2002) *Health and Physical Assessment*, 3rd edn. London: Mosby

Bickley, L. & Szilagyi P. (2007) *Bates' Guide to Physical Examination*, 5th edn. Philadelphia: Lippincott

Brown, E., Collis, W., Leung, T. & Salmon, A. (2002) *Heart Sounds Made Easy*. Edinburgh: Churchill Livingstone

Epstein, O., Perkin, G., de Bono, D. & Cookson, J. (2003) *Clinical Examination*, 3rd edn. London: Mosby

Epstein, O., Perkin, G., de Bono, D. & Cookson, J. (2008) *Clinical Examination*, 4th edn. London: Mosby

Hatchett, R. & Thompson, D. (2007) The sociological and human impact of coronary heart disease. In: *Cardiac Nursing a Comprehensive Guide*, 2nd edn, (eds R. Hatchett & D. Thompson). Edinburgh: Churchill Livingstone

Hatton, C. & Blackwood, R. (2003) *Lecture Notes on Clinical Skills*, 4th edn. Oxford: Blackwell Science

RCN (2008) Advanced Nurse practitioners – an RCN guide to the advanced nurse practitioner role, competencies and programme accreditation. London: Royal College of Nursing

Riley, J. (2002) The ECG: its role and practical application. In: *Cardiac Nursing a Comprehensive Guide* (eds R. Hatchett & D. Thompson). Edinburgh: Churchill Livingstone

Swartz, M. (2006) *Physical Diagnosis, History and Examination*, 5th edn. London: W. B. Saunders

Talley, N. & O'Connor, S. (2006) *Clinical Examination: a Systematic Guide to Physical Diagnosis*, 5th edn. London: Churchill Livingstone

Chapter 5

Bickley, L. & Szilagyi, P. (2007) *Bates' Guide to Physical Examination*, 5th edn. Philadelphia: Lippincott

Dains, J., Baumann, L. & Scheibel, P. (2007) *Advanced Health Assessment and Clinical Diagnosis in Primary Care*, 3rd edn. London: Mosby

Douglas, G., Nicol, F. & Robertson, C. (eds) (2005) *Macleod's Clinical Examination*, 11th edn. Edinburgh: Elsevier

Epstein, O., Perkin, G., de Bono, D. & Cookson, J. (2008) *Clinical Examination*, 4th edn. London: Mosby

Gleadle, J. (2007) *History and Examination at a Glance*, 2nd edn. New York: Wiley

Talley, N. & O'Connor, S. (2006) *Clinical Examination: A Systematic Guide to Physical Diagnosis*, 5th edn. Edinburgh: Churchill Livingstone

Chapter 6

Bickley, L. & Szilagyi, P. (2007) *Bates' Guide to Physical Examination*, 5th edn. Philadelphia: Lippincott

Dains, J., Baumann, L. & Scheibel, P. (2007) *Advanced Health Assessment and Clinical Diagnosis in Primary Care*, 3rd edn. London: Mosby

Douglas, G., Nicol, F. & Robertson, C. (eds) (2005) *Macleod's Clinical Examination*, 11th edn. Edinburgh: Elsevier

Epstein, O., Perkin, G., de Bono, D. & Cookson, J. (2008) *Clinical Examination*, 4th edn. London: Mosby

Gleadle, J. (2007) *History and Examination at a Glance*, 2nd edn. New York: Wiley

Talley, N. & O'Connor, S. (2006) *Clinical Examination: A Systematic Guide to Physical Diagnosis*, 5th edn. Edinburgh: Churchill Livingstone

Chapter 16

Ashford, R. & Evans, N. (2001) *Surgical Critical Care*. London: Greenwich Medical Media

Esmond, G. (2001) *Textbook of Respiratory Care*. Edinburgh: Churchill Livingstone

Grainger, R. (2001) *Grainger and Allison's Diagnostic Radiology: A Textbook of Medical Imaging*, 4th edn. London: Churchill Livingstone

Hatchett, R. & Thompson, D. (2007) The sociological and human impact of coronary heart disease. In: Hatchett, R. & Thompson, D. (eds) *Cardiac Nursing a Comprehensive Guide*, 2nd edn. , Edinburgh: Churchill Livingstone

Hatton, C. & Blackwood, R. (2003) *Lecture Notes on Clinical Skills*, 4th edn. Oxford: Blackwell Science

Jones, S. (2006) *Imaging for Nurses.* Oxford: Blackwell

Chapter 17

Riley, J. (2002) The ECG: its role and practical application. In: Hatchett, R. & Thompson, D. (eds) *Cardiac Nursing: A Comprehensive Guide.* Edinburgh: Churchill Livingstone

Chapter 20

British Thoracic Society (2001) British Thoracic Society guidelines for the management of community acquired pneumonia in adults. *Thorax*, **56** (suppl 4).

British Thoracic Society (2004) British Thoracic Society guidelines for the management of community acquired pneumonia in adults – update. Available at: https://britthoracic.org.uk/portals/0/cliinical%information/pneumonia/Guidelines/MACAprevisedApr04.pdf.

British Thoracic Society and Scottish Intercollegiate Guideline Network (2008) *British Guidelines on the Management of Asthma: A National Clinical Guide.* London: British Thoracic Society

Department of Health (2007) *National Stroke Strategy.* London: DH Publications

Kumar, P. & Clarke, M. (2005) *Clinical Medicine*, 6th edn. London: Saunders

Royal College of Physicians and the British Thoracic Society (2008) *Non-Invasive Ventilation in Chronic Obstructive Pulmonary Disease: Management of Acute Type 2 Respiratory Failure.* London: Royal College of Physicians

Index